Pruritus

Editor

GIL YOSIPOVITCH

DERMATOLOGIC CLINICS

www.derm.theclinics.com

Consulting Editor
BRUCE H. THIERS

July 2018 • Volume 36 • Number 3

ELSEVIER

1600 John F. Kennedy Boulevard • Suite 1800 • Philadelphia, Pennsylvania, 19103-2899

http://www.theclinics.com

DERMATOLOGIC CLINICS Volume 36, Number 3
July 2018 ISSN 0733-8635, ISBN-13: 978-0-323-61080-3

Editor: Jessica McCool
Developmental Editor: Sara Watkins

Dermatologic Clinics (ISSN 0733-8635) is published quarterly by Elsevier Inc., 360 Park Avenue South, New York, NY 10010-1710. Months of publication are January, April, July, and October. Business and editorial offices: 1600 John F. Kennedy Blvd., Suite 1800, Philadelphia, PA 19103-2899. Customer service office: 11830 Westline Drive, St. Louis, MO 63146. Periodicals postage paid at New York, NY, and additional mailing offices. Subscription prices are USD 392.00 per year for US individuals, USD 701.00 per year for US institutions, USD 451.00 per year for Canadian individuals, USD 855.00 per year for Canadian institutions, USD 505.00 per year for international individuals, USD 855.00 per year for international institutions, USD 100.00 per year for US students/residents, and USD 240.00 per year for Canadian and international students/residents. International air speed delivery is included in all *Clinics* subscription prices. All prices are subject to change without notice. **POSTMASTER:** Send address changes to *Dermatologic Clinics*, Elsevier Health Sciences Division, Subscription Customer Service, 3251 Riverport Lane, Maryland Heights, MO 63043. **Customer Service: 1-800-654-2452 (U.S. and Canada); 314-447-8871 (outside U.S. and Canada). Fax: 314-447-8029. E-mail: journalscustomerservice-usa@elsevier.com (for print support); journalsonlinesupport-usa@elsevier.com (for online support).**

Reprints. For copies of 100 or more, of articles in this publication, please contact the Commercial Reprints Department, Elsevier Inc., 360 Park Avenue South, New York, New York 10010-1710. Tel.: 212-633-3874; Fax: 212-633-3820; Email: reprints@elsevier.com.

The *Dermatologic Clinics* is covered in *MEDLINE/PubMed (Index Medicus), Current Contents/Clinical Medicine, Excerpta Medica, Chemical Abstracts,* and *ISI/BIOMED.*

Contributors

CONSULTING EDITOR

BRUCE H. THIERS, MD
Professor and Chairman Emeritus,
Department of Dermatology and
Dermatologic Surgery, Medical University
of South Carolina, Charleston,
South Carolina, USA

EDITOR

GIL YOSIPOVITCH, MD
Professor, Department of Dermatology and
Cutaneous Surgery, Miami Itch Center,
University of Miami Miller School of Medicine,
University of Miami Hospital, Miami, Florida,
USA

AUTHORS

YAHYA ARGOBI, MD
Assistant Professor, Department of
Dermatology, King Khalid University, College
of Medicine, Abha, Saudi Arabia

MARK A. BECHTEL, MD
Professor of Medicine, Director, Division
of Dermatology, The Ohio State
University College of Medicine, Columbus,
Ohio, USA

CHARLOTTE BERNIGAUD, MD
Dermatology Department, AP-HP, Hôpital
Henri Mondor, Université Paris Est, Research
Group Dynamyc, Ecole nationale vétérinaire
d'Alfort, Maisons-Alfort, Université Paris-Est
Créteil, Créteil, France

EMILIE BRENAUT, MD
Dermatology Department, University Hospital
of Brest, Laboratory on Interactions Neurons-
Keratinocytes (LINK), University of Western
Brittany, Brest, France

ANNA BUTEAU, MD
Resident, Internal Medicine, Dell Medical
School, The University of Texas at Austin,
Austin, Texas, USA

TAIGE CAO, MD
National Skin Centre, Singapore, Singapore

OLIVIER CHOSIDOW, MD, PhD
Dermatology Department, AP-HP, Hôpital
Henri Mondor, Université Paris-Est, EpiDermE,
Epidémiologie en Dermatologie et Evaluation
des Thérapeutiques, Université Paris-Est
Créteil, Créteil, France

MIRIAM M. DÜLL, MD
Department of Medicine 1, Friedrich-
Alexander-University Erlangen-Nürnberg,
Erlangen, Germany

SARINA B. ELMARIAH, MD, PhD
Assistant Physician, Massachusetts General
Hospital, Instructor, Harvard Medical School,
Boston, Massachusetts, USA

STEPHEN ERICKSON, BS
Division of Dermatology, Department of
Medicine, Washington University School
of Medicine in St. Louis, St Louis,
Missouri, USA

ELIZABETH M. FITE, MD
Department of Dermatology, The University of
Tennessee Health Science Center, Memphis,
Tennessee, USA

ANNA CHIARA FOSTINI, MD
Department of Dermatology and Cutaneous
Surgery, Miami Itch Center, University of Miami
Miller School of Medicine, Miami, Florida, USA;
Department of Medicine, Section of
Dermatology, University of Verona, Verona, Italy

JOAN GUITART, MD, FAAD
Professor of Dermatology and Pathology,
Department of Dermatology, Northwestern
University, Feinberg School of Medicine,
Chicago, Illinois, USA

ARNAUD JANNIC, MD
Dermatology Department, AP-HP, Hôpital
Henri Mondor, Université Paris-Est, Research
Group Dynamyc, Ecole nationale vétérinaire
d'Alfort, Maisons-Alfort, Université Paris-Est
Créteil, Créteil, France

BRIAN S. KIM, MD, MTR
Division of Dermatology, Departments of
Medicine, Pathology and Immunology, and
Anesthesiology, Center for the Study of Itch,
Washington University School of Medicine in
St. Louis, St Louis, Missouri, USA

ANDREAS E. KREMER, MD, PhD, MHBA
Department of Medicine 1, Friedrich-
Alexander-University Erlangen-Nürnberg,
Erlangen, Germany

MARIO E. LACOUTURE, MD
Director, Oncodermatology Program,
Dermatology Service, Department of Medicine,
Memorial Sloan Kettering Cancer Center,
Associate Professor, Department of Medicine,
Weill Cornell Medical College, New York,
New York, USA

ETHAN A. LERNER, MD, PhD
Associate Professor of Dermatology, Harvard
Medical School, Massachusetts General
Hospital, Boston, Massachusetts, USA

**MARIA ESTELA MARTINEZ-ESCALA,
MD, PhD**
Post Doctoral Clinical Research Fellow,
Department of Dermatology, Northwestern
University, Feinberg School of Medicine,
Chicago, Illinois, USA

MATTHEW W. McEWEN, BS
College of Medicine, The University of
Tennessee Health Science Center, Memphis,
Tennessee, USA

ZACHARY NAHMIAS, MD
Division of Dermatology, Department of
Medicine, Washington University School
of Medicine in St. Louis, St Louis,
Missouri, USA

TEJESH PATEL, MD
Amonette-Rosenberg Endowed Chair,
Associate Professor, Kaplan-Amonette
Department of Dermatology, The University
of Tennessee Health Science Center,
Memphis, Tennessee, USA

RITA O. PICHARDO, MD
Department of Dermatology, Wake Forest
University School of Medicine,
Winston-Salem, North Carolina, USA

JASON REICHENBERG, MD
Associate Professor, Dermatology, Dell
Medical School, The University of Texas at
Austin, Austin, Texas, USA

RADOMIR RESZKE, MD
Department of Dermatology, Venereology and
Allergology, Wroclaw Medical University,
Wrocław, Poland

JORDAN DANIEL ROSEN, BS
Department of Dermatology and Cutaneous
Surgery, Miami Itch Center, University of
Miami Miller School of Medicine, Miami,
Florida, USA

ILANA S. ROSMAN, MD
Division of Dermatology, Departments
of Medicine and Pathology and Immunology,
Director, Washington University
Dermatopathology Center, Washington
University School of Medicine in St. Louis,
St Louis, Missouri, USA

JESSICA A. SAVAS, MD
Department of Dermatology, Wake Forest
University School of Medicine, Winston-Salem,
North Carolina, USA

LINDA SERRANO, MD
Post Doctoral Clinical Research Fellow,
Department of Dermatology, Northwestern
University, Feinberg School of Medicine,
Chicago, Illinois, USA

GIDEON P. SMITH, MD, MPH, PhD
Director, Department of Dermatology,
Connective Tissue Diseases Clinic,
Massachusetts General Hospital, Boston,
Massachusetts, USA

SONJA STÄNDER, MD
Professor of Dermatology and
Neurodermatology, Department of Dermatology,
Center for Chronic Pruritus, University Hospital
Münster, Münster, Germany

JACEK C. SZEPIETOWSKI, MD, PhD
Professor, Department of Dermatology,
Venereology and Allergology,
Wroclaw Medical University, Wrocław,
Poland

HONG LIANG TEY, MD
National Skin Centre, Lee Kong Chian School
of Medicine, Nanyang Technological
University, Singapore, Singapore

JENNIFER WU, MD
Visiting Investigator, Dermatology Service,
Department of Medicine, Memorial Sloan
Kettering Cancer Center, New York, New York,
USA; Attending Physician, Department of
Dermatology, Drug Hypersensitivity Clinical
and Research Center, Chang Gung Memorial
Hospital, College of Medicine Chang Gung
University, Keelung, Linkou, and Taipei, Taiwan

GIL YOSIPOVITCH, MD
Professor, Department of Dermatology and
Cutaneous Surgery, Miami Itch Center,
University of Miami Miller School of Medicine,
University of Miami Hospital, Miami, Florida, USA

CLAUDIA ZEIDLER, MD
Department of Dermatology, Center for
Chronic Pruritus, University Hospital Münster,
Münster, Germany

XIAOLONG A. ZHOU, MD
Instructor, Department of Dermatology,
Northwestern University, Feinberg School of
Medicine, Chicago, Illinois, USA

Contents

Chronic itch is a clinically challenging yet scientifically remarkable and complex process. Increasing understanding of the pathophysiology of chronic itch is leading to targeted therapeutic approaches that are now dramatically improving quality of life. This improvement will accelerate as the tools of basic and clinical research continue to be applied to this previously intractable problem.

Pruritus is a common and troubling symptom associated with many dermatologic, systemic, neurologic, or psychiatric disorders. This article reviews the current understanding of the pathogenesis of itch and offers a differential diagnosis for the causes of chronic pruritus. The article discusses key diagnostic steps and considerations when evaluating patients with chronic pruritus.

Prurigo nodularis occurs with chronic pruritus and the presence of single to multiple symmetrically distributed, hyperkeratotic, and intensively itching nodules. Diverse dermatologic, systemic, neurologic, or psychiatric conditions can lead to prurigo nodularis. Structural analysis demonstrated a reduced intraepidermal nerve fiber density and increased dermal levels of nerve growth factor and neuropeptides, such as substance P and calcitonin gene-related peptide. Novel therapy concepts such as inhibitors at neurokinin-1, opioid receptors, and interleukin-31 receptors have been developed. The mainstays of prurigo nodularis therapy comprise topical steroids, capsaicin, calcineurin inhibitors, phototherapy, and the systemic application of anticonvulsants, μ-opioid receptor antagonists, or immunosuppressants.

Chronic pruritus (>6 weeks' duration) in the geriatric population (≥65 years old) is an increasing health care problem. The pathophysiologic predisposing factors are abnormalities of the epidermal barrier, immune system, and nervous system. Causes can be dichotomized into histaminergic and nonhistaminergic pruritus. Topical treatments are generally safe. Systemic treatments are chosen depending on the condition, comorbid diseases, and drug interactions. Treatment options are limited. Progress has been made in identifying itch-selective mediators over the last decade.

Numerous new medications are currently undergoing clinical trials, and they are anticipated to enter the clinics in the near future.

Neuropathic pruritus is a challenging condition that can be caused by injury or dysfunction in any part of the nervous system. A vast array of clinical pictures exists, including both localized and generalized pruritus, and their principal entities are described in this article. Diagnosis is often difficult and depends on patient history, imaging, and neurophysiologic studies. Other causes of chronic itch should be excluded. The management of neuropathic itch is demanding, and most interventions are not curative. The best treatment options include anticonvulsants, topical anesthetics, and capsaicin.

Vulvar pruritus is a common complaint among young girls and women presenting to primary care physicians, gynecologists, and dermatologists. Female genital itch is especially disruptive because of its interference with sexual function and intimacy. Causes of vulvar itch are vast and may be inflammatory, environmental, neoplastic, or infectious, often with several causes coexisting simultaneously. Diagnosis may be difficult because of the unique anatomy and inherent properties of genital and perianal skin. Treatment is aimed at eliminating outside irritants, restoring epidermal barrier function, and suppressing inflammation.

Pruritus is a common symptom in cutaneous T-cell lymphoma (CTCL) and critically affects the quality of life of patients. Understanding the pruritogenesis has led to the development of new therapeutic agents with promising outcomes in the management of this recalcitrant symptom. Clinical assessments are warranted to aid in the evaluation of treatment response or disease recurrence. Severe pruritus scores may require further investigation of emotional distress for a better patient approach. Dermatologists play a key role in the treatment of CTCL pruritus by guiding the patient in the importance of preserving the integrity of the skin barrier.

Pruritus in pregnancy can be a source of significant discomfort in the pregnant patient. Some cases are associated with pregnancy-specific dermatoses, although some patients experience a flare of a preexisting dermatosis. Severe pruritus may be a manifestation of a pregnancy-specific dermatosis associated with increased fetal risks and complications. Early accurate diagnosis and appropriate management are important. Examination often reveals important clinical findings, aiding accurate diagnosis. Pemphigoid gestationis often presents with periumbilical involvement, whereas polymorphic eruption of pregnancy spares the umbilicus and presents in the striae distensae. Intrahepatic cholestasis of pregnancy is associated with intense pruritus of the palms.

Psychogenic pruritus is defined as itch not related to dermatologic or systemic causes. When a patient presents with pruritus, regardless of the presumed cause, the standard workup should include a thorough history, dermatologic examination, and laboratory examinations or biopsies as needed. If no medical source is found, the provider must work in partnership with the patient to explore other causes and that may include acknowledging and treating underlying psychiatric conditions.

Targeted anticancer therapies have significantly increased the survival of patients with a variety of malignancies, improving tolerability and treatment duration. The increased lifespan and the expanded use of targeted agents have led to a variety of treatment-related adverse events. Pruritus, a common dermatologic adverse event with various incidences ranging from 2.2% to 47% across different categories of targeted anticancer therapies, has been overlooked. This article reviews the incidence, accompanying skin conditions, possible pathomechanism, and proposed management algorithms of pruritus associated with targeted therapies, including immunotherapies.

Chronic pruritus, or itch lasting greater than 6 weeks, is an increasingly common and debilitating medical problem. Recent studies have unveiled previously unrecognized neuroimmune axes whereby inflammatory cytokines act directly on the nervous system to promote itch. Thus, the emergence of newer targeted biologic therapies has generated the possibility of novel treatment strategies for chronic itch disorders. This article reviews the pathophysiology of multiple chronic itch disorders, including atopic dermatitis, chronic idiopathic pruritus, chronic urticaria, and prurigo nodularis. Furthermore, new and emerging immunomodulatory therapies that will likely alter current treatment paradigms are discussed.

Chronic pruritus is a common condition that has a detrimental impact on quality of life. As the molecular pathogenesis of itch is elucidated, novel therapies that disrupt itch pathways are being investigated. Emerging treatments include drugs targeting the neural system, drugs targeting the immune system, antihistamines, bile acid transport inhibitors, and topical drugs that work through a variety of mechanisms such as phosphodiesterase-4 inhibition or targeting of nerve ion channels. Many of these therapies show promising results in the treatment of chronic itch of various etiologies, such as atopic dermatitis, psoriasis, uremic pruritus, and cholestatic pruritus.

DERMATOLOGIC CLINICS

ISSUE OF RELATED INTEREST

Immunology and Allergy Clinics of North America, February 2017 (Vol. 37, No. 1)
Allergic Skin Diseases
Peck Y. Ong and Peter Schmid-Grendelmeier, *Editors*
Available at: http://immunology.theclinics.com/

THE CLINICS ARE AVAILABLE ONLINE!
Access your subscription at:
www.theclinics.com

Erratum

"The Role of Systemic Retinoids in the Treatment of Cutaneous T-Cell Lymphoma," by Dr. Auris O. Huen and Dr. Ellen J. Kim, published in Dr. Elise A. Olsen's October 2015 issue of *Dermatologic Clinics* devoted to Cutaneous Lymphoma (Volume 33, Issue 4), has been updated to correct an incorrectly quoted reference.

Reference 43, "Prospective Randomized Multicenter Clinical Trial on the Use Of Interferon -2a Plus Acitretin Versus Interferon -2a Plus PUVA in Patients with Cutaneous T-Cell Lymphoma Stages I and II" by Stadler R, Otte H.G., Luger T., et al, describes a clinical trial comparing PUVA + IFN vs Acitretin+IFN, rather than PUVA + Acitretin, as stated in the article. As such, the following paragraph on Page 719 should be disregarded.

- "PUVA also was combined with acitretin in 42 patients with CTCL, producing a CR rate of 38%. This was significantly lower compared with the comparator arm of PUVA with IFN, which had a CR rate at 70%.[43]"

The author would like to amend this error by including the following update on the same page of the article.

- "Acitretin has also been combined with interferon alpha in a prospective randomized controlled clinical trial where 42 early stage CTCL patients achieved a CR rate of 38% (in contrast to the 70% CR rate in the comparator arm of PUVA with IFN).[43]"

Dermatol Clin 36 (2018) xiii
https://doi.org/10.1016/j.det.2018.02.018

Preface
Chronic Itch: A Disease in Its Own Right

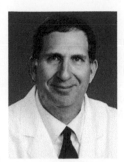

Gil Yosipovitch, MD

Editor

Experienced by millions of people worldwide, chronic pruritus is a debilitating symptom associated with numerous skin, neural, systemic, and psychogenic causes. In the last decade, a revolution in basic itch research has led to new therapeutic targets beyond the "good old antihistamines and corticosteroids that have limited efficacy." Although the pathophysiology of pruritus of many diseases remains poorly understood, we have increased our knowledge of its characteristics and management. The goal of the current issue of *Dermatologic Clinics* is to cover the cause, manifestations, and therapeutic strategies for a variety of pruritic conditions, many of which have not been extensively covered. I hope that this issue provides the general dermatologist with practical tools to assess and manage chronic pruritus patients in daily clinical practice and awareness of new and emerging therapies.

The pathophysiology of chronic itch differs markedly from the physiology of acute itch, and there are many types of chronic itch with different treatment targets. Lerner provides a concise review of the many advances that have been made in understanding the basic mechanisms that cause pruritus. Elmariah provides algorithms of diagnosing pruritus, with and without primary skin rash, and other types of chronic itch. Zeidler and colleagues provide a practical workup and management of prurigo nodularis, which undoubtedly is one of the most severe types of chronic itch. They describe new treatments targeting the neural system.

Cao and colleagues discuss the unmet need to treat pruritus in aging skin that requires recognition of the physiologic changes in epidermal barrier, immune system, and nervous system. Rosen and colleagues describe the numerous neuropathic itch syndromes in the peripheral and central nervous system and its management with drugs targeting the neural system. Savas and Pichardo-Geisenger provide a succinct article discussing the diagnosis and management of pruritic vulvar dermatoses that are all too often underdiagnosed and undertreated.

Serrano and colleagues review the pathogenesis and management of cutaneous T-cell lymphoma–associated pruritus, an extremely challenging condition in Sezary and erythrodermic types. Bechtel reviews pruritus in pregnancy, reported in 14% to 20% of pregnancies. He describes the clinical presentation of the different pruritic entities common in pregnancy, including the pregnancy-specific dermatosis, and provides useful diagnostic pearls and safe treatments. Smith and Argobi address the most common triggers for pruritus in connective tissue diseases. Of note, pruritus is a prominent feature in dermatomyositis and can present as an initial symptom.

Reszke and Szepietowski provide a detailed review on end-stage renal disease chronic itch, which continues to be the leading cause of systemic itch. They provide extensive recommendations for both topical and systemic treatments. The article by Düll and Kremer discusses the management of hepatic itch, which occurs in almost all liver diseases,

Dermatol Clin 36 (2018) xv–xvi
https://doi.org/10.1016/j.det.2018.02.017
0733-8635/18/© 2018 Published by Elsevier Inc.

particularly those with cholestatic features. Jannic and colleagues provide a review of scabies and its management. Scabies is the itchiest infectious disease, and it affects 100 to 130 million people yearly. Buteau and Reichenberg discuss psychogenic causes of chronic itch, providing three categories of psychogenic pruritus with diagnosis and management strategies for the different types. Wu and Lacouture describe the incidence and clinical presentations of pruritus associated with all the new targeted anticancer therapies and management of this type of itch. Erickson and colleagues review the pathophysiology of itch with underlying immune involvement of Th2 cytokines. Blocking the neuroimmune axis has emerged as a novel immunomodulatory approach to treat chronic itch disorders. The final article, by McEwen and colleagues, discusses the emerging topical and systemic therapies both on the market and in the pipeline for the treatment of chronic itch.

I wish to express my sincere thanks to the international group of experts who collectively contributed their insightful reviews to this issue.

Gil Yosipovitch, MD
Department of Dermatology and Cutaneous Surgery
and Miami Itch Center
Miller School of Medicine
University of Miami
1475 Northwest 12th Avenue
Miami, FL 33136, USA

E-mail address:
yosipog@gmail.com

Pathophysiology of Itch

Ethan A. Lerner, MD, PhD*

KEYWORDS

- Atopic dermatitis • Central sensitization • Chronic itch • Epigenetics • Pruritus

KEY POINTS

- Chronic itch has a major negative impact on quality of life.
- There are chronic itches, not just 1 chronic itch.
- The pathophysiology of chronic itch is becoming increasingly understood.
- This understanding is being driven by findings in basic and clinical research combined with clinical responses to new classes of therapeutic agents that specifically target cytokines, receptors and channels.

The pathophysiology of chronic itch differs markedly from the physiology of acute itch. Acute itch physiology is encompassed by stimulation of sensory neural fibers in the skin resulting in a signal sent to the brain that is interpreted as itch followed by a motor response to scratch such that the stimulus that initiated the cycle is removed.[1] Chronic itch is filled with complexity, redundancy, and dynamic processes.[2] There is no single chronic itch but rather distinct and overlapping chronic itches. A detailed understanding of the pathophysiology that underlies chronic itches is now leading to targeted therapeutic approaches for distinct itches and is making a difference in the clinic.

At the clinical level, chronic itches are defined as those lasting 6 weeks or longer. Everyone with atopic dermatitis itches. Although there are commonalities between their itches, the itches also differ by a variety of measures. These include the quality and severity of the sensation and components of burning, pricking, stinging, and pain.[3] Scratching can be pleasurable and may or may not relieve the itch until pain is generated on account of localized removal of the epidermis. In chronic urticaria, itch is a given although scratching is neither pleasurable nor helpful with the response primarily related to rubbing. In other inflammatory conditions, such as psoriasis, itch may or may not be a feature. In systemic conditions that are not necessarily considered inflammatory, such as chronic liver and chronic kidney diseases, itch can be intense but may not be associated with specific skin manifestations and neither the sensation of itch nor its location is uniform. Add to these the itches, not entirely understood and for which no therapeutic approaches are regularly beneficial, that result from the emerging use of immune checkpoint inhibitors to treat cancer.[4] Next are the neurogenic or neuropathic itches, including brachioradial pruritus and notalgia paresthetica which can be associated with nerve compression while herpes zoster is associated with neurogenic inflammation. Finally, there are psychogenic itches. These itches are associated with conditions ranging from depression or obsessions to delusions of parasitosis, in which the entire process may be localized in the brain, raising the question of whether targeting the periphery can have an impact. Chronic itch is thus associated with a broad range of clinical entities that can arise in distinct anatomic locations. Therapeutic approaches that restore homeostasis or interrupt the flow of immunologic or neurosensory information in the area may be of benefit for particular itches.

Disclosure Statement: The author has nothing to disclose.
Department of Dermatology, Harvard Medical School, Massachusetts General Hospital, Boston, MA 02114, USA
* Massachusetts General Hospital, 149, 13th Street, Charlestown, MA 02129.
E-mail address: ELERNER@mgh.harvard.edu

Dermatol Clin 36 (2018) 175–177
https://doi.org/10.1016/j.det.2018.02.001
0733-8635/18/

At the environmental, biochemical, molecular, and cellular levels, a vast number of waypoints exist between the skin and brain. At the wide entrance to the funnel are exogenous agents, including components of the microbiome, and larger environmental stimuli, such as arthropods and plants, in addition to irritants and materials with different pH, moisture content, and temperature. These interface with endogenous components comprising the skin barrier, keratinocytes, and a plethora of immune cells, each of which has an interactive conversation with one another and with sensory fibers that transmit histamine-dependent and histamine-independent itch. This conversation includes direct cell-cell communication and selective granule release as well as numerous mediators, receptors, and channels that can be shared directly or through family members across the many different cell types. The sensory fibers extend to dorsal root ganglia outside of the spinal cord and then synapse with second order neurons in the spinal cord. Although the funnel may be squeezed at this point, that view is again simplistic given the extensive excitatory and inhibitory neural circuitry, together with the contribution of microglia, in the spinal cord. These conversations in the spinal cord converge to brain regions, with the funnel ultimately narrowing as the sensation as itch is interpreted.[5] With the possible exception of histamine accounting for urticaria in some patients, however, there are no examples in which either the mediators of chronic itch or biomarkers have been definitively correlated with a particular itch. The lack of clarity with respect to the contribution of individual components to chronic itch presents an opportunity ripe for analysis via the application of proteomic, metabolomic, and next-generation sequencing approaches. It is logical to posit that comparative proteomics and metabolomics if applied to populations of patients with itchy and nonitchy primary biliary cirrhosis or chronic kidney disease might allow for the mediators to be determined. Chronic itch is thus associated with distinct but interacting environmental, biochemical, molecular, and cellular components. Again, therapeutic approaches that restore homeostasis or effectively interrupt the flow of information between these components may be of benefit for particular itches.

At the conceptual level, chronic itch may result from *peripheral sensitization* or *central sensitization*,[6] terms borrowed from the chronic pain field. In peripheral sensitization, chronic itch develops from activation of pruriceptors, akin to nociceptors that respond to pain. Chronic exposure to pruritogens or inflammatory mediators that are associated with itch enhances the responsiveness of pruriceptive nerve fibers. Peripheral sensitization leads to increased action potential firing and transmitter release in the dorsal horn of the spinal cord, where somatosensory information is processed. Mediators released from microglia in the dorsal horn modulate the activity of neurons in the vicinity. The heightened activity of dorsal horn neurons leads to heightened excitability—central sensitization. It is possible that sensitization is a parallel to long-term potentiation associated with learning and memory. Sensitization is considered responsible for exaggerated responses to itchy stimuli and is termed, *hyperknesis*. Sensitization contributes to itch elicited by normally nonpruritic stimuli, or *alloknesis*. Peripheral and central sensitization may well be associated with epigenetic changes but such changes have not yet been reported. Therapeutic approaches that allow for reversal or modulation of epigenetic changes are likely to be of benefit in chronic itch associated with sensitization.

The information above is purposely general. There are extensive lists of components that are considered part of the itch pathways.[7] These lists reveal the current state of knowledge but are not yet complete enough to generate a convincing gestalt as to the physiology of itch and thus the pathophysiology. That does not imply a lack of progress. The literature is replete with in vitro studies that replicate portions of itch pathways. In in vivo studies, especially those that use state-of-the-art genetic models in mice, spontaneous itch develops or, when stimuli are provided over a few days to a few weeks, scratching bouts are counted and the models considered to represent chronic itch. These models are limited with respect to clinical correlates because none accurately recapitulates chronic itch in patients although they do reveal that a plethora of channels, receptors, and mediators contribute to chronic itch that is associated with cutaneous inflammation or neural pathways. A limited selection of this plethora includes transient receptor potential channels, sodium channels, ligand-gated ionotropic and metabotropic receptors, toll-like receptors, cytokine receptors, and a series of G-protein coupled receptors (GPCRs), including the gastrin-releasing peptide receptor, neurokinin 1 receptor, members of the mas-related GPCR family, the neuropeptide Y, opiate receptors, and, when known, their respective ligands. All these contribute to itch and, in certain cases, its modulation.

As might be expected, treatment approaches that correct or interrupt the flow of information between the skin and dorsal root ganglia have been shown effective for the chronic itches associated with inflammatory skin diseases. Corticosteroids have long been used to reduce inflammation with the benefit of relieving itch, demonstrating a link between the immune and nervous systems. Blocking the activity of interleukin (IL)-31 rapidly alleviates itch in patients with atopic dermatitis while inflammation is maintained, perhaps allowing for unlinking the immune and nervous systems.[8] Blocking the IL-4/IL-13 pathway is effective at treating the inflammatory aspects of many, but not all, patients with atopic dermatitis.[9] The relief of itch from this therapeutic approach may result from the anti-inflammatory activity as well as blockade of IL-4 receptors expressed on sensory nerves. This possibility is supported by the demonstration that an inhibitor of Janus-associated kinases, which are downstream of IL-4 receptor activation, seems effective in examples of chronic idiopathic pruritus.[10]

Finely targeted approaches are increasingly available for some chronic itches of inflammatory skin disease. Less targeted approaches are used for the treatment of neurogenic, neuropathic, or psychogenic itches. This therapeutic paucity will change as more is learned about the processes underlying these conditions. In summary, detailed understanding of the pathophysiology of chronic itch is becoming achievable. This understanding should lead to safe, effective, and targeted therapeutics. To paraphrase Winston Churchill, we are near the end of the beginning of understanding chronic itch.

REFERENCES

1. Green D, Dong X. The cell biology of acute itch. J Cell Biol 2016;213:155–61.
2. LaMotte RH, Dong X, Ringkamp M. Sensory neurons and circuits mediating itch. Nat Rev Neurosci 2014; 15:19–31.
3. Sikand P, Shimada SG, Green BG, et al. Similar itch and nociceptive sensations evoked by punctate cutaneous application of capsaicin, histamine and cowhage. Pain 2009;144:66–75.
4. Ensslin CJ, Rosen AC, Wu S, et al. Pruritus in patients treated with targeted cancer therapies: systematic review and meta-analysis. J Am Acad Dermatol 2013;69:708–20.
5. Mu D, Deng J, Liu KF, et al. A central neural circuit for itch sensation. Science 2017;357:695–9.
6. Schmelz M. Itch and pain differences and commonalities. Handb Exp Pharmacol 2015;227: 285–301.
7. Meng J, Steinhoff M. Molecular mechanisms of pruritus. Curr Res Transl Med 2016;64:203–6.
8. Ruzicka T, Hanifin JM, Furue M, et al. Anti-interleukin-31 receptor A antibody for atopic dermatitis. N Engl J Med 2017;376:826–35.
9. Simpson EL, Bieber T, Guttman-Yassky E, et al. Two phase 3 trials of dupilumab versus placebo in atopic dermatitis. N Engl J Med 2016;375: 2335–48.
10. Oetjen LK, Mack MR, Feng J, et al. Sensory neurons co-opt classical immune signaling pathways to mediate chronic itch. Cell 2017;171:217–28.

Diagnostic Work-up of the Itchy Patient

Sarina B. Elmariah, MD, PhD*

KEYWORDS

• Pruritus • Itch • Diagnosis • Evaluation • Pruriceptive • Neuropathic • Systemic

KEY POINTS

• Itch is a symptom of many dermatologic, systemic, neurologic, or psychiatric disorders.
• Chronic or severe itch has a negative impact on the quality of life of affected individuals.
• The most important and fundamental factor in ultimately diagnosing the cause of itch remains a detailed history and physical examination.
• In the absence of primary inflammation, a work-up for other systemic or neurologic causes may be necessary.

INTRODUCTION

Itch, also called pruritus, is defined as a sensation that provokes the urge to scratch. Pruritus arises commonly in the setting of numerous dermatologic, systemic, neurologic, and psychiatric disorders, affecting all age groups, races, and both genders. Pruritus is considered chronic when symptoms arise regularly for more than 6 weeks. At any given time, approximately 25% to 38% of the general population may be affected by pruritus. Rates of moderate to severe itch may be much higher in specific populations, such as those with inflammatory or allergic skin disease, or individuals with chronic medical disorders (eg, chronic renal failure, cholestasis, or malignancy).[1–3]

Chronic pruritus has a significant and negative impact on patient quality of life. Similar to chronic pain, patients with chronic or severe itch experience reduction in time and quality of sleep, impaired memory and attention, physician-diagnosed depression and anxiety, and social isolation and withdrawal.[4–12]

Because itch is a symptom that may arise in the setting of many conditions and is not itself a singular disease, identifying the cause of a patient's pruritus is often challenging. It is thus important to have a framework for how to approach the diagnostic evaluation of the chronically itchy patient. This article reviews basic pathophysiology of itch signaling, discusses the broad differential diagnosis for chronic pruritic disorders, and outlines an approach to the clinical assessment of patients with chronic itch in the presence or absence of primary skin findings.

ANATOMIC ITCH CLASSIFICATION

Chronic itch is often classified into several subtypes typically reflecting anatomic basis of disease activity. In one scheme proposed by Twycross and colleagues,[13] pruritus subgroups include pruriceptive or dermatologic itch (arising in the skin), neuropathic itch (arising along the neural pathways caused by injury or damage), neurogenic itch (arising from abnormal activation of undamaged nerves because of endogenous or exogenous agents), and psychogenic itch (arising in the context of psychiatric disease). Building on this scheme, the International Forum for the Study of

Disclosure Statement: The author has nothing to disclose.
Massachusetts General Hospital, Boston, MA 02114, USA
* Cutaneous Biology Research Center, Department of Dermatology, Massachusetts General Hospital, 149 Thirteenth Street, Charlestown, MA 02129.
E-mail address: sbelmariah@mgh.harvard.edu

Dermatol Clin 36 (2018) 179–188
https://doi.org/10.1016/j.det.2018.02.002

Itch (IFSI) designed a two-tiered classification system that allows a physician to categorize itch based on clinical features alone (in the absence of a known or definitive anatomic target) or once diagnostic data have been obtained that suggest the underlying cause.[14] In the first tier, the IFSI scheme divides itch into three major types based on patient history and physical examination including Group I (pruritus on diseased skin including autoimmune or allergic disorders, drug rashes), Group II (pruritus on nondiseased or noninflamed skin including itch caused by systemic, neurologic, or psychiatric disorders, diseases of pregnancy, and drug-induced itch without a rash), or Group III (pruritus presenting with secondary scratch lesions, such as prurigo nodularis, lichen simplex chronicus, or hyperpigmentation). If clinical evaluation and diagnostic tests suggest a cause for the patient's pruritus, further categorization into one of the following six groups may be possible: (1) dermatologic diseases; (2) systemic diseases including diseases of pregnancy and drug-induced pruritus; (3) neurologic; (4) psychiatric/psychosomatic diseases; (5) mixed, when more than one underlying disease may contribute to itch; and (6) other, when no cause is identified.[14]

DIFFERENTIAL DIAGNOSIS OF ITCH

Itch in dermatologic disease or pruritoceptive itch results from the elaboration of inflammatory mediators in the skin in the setting of allergic diseases, infections, autoimmune or connective tissue diseases, cutaneous neoplasms, and genodermatoses. Commonly encountered primary inflammatory dermatoses that are associated with itch include atopic dermatitis, psoriasis, allergic or irritant contact dermatitis, urticaria, bullous pemphigoid, dermatophytosis, scabies and other infestations, xerosis, and many other conditions. Itch may be localized (as in the case of allergic contact dermatitis) or widespread (as in the case of scabies, atopic dermatitis). In many of the previously mentioned conditions, the presence of primary inflammatory lesions allows for immediate diagnosis by the trained clinician. In some cases, however, secondary changes of the skin may obscure primary lesions and further evaluation may be required.

Generalized pruritus may manifest in the context of numerous systemic diseases, including malignancy, renal and hepatic dysfunction, metabolic and endocrine disorders, infectious syndromes, and as a side effect of systemic medications (Table 1). In the IFSI classification, pruritic disorders of pregnancy are also included in this category. The exact mechanism by which such disorders provoke itch is unknown. In general, it is believed that damage, dysfunction, or neoplasia of specific organs results in the production of one or more byproducts that function as pruritogens that directly activate peripheral or central nerves. In some scenarios, acquired dysfunction of the nerves or neuropathy may lead to abnormal sensations of itch, similar to pain. Because of the highly variable nature of how pruritus arises in systemic disease, itch may manifest early in disease and can precede other systemic symptoms (eg, paraneoplastic itch in Hodgkin lymphoma), or may arise late in disease (eg, in chronic kidney disease). When chronic pruritus arises in the setting of systemic disease, only secondary lesions, such as excoriations, lichenification, prurigo nodules, and hyperpigmentation are observed on examination. Occasionally, other cutaneous stigmata of disease may be present and help the clinician hone in on a possible diagnosis (eg, jaundice, palmar erythema, and periumbilical varicosities in the setting of liver failure; acanthosis nigracans in diabetes or metabolic disorders; diffuse petechiae or purpura in the setting of various hematologic malignancies; nail changes in liver or kidney disease).

Itch that results from injury, degeneration, or acquired dysfunction of the afferent pruritoceptive pathways is considered neuropathic in origin (Table 2). Examples of neuropathic pruritus include localized pruritus syndromes, such as brachioradialis pruritus, notalgia or meralgia paresthetica, and postherpetic itch. Widespread or generalized neuropathic itch may develop in the context of neurodegenerative disorders, such as multiple sclerosis or because of small fiber neuropathies. Similar to what is observed in systemic itch, clinical findings in patients with neuropathic itch conditions consist of secondary lesions including excoriations, hyperpigmentation, and lichenification. Some systemic diseases may compromise neural pathways resulting in itch and may thus reflect a neuropathic cause. However, because neural compromise in these situations is secondary to another underlying disorder, such itches are currently classified under the systemic rubric.

Individuals with psychiatric or psychosomatic diseases may experience itch, formication and other tactile hallucinations, self-injurious or picking behaviors, and neurotic excoriations. One study estimated that approximately 40% of individuals admitted for inpatient psychiatric care experienced generalized itch.[15] Although skin picking is common in the general population, it frequently accompanies affective and anxiety

Table 1
Common systemic diseases that cause itch

Condition	Cutaneous Manifestations of Underlying Disease	Diagnostic Findings
Renal disorders		
End-stage chronic renal failure	Skin findings: butterfly sign (sparing of central back surrounded by hyperpigmentation and excoriations on "reachable" areas of back) Systemic findings/association: N/A	Clinical history/physical examination: suggestive, but need pathologic and/or serologic confirmation of underlying disease Pathology (skin): nondiagnostic Diagnostic work-up: BUN/Cr, CBC, ferritin
Reactive perforating collagenosis	Skin findings: dome-shaped flesh-colored or hyperpigmented papules with an adherent keratotic plug Systemic findings/association: chronic renal insufficiency, anemia	Clinical history/physical examination: suggestive, but need pathologic and/or serologic confirmation of skin lesions Pathology (skin): epidermal hyperplasia or cup-shaped depression with keratin plug containing parakeratosis, inflammatory debris, and basophilic collagen fibers in dermis and extruding through epidermis Diagnostic work-up: BUN/Cr, ferritin, fasting serum glucose
Hepatobiliary disease		
Primary biliary cirrhosis	Skin findings: palmar pruritus with or without erythema, hyperpigmentation, xanthelasma/xanthomas, spider nevi, jaundice Systemic findings/association: HSM ± ascites, peripheral edema, fatigue, abdominal discomfort	Clinical history/physical examination: suggestive, but need pathologic and/or serologic confirmation of underlying disease Pathology (skin): nondiagnostic Diagnostic work-up: elevated alkaline phosphatase, γ-glutamyl transpeptidase, IgM, AST/ALT, elevated bilirubin, ± thrombocytopenia, + antinuclear antibodies and antimitochondrial antibodies
Hepatitis C	Skin findings: xerosis, jaundice, peripheral edema, spider nevi, purpura, lichen planus, porphyria cutanea tarda Systemic findings/association: HSM ± ascites, peripheral edema, fatigue, abdominal discomfort, Raynaud disease	Clinical history/physical examination: suggestive, but need pathologic and/or serologic confirmation of underlying disease Pathology (skin): nondiagnostic Diagnostic work-up: Hepatitis C antibody, qualitative and quantitative assays for hepatitis C virus RNA, genotyping, hepatitis B Ag/Ab, HIV, CBC, TSH, LFTs
Cholestatic jaundice, also cholestasis of pregnancy	Skin findings: jaundice, telangiectasia/spider angiomas, palmar erythema, xanthelasma; alopecia Systemic findings/association: chronic hepatic insufficiency, peripheral edema, numerous sequelae depending on the cause of cholestasis	Clinical history/physical examination: suggestive, but need pathologic and/or serologic confirmation of underlying disease Pathology (skin): nondiagnostic Diagnostic work-up: elevated alkaline phosphatase, γ-glutamyl transpeptidase, AST/ALT, elevated bilirubin; cholangiography to help discern potential causes

(continued on next page)

Table 1
(continued)

Condition	Cutaneous Manifestations of Underlying Disease	Diagnostic Findings
Hematopoeitic disease		
Polycythemia vera	Skin findings: ecchymoses, mucosal bleeding Systemic findings/association: headache, splenomegaly, hepatomegaly, hypertension	Clinical history/physical examination: suggestive, but diagnosis of exclusion Pathology (skin): nondiagnostic Diagnostic work-up: hemoglobin >16.5; bone marrow biopsy showing hypercellularity with trilinear growth; JAK2V617F or JAK2 exon 12 mutation
Iron-deficiency anemia	Skin findings: pallor, nail bed pallor and spoon-shaped nail (koilonychia) atrophy of the lingual papillae on tongue, angular stomatitis Systemic findings/association: fatigue, cold intolerance, muscle cramps, splenomegaly, rarely pseudotumor cerebri	Clinical history/physical examination: suggestive, but diagnosis of exclusion after serologic confirmation of underlying anemia Pathology (skin): nondiagnostic Diagnostic work-up: low hemoglobin, hematocrit, MCV, and MCHC; low serum iron and ferritin, elevated TIBC; stool Hemoccult test; bone marrow aspiration
Hodgkin lymphoma	Skin findings: excoriations secondary to pruritus, new onset of eczema, xerosis Systemic findings/association: weight loss, fatigue, fever, sweats, asymptomatic lymphadenopathy, splenomegaly, hepatomegaly	Clinical history/physical examination: suggestive, but need pathologic and/or serologic confirmation of underlying disease Pathology (skin): nondiagnostic Diagnostic work-up: CBC with diff, ESR, LDH; chest, abdomen, pelvic CT + PET; lymph node biopsy needed to confirm
Non-Hodgkin lymphoma	Skin findings: in some cases, primary cutaneous papules, nodules, patches, plaques or tumors; pallor, purpura, ecchymoses Systemic findings/association: bulky lymphadenopathy, splenomegaly, hepatomegaly, abdominal or testicular masses	Clinical history/physical examination: suggestive but need pathologic and/or serologic confirmation of underlying disease Pathology (skin): nondiagnostic Diagnostic work-up: CBC with diff may show abnormalities, elevated β_2-microglobulin, LDH; chest, abdomen, pelvic CT + PET; lymph node or bone marrow biopsy needed to confirm
Multiple myeloma	Skin findings: pallor, purpura, ecchymoses Systemic findings/association: bone tenderness, neuropathy, hepatomegaly, splenomegaly, cardiomegaly	Clinical history/physical examination: suggestive, but need pathologic and/or serologic confirmation of underlying disease Pathology (skin): nondiagnostic Diagnostic work-up: SPEP and UPEP with immunofixation; bone marrow biopsy; CBC with diff may show abnormalities, elevated β_2-microglobulin, LDH; spine MRI

(continued on next page)

Table 1
(continued)

Condition	Cutaneous Manifestations of Underlying Disease	Diagnostic Findings
Endocrine and metabolic syndromes		
Hyperthyroidism	Skin findings: pretibial myxedema, erythema, edema, velvety skin, flushing and hyperhidrosis Systemic findings/association: anxiety, heat intolerance, palpitations, tachycardia, hypertension, tremors, muscle weakness	Clinical history/physical examination: suggestive, but need pathologic and/or serologic confirmation of underlying disease Pathology (skin): nondiagnostic Diagnostic work-up: suppressed TSH, elevated T3, T4; + autoantibodies - anti-TPO, anti-TSab
Hypothyroidism	Skin findings: xerosis, rough skin, coarse or brittle hair, alopecia, macroglossia, periorbital edema, pallor, jaundice Systemic findings/association: weight gain, fatigue, depression, bradycardia, altered blood pressure	Clinical history/physical examination: suggestive, but need pathologic and/or serologic confirmation of underlying disease Pathology (skin): nondiagnostic Diagnostic work-up: elevated TSH, decreased T3, T4; + autoantibodies -anti-thyroid peroxidase and antithyroglobulin antibodies; thyroid imaging
Diabetes	Skin findings: acanthosis nigricans, necrobiosis lipoidica diabeticorum, granuloma annulare, diabetic dermopathy, waxy skin syndrome, diabetic bullae, xerosis Systemic findings/association: retinopathy, neuropathy, chronic kidney disease, increased cardiovascular morbidity and mortality	Clinical history/physical examination: suggestive, but need pathologic and/or serologic confirmation of underlying disease Pathology (skin): nondiagnostic for itch, but may have reduced IENF density Diagnostic work-up: elevated fasting glucose, 2-h oral tolerance test, and HgbA$_{1c}$; UA; may have altered QST or QSART
Infectious disease		
HIV infection	Skin findings: coarse or xerotic skin, erythematous papules or folliculitis, history of recurrent infections, eczema Systemic findings/association: flulike illness, generalized lymphadenopathy, opportunistic infections, weight loss, dementia if severe	Clinical history/physical examination: suggestive, but need pathologic and/or serologic confirmation of underlying disease Pathology (skin): eosinophilic folliculitis reveals dermal eosinophils around the hair follicles and sebaceous glands Diagnostic work-up: ELISA or Western blot for HIV 1/2; p24 antigen detection; viral load; CD4 T-cell count

Abbreviations: ALT, alanine transaminase; AST, aspartate transaminase; BUN/Cr, blood, urea, nitrogen, creatinine; CBC, complete blood count; CSF, cerebrospinal fluid; CT, computed tomography; CVA, cerebrovascular incident; ELISA, enzyme-linked immunosorbent assay; ESR, erythrocyte sedimentation rate; HgbA$_{1c}$, hemoglobulin A$_{1c}$; HIV, human immunodeficiency virus; HSM, hepatosplenomegaly; IENF, intraepidermal nerve fiber; IF, immunofluorescence; LDH, lactate dehydrogenase; LFT, liver function tests; MCHC, mean corpuscular hemoglobin concentration; MCV, mean corpuscular volume; QSART, quantitative pseudomotor axon reflex testing; QST, quantitative sensory testing; SPEP, protein electrophoresis study from serum; TIBC, total iron binding capacity; TPO, thyroperoxidase; TSAB, thyroid-stimulating antibody; TSH, thyroid-stimulating hormone; UA, urine analysis; UPEP, protein electrophoresis study from urine.

disorders, eating and substance abuse disorders, and impulse control disorders. Psychiatric or psychogenic itch is a diagnosis of exclusion, and must be rendered once dermatologic, systemic, or neurologic causes of itch have been excluded. It is important to recognize that itch may result from medications used to treat psychiatric or neurologic diseases and that emotional stress

Table 2
Neuropathic itch

Condition	Cutaneous Manifestations of Underlying Disease	Diagnostic Findings
Brachioradial pruritus	Skin findings: excoriations on lateral aspect of arms and shoulders; may be generalized Systemic findings/association: neck, shoulder injury, photosensitivity	Clinical history/physical examination: sufficient for diagnosis in some cases Pathology (skin): nondiagnostic Diagnostic work-up: radiograph, CT, or MRI of cervical spine may demonstrate abnormalities
Notalgia or meralgia paresthetica	Skin findings: hyperpigmented patches on upper middle aspect of back, T2-T6 (notalgia), or outer thigh, lateral femoral cutaneous (meralgia); frequently unilateral Systemic findings/association: obesity, pregnancy	Clinical history/physical examination: sufficient for diagnosis in most of cases Pathology (skin): nondiagnostic Diagnostic work-up: radiograph, CT, or MRI of spine may demonstrate abnormalities
Postherpetic neuralgia	Skin findings: hyperpigmentation, lichenification or excoriations limited to previously affected dermatomes Systemic findings/association: prior herpes zoster eruption	Clinical history/physical examination: sufficient for diagnosis in most cases Pathology (skin): nondiagnostic Diagnostic work-up: CSF may show pleocytosis, elevated protein, or VZV DNA; increased anti-VZV antibody titers may be present
Multiple sclerosis	Skin findings: xerosis, localized or widespread secondary skin changes (hyperpigmentation, lichenification, excoriatons) Systemic findings/association: ataxia, double vision, Lhermitte sign (electrical spine pain when bending neck), sensory loss, parasthesias, dysesthesia	Clinical history/physical examination: suggestive, but diagnosis of exclusion Pathology (skin): may have reduced IENF density on protein gene product 9.5 biopsy Diagnostic work-up: MRI of brain and spinal cord, CSF electrophoresis, visual and sensory evoked potentials; may observe altered QST and QSART
Cerebrovascular accident	Skin findings: localized or widespread secondary skin changes (hyperpigmentation, lichenification, excoriatons); may also have cutaneous findings of purpura, petechia, Janeway lesions, Osler nodes Systemic findings/association: sensory loss, weakness, ataxia	Clinical history/physical examination: suggestive, but diagnosis of exclusion Pathology (skin): nondiagnostic Diagnostic work-up: imaging as part of CVA assessment

Abbreviations: CSF, cerebrospinal fluid; CT, computed tomography; CVA, cerebrovascular incident; IENF, intraepidermal nerve fiber; QSART, quantitative pseudomotor axon reflex testing; QST, quantitative sensory testing; VZV, varicella zoster virus.

and psychological factors may impact itch severity in the setting of pre-existing dermatologic or systemic disease.

DIAGNOSTIC EVALUATION OF THE ITCHY PATIENT

Because the differential diagnosis is so broad, it is necessary to take a systematic approach to evaluating the patient with chronic pruritus. The foundation of any successful diagnostic evaluation is a detailed history that elicits the onset, distribution (localized vs generalized), and progression of symptoms and whether symptoms are accompanied by a rash. The quality of the sensory disturbance may also be helpful. For example, burning in association with itch is characteristic of hives, but may also manifest with patients with atopic dermatitis, photodermatoses, or peripheral neuropathy. Identifying exposures, locations, or activities that provoke or aggravate itch may help narrow the differential diagnosis (eg, as in the case of an environmental or contact allergy, aquagenic pruritus, or cholinergic urticaria). Eliciting a history of new topical or systemic medications, personal care items (eg, detergents, fragrances, lotions), household items (eg, furniture, carpets, mattresses), or new household pets may suggest an allergy. A recent history of travel might suggest exposure to scabies, lice, or other parasitic infections. To elicit symptoms of systemic, neurologic, or psychiatric disease, a detailed review of symptoms should also be performed. Patients should be questioned about recent emotional stress, febrile illness, weight loss, abdominal discomfort, diarrhea or other gastrointestinal symptoms, numbness or paresthesias, dizziness, weakness, arthritis, allergic symptoms (conjunctivitis, rhinitis, angioedema), or other constitutional symptoms.

A comprehensive physical examination should be performed at the initial evaluation and should be repeated at subsequent visits as symptoms persist or evolve. The presence of primary lesions including xerosis, ichthyosis, macular or papular erythema, vesicles, bullae, or wheals suggests an underlying dermatologic disease. When pruritus is severe, primary lesions may be deeply excoriated or lichenified, obscuring characteristic lesional architecture and making a clinical diagnosis based on lesion morphology more challenging. Scratching the skin to elicit dermatographism may be helpful when allergic conditions, atopy, urticarial, or hypersensitivity reactions are suspected. Moreover, if the patient history suggests that exercise, heat, or cold can induce pruritus, consideration should be given to examining the patient for potential skin changes (eg, urticaria) following physical activity (eg, running in place for 1 minute), and application of a warm wash cloth or an ice cube. Examination of ocular, oral, and if symptomatic genital mucosa may also reveal inflammation, dehydration, or evidence of systemic or autoimmune diseases. In addition, physicians should seek out cutaneous signs of systemic diseases that might contribute to the patient's itch (eg, acanthosis nigricans in the undiagnosed patients with diabetes; jaundice, spider angioma, xanthelasma, purpura, or nail changes in a patient with chronic hepatic failure). Palpation of the thyroid for thyromegaly, nodularity, or tenderness (suggestive of Graves disease or Hashimoto thyroiditis); abdominal tenderness or organ enlargement (suggestive of hepatobiliary or splenic disease); and evaluation for lymphadenopathy (suggestive of malignancy or infection) should be performed.

If neuropathic disease is suspected, evaluation for abnormalities in pain or temperature (pathways that parallel and interact with itch pathways) should be performed. In a typical dermatology clinic setting, testing pain responses to a pinprick stimulus could be performed with the edge of single-use, disposable needle (26–30 gauge) or the broken edge of a wooden swab stick or tongue depressor. Temperature sensation may be assessed using the end of any metal instrument kept at room temperate. Sensory testing should begin on the distal first toe if a widespread neuropathy is suspected and then work proximally up the leg to assess the extent of sensory loss. If localized or dermatomal sensory disturbance is suspected, test at the distal and then proximal aspect of the area of concern and the corresponding contralateral area of the body for comparison. In general, it is helpful to have patients close their eyes during neurologic evaluation.

If a diagnosis is made following history and physical examination, further evaluation may or may not be necessary. When a nonspecific dermatitis or heavily excoriated primary lesions are observed on the initial examination, a skin biopsy may be helpful to confirm a suspected diagnosis. In the absence of an obvious primary dermatitis, when an immediate diagnosis cannot be made, the author suggests a trial of empiric therapy for 2 to 3 weeks. This effort may consist of regular use of bland emollients and midpotency topical corticosteroids, and avoidance of harsh detergents, fragrances, and any identifiable triggers (**Fig. 1**). In patients who are dermatographic or in whom the clinician is suspecting an allergic trigger, a trial of long-acting, oral antihistamines should be pursued. If a hypersensitivity reaction to a particular medication or supplement is suspected, then a trial of drug avoidance for a minimum of 2 to 3 months should be pursued if possible.

When a patient with chronic itch has failed a reasonable trial of empiric therapy, further diagnostic evaluation should be pursued (see **Fig. 1**). First, the clinician should perform a skin biopsy of lesional or actively pruritic skin for standard hematoxylin and eosin staining to evaluate for subclinical inflammation. Special stains to evaluate for an increase in the number of specific inflammatory cells (eg, mast cells, eosinophils) or the presence of fungal elements may be necessary. An additional biopsy may be sent for direct immunofluorescence to assess for autoimmune inflammation (eg, bullous pemphigoid, dermatitis herpetiformis) if clinical suspicion warrants.

If an allergic reaction is suspected based on clinical examination or suggested by skin biopsy, patch testing for type IV delayed hypersensitivity reactions should be performed to common allergens including preservatives, fragrances, metals, and to the patient's own personal care products (eg, soaps, detergents, lotions). The relevance of any identified allergens must then be determined

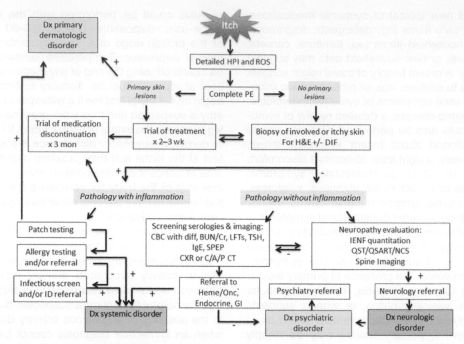

Fig. 1. Diagnostic approach to the itchy patient. BUN/Cr, blood, urea, nitrogen, creatinine; C/A/P CT, chest, abdomen, pelvis computed tomography; CBC, complete blood count; CXR, chest radiograph; DIF, direct immuno-fluorescence; GI, gastrointestinal; H&E, hematoxylin and eosin; HPI, history of present illness; ID, infectious disease; IENF, intraepidermal nerve fiber quantitation; LFT, liver function tests; NCS, nerve conduction studies; Onc, oncology; PE, physical exam; QSART, quantitative sudomotor axon reflex testing; QST, quantitative sensory testing; ROS, review of systems; SPEP, protein electrophoresis study from serum; TSH, thyroid stimulating hormone. (*Adapted from* Fleurant A, Elmariah SB. Evaluation of the itchy patient. Curr Dermatol Rep 2018;8. https://doi.org/10.1007/s13671-018-0208-y; with permission.)

by having the patient avoid them for at least 3 months. Additional allergy testing for type I IgE-mediated hypersensitivity reactions performed by an allergist may be warranted in patients who fail patch testing or have chronic or seasonal urticarial dermatoses.

When chronic itch arises in the setting of urticaria, new-onset dermatographism, or pathologic evidence of eosinophils and/or blood eosinophilia in the absence of an identifiable allergic cause, patients should undergo evaluation for intestinal parasitic infection by helminths and/or protozoa. Such studies are also indicated when patients with chronic pruritus report having traveled outside of the United States or been camping before the onset of their symptoms; after consuming undercooked meats; and in any patient who reports having abdominal symptoms, diarrhea, and/or has evidence of unexplained nutritional deficiencies (eg, vitamin B_{12} or iron deficiency). Initial screening consists of examination of stool smears collected over 3 days for ova or parasites.[16] Serologic screening for antibodies to strongyloides is advised by some experts. Similarly, screening for peripheral blood antibodies or

detection of antigens directly in the stool using such techniques as enzyme-linked immunosorbent assay, immunoblot, or polymerase chain reaction assays may be helpful to evaluate for helminths that are not readily identified in stool samples (eg, *Toxocara* sp, schistosomes, filariae, and trichinella).[17] When the clinical suspicion for a parasitic infection is high, empiric antihelminthic therapy may be considered and the patient should be referred to an infectious disease specialist.

In the absence of clinical or pathologic inflammation of the skin, patients with chronic pruritus should undergo diagnostic work-up for systemic or neurologic causes of itch. The initial serologic screening should include complete blood count with differential; liver function tests including aspartate transaminase, alanine transaminase, alkaline phosphatase, and total and direct bilirubin; lactate dehydrogenase; thyroid-stimulating hormone; and a total IgE level.[3] Further serologic testing should be performed based on individual risk factors or concomitant symptoms. For example, in sexually active individuals and/or those with intravenous drug use or transfusion history, unexplained weight loss, or febrile illness, screening for infectious causes, such as human immunodeficiency virus (HIV), hepatitis B or C, or syphilis, may be warranted. In patients with an exposure history and systemic complaints, screening for Lyme disease or tuberculosis should be pursued because late or latent stages of these diseases may be accompanied by itch with or without a rash. Protein electrophoresis studies from serum or urine with immunofixation, peripheral blood smear, chest radiograph, colonoscopy, and prostate or breast examination (as appropriate) may be indicated in chronically itchy patients that are older or experiencing constitutional symptoms.[18] Serologic or stool studies if parasite infection is suspected may be performed as outlined previously.

When the initial systemic work-up suggests an underlying cause, a referral to one or more specialists in the indicated fields should be made. Most commonly, patients with chronic itch may benefit from being seen by allergy/immunology, rheumatology, hematology/oncology, endocrinology, and/or infectious disease specialists for further diagnostic evaluation. An allergist may perform a series of tests to evaluate ingested, inhaled, or other environmental allergens and the potential for a mast cell disorder. Allergy skin tests including prick, puncture, or intradermal testing or serologic radioallergosorbent tests is highly recommended when an environmental trigger is suspected. Patients with refractory pruritus who also experience hives, angioedema, heat intolerance, flushing, dizziness, gastrointestinal upset, pulmonary, or cardiac symptoms, or have a history of anaphylaxis should undergo further evaluation for mast cell disease. Screening consists of evaluating total serum tryptase and histamine levels, 24-hour urinary excretion of histamine, N-methylhistamine or N-methylimidazoleacetic acid, leukotrienes, or prostaglandin isoforms (eg, leukotriene E_4, prostaglandin D_2, 11-beta-prostaglandin F_2).[19,20] Screening for genetic mutations in c-kit from peripheral blood or bone marrow may be helpful in working up a possible proliferative disorder involving mast cells.[19,20]

When a patient with chronic itch has evidence of hematologic disease including anemia or polycythemia, thrombocytopenia or thrombocytosis, leukocytosis, unexplained eosinophilia, or a protein electrophoresis study from serum suggestive of a gammopathy on his or her initial screening, the patient should be referred to a hematologist for bone marrow examination. In some cases, genetic screening for malignancy-associated mutations may be performed using peripheral blood.

Several different options exist when approaching the diagnostic evaluation of pruritus in a patient in whom neuropathic itch is suspected or

systemic work-up has been unrevealing. If clinical suspicion for neuropathy is high, a trial of treatment with neuromodulators may be attempted. When pruritus is limited to a localized area of skin, mononeuropathy or multifocal neuropathy of a local cause (eg, trauma, compression, or entrapment) may be confirmed by computed tomography or MRI of the corresponding area of the spine or proximal joint. If pruritus is generalized and/or accompanied by other sensory symptoms (eg, burning, pain, tingling, prickling, or sensory loss), the patient should undergo evaluation for a polyneuropathy that affects multiple peripheral nerves simultaneously. A reasonable first step in this scenario is to evaluate the intraepidermal nerve fiber density and patterns of cutaneous innervation by examining skin obtained from the distal lower leg. Skin samples intended for this type of study require that the tissue be preserved in a paraformaldehyde-based fixative, that the pathology service can perform immunofixation or immunohistochemistry for protein gene product 9.5 to identify neural processes, and a pathologist who is familiar with reading such samples.[21] A reduction in intraepidermal nerve fiber density suggests a small fiber polyneuropathy and warrants referral to a neurologist for quantitative sensory and/or sudomotor reflex testing.[22] Similar to pruritus, polyneuropathy is associated with a large number of systemic and/or neurologic processes. Screening for some of the more common causes (eg, diabetes, HIV, nutritional deficiencies, alcohol abuse or drug toxicities, autoimmune disease) should include fasting serum glucose, glucose tolerance testing or HgbA$_{1c}$, vitamin B$_{12}$ levels, protein electrophoresis studies from serum or urine with immunofixation, thyroid-stimulating hormone, antinuclear antibodies, erythrocyte sedimentation rate, rheumatoid factor, and HIV.[22] Screening for Lyme disease and more specific testing for autoimmune disorders or infectious agents may also be performed if indicated by history or physical examination.

If the diagnostic work-up suggested previously is unrevealing, the author advocates a trial of empiric neuromodulator therapy if it has not previously been attempted. If such an intervention attenuates pruritus, it is up to the clinician's discretion as to whether a diagnosis of neuropathic or psychogenic itch may be appropriate. Whether the patient's itch is psychiatric in nature or simply exacerbated by stress, the influence of chronic and severe pruritus on an individual's quality of life should not be underestimated. The author advocates that all patients with chronic itch who are suffering from associated anxiety, depression, or social isolation may benefit from seeing a psychiatrist, psychologist, or mind-body specialist, and/or taking part in a support group.

SUMMARY

Pruritus is a common and at times disabling symptom that arises in the setting of countless dermatologic, systemic, neurologic, or psychiatric disorders. Although it may be trivial to diagnose the cause of pruritus in cases of primary dermatologic disease, identifying causes of chronic pruritus in the absence of an eruption may be far more challenging. Obtaining a detailed history, review of systems, and performing a complete physical examination are critical first steps in evaluating the chronically itchy patient, and invariably direct the clinician's diagnostic work-up. A skin biopsy of actively itchy skin is helpful when trying to confirm or exclude primary inflammation. If inflammation is observed, patients may undergo evaluation for allergic, infectious, malignant, or autoimmune pathology that would fuel such inflammation. In the absence of primary inflammation, systemic or neurologic causes must be evaluated. Referral to other medical subspecialties should be considered only after initial screening has been attempted or the history and physical suggest another underlying primary diagnosis.

REFERENCES

1. Pereira MP, Kremer AE, Mettang T, et al. Chronic pruritus in the absence of skin disease: pathophysiology, diagnosis and treatment. Am J Clin Dermatol 2016;17:337–48.

2. Stander S, Schäfer I, Phan NQ, et al. Prevalence of chronic pruritus in Germany: results of a cross-sectional study in a sample working population of 11,730. Dermatology 2010;221:229–35.

3. Yosipovitch G, Bernhard JD. Clinical practice. Chronic pruritus. N Engl J Med 2013;368:1625–34.

4. Dalgard F, Svensson A, Holm JO, et al. Self-reported skin morbidity among adults: associations with quality of life and general health in a Norwegian survey. J Investig Dermatol Symp Proc 2004;9:120–5.

5. Pisoni RL, Wikström B, Elder SJ, et al. Pruritus in haemodialysis patients: International results from the Dialysis Outcomes and Practice Patterns Study (DOPPS). Nephrol Dial Transplant 2006;21:3495–505.

6. Stumpf A, Ständer S, Warlich B, et al. Relations between the characteristics and psychological comorbidities of chronic pruritus differ between men and women: women are more anxious than men. Br J Dermatol 2015;172:1323–8.

7. Kini SP, DeLong LK, Veledar E, et al. The impact of pruritus on quality of life: the skin equivalent of pain. Arch Dermatol 2011;147:1153–6.

8. Ross SE, Hachisuka J, Todd AJ. Spinal Microcircuits and the Regulation of Itch. In: Carstens E, Akiyama T, editors. Itch: Mechanisms and Treatment. Boca Raton (FL): CRC Press/Taylor & Francis; 2014. Chapter 20.

9. Azimi E, Xia J, Lerner EA. Peripheral mechanisms of itch. Curr Probl Dermatol 2016;50:18–23.

10. Wilson SR, Thé L, Batia LM, et al. The epithelial cell-derived atopic dermatitis cytokine TSLP activates neurons to induce itch. Cell 2013;155:285–95.

11. Gangemi S, Quartuccio S, Casciaro M, et al. Interleukin 31 and skin diseases: a systematic review. Allergy Asthma Proc 2017;38:401–8.

12. Akiyama T, Lerner EA, Carstens E. Protease-activated receptors and itch. Handb Exp Pharmacol 2015;226:219–35.

13. Twycross R, Greaves MW, Handwerker H, et al. Itch: scratching more than the surface. QJM 2003;96:7–26.

14. Stander S, Weisshaar E, Mettang T, et al. Clinical classification of itch: a position paper of the International Forum for the Study of Itch. Acta Derm Venereol 2007;87:291–4.

15. Kretzmer GE, Gelkopf M, Kretzmer G, et al. Idiopathic pruritus in psychiatric inpatients: an explorative study. Gen Hosp Psychiatry 2008;30:344–8.

16. Micheletti RG, Dominguez AR, Wanat KA. Bedside diagnostics in dermatology: parasitic and noninfectious diseases. J Am Acad Dermatol 2017;77:221–30.

17. Buonfrate D, Formenti F, Perandin F, et al. Novel approaches to the diagnosis of Strongyloides stercoralis infection. Clin Microbiol Infect 2015;21:543–52.

18. Yosipovitch G. Chronic pruritus: a paraneoplastic sign. Dermatol Ther 2010;23:590–6.

19. Akin C, Valent P, Metcalfe DD. Mast cell activation syndrome: proposed diagnostic criteria. J Allergy Clin Immunol 2010;126:1099–104.e4.

20. Onnes MC, Tanno LK, Elberink JN. Mast cell clonal disorders: classification, diagnosis and management. Curr Treat Options Allergy 2016;3:453–64.

21. Myers MI, Peltier AC. Uses of skin biopsy for sensory and autonomic nerve assessment. Curr Neurol Neurosci Rep 2013;13:323.

22. Terkelsen AJ, Karlsson P, Lauria G, et al. The diagnostic challenge of small fibre neuropathy: clinical presentations, evaluations, and causes. Lancet Neurol 2017;16:934–44.

Prurigo Nodularis and Its Management

Claudia Zeidler, MD[a],*, Gil Yosipovitch, MD[b], Sonja Ständer, MD[a]

KEYWORDS

- Prurigo nodularis • Chronic pruritus • Itch • Pruritus • Scratch lesions • Therapy

KEY POINTS

- Prurigo nodularis occurs along with single or multiple distributed hyperkeratotic intensively itchy nodules.
- Prurigo nodularis is difficult to treat and causes a high disease burden.
- New treatments that target the neural system offer significant hope for this intractable itch.

INTRODUCTION

Many patients with chronic pruritus suffer from prurigo nodularis (PN), an intensely pruritic, chronic disease that occurs as a result the so-called vicious itch–scratch cycle.[1] PN is a subtype of chronic prurigo CPG that was recently defined as being its own disease entity.[2]

It is thought that 50% of patients with PN suffer from an atopic disposition.[3] Besides dermatoses, several systemic diseases, infections, and psychiatric and neurologic disorders are known to trigger PN and the frequently treatment-refractory itch–scratch cycle.[4] PN is regarded as having the highest itch intensity among the many diverse types of chronic pruritus.[4,5] It can not only cause sleep disturbances and psychiatric comorbidities, but also a diminished quality of life.[6]

EPIDEMIOLOGY

There is a severe lack of epidemiologic data detailing the prevalence and incidence of PN. Findings based on case series indicate that all age groups, including children,[7] can be affected by PN; however, the elderly were found to be the most frequently affected patient group.[4] Increased numbers of PN lesions are also associated with African Americans suffering from atopic eczema more than any other racial group.[8] Conclusions have not been made regarding gender differences owing to a lack of consistent reporting.[4]

PATHOPHYSIOLOGY

Although the detailed pathogenesis remains nearly unclear, cutaneous inflammation and neuronal plasticity seem to play a crucial role in PN.[9] The neural dermal hyperplasia (Pautrier's neuroma) associated with PN was already observed by Pautrier in 1934.[10] Histopathologic studies have established that changes occur in nearly all types of skin cells, including collagen fibers, epidermal keratinocytes, mast cells, dendritic cells, endothelial cells, eosinophils, and the epidermal and dermal nerve fibers.[11,12] An increased quantity of fibroblasts and capillaries, a papillary dermal fibrosis, and dense dermal interstitial and perivascular infiltrate with elevated numbers of T cells, mast cells, and eosinophil granulocytes has been observed

Disclosure Statement: The authors have nothing to disclose.
[a] Department of Dermatology, Center for Chronic Pruritus, University Hospital Münster, Von- Esmarch-Strasse 58, Münster DE-48149, Germany; [b] Department of Dermatology and Itch Center, Miller School of Medicine, University of Miami, University of Miami Hospital, 1295 Northwest 14th Street, South Building, Suites K-M, Miami, FL, USA
* Corresponding author.
E-mail address: Claudia.zeidler@ukmuenster.de

Dermatol Clin 36 (2018) 189–197
https://doi.org/10.1016/j.det.2018.02.003

derm.theclinics.com

in the dermis of PN lesions. In the epidermis, an irregular epidermal hyperplasia or pseudoepitheliomatous hyperplasia, a thick compact orthohyperkeratosis, focal parakeratosis, and hypergranulosis can be observed. However, the altered nerve fibers structure seems to be of the greatest importance.[12]

Skin cells can trigger inflammation and pruritus via releasing the substances interleukin (IL)-31, tryptase, eosinophil cationic protein, histamine, prostaglandins, and various neuropeptides such as nerve growth factor, substance P (SP), and calcitonin gene-related peptide.[13–16] From a comparison of skin biopsies from patients with PN and healthy skin, it was found that a 50-fold upregulation of IL-31 messenger RNA occurred in the PN biopsies.[17] Recent studies have determined that the T-cell–derived cytokine IL-31 produces severe pruritus in mouse models via binding to a heterodimeric IL-31 receptor A and oncostatin M receptor, which is expressed on epithelial cells, including keratinocytes and on IL-31RA(+)/TRPV1(+)/TRPA1(+) neurons and eosinophils.[18–20]

SP is produced and secreted by neurons, binding to the neurokinin-1 receptor expressed in the skin and central nervous system.[21] After binding in the skin, neurogenic inflammation, brief vasodilation, plasma extravasation, and mast cell degranulation develop.[21] An increased expression of this neuropeptide in PN has previously been observed by researchers,[22] possibly indicating the discovery of a causal proinflammatory signal important to the development of PN. The SP antagonist (an neurokinin-1 antagonist) aprepitant has demonstrated positive effects on pruritus in patients with PN.[23] These findings underline the importance of SP for PN. Calcitonin gene-related peptide is also overexpressed in PN.[24] This neuropeptide has a similar mechanism resulting in neurogenic inflammation via the regulation of inflammatory cells such as eosinophils and mast cells.[24] In addition to neuropeptides, increased numbers of neutrophins are also found in the nerve fibers of those with PN.[15]

When compared with findings in the dermis, the epidermis of skin affected by PN, as well as its interlesional skin, revealed hypoplasia of the sensory nerves.[13,24] Furthermore, biopsies of healed nodules displayed a recovering epidermal nerve fiber density.[25] A functional small fiber neuropathy was, however, undetectable in patients with PN.[26] It is, therefore, likely that the reduced epidermal nerve fiber density is a consequence of recurrent scratching rather than the result of a small fiber neuropathy.[26]

CLINICAL PRESENTATION

Crusted or excoriated, hyperkeratotic, light to bright red papules, nodules, or plaques with hyperpigmented margins are distinguishing characteristics of PN. Skin lesions can range from either a few millimeters to 2 to 3 cm in size and in number from just a few to hundreds of lesions. Patients can be graded into mild (≤20 lesions), moderate (20–100 lesions) to severe (>100 lesions) forms of PN (unpublished data, Jasmin Pölkin, 2018). On top of the lesions, independent of their number, excoriations and crusts can be present, pointing to ongoing scratching. In most cases, the lesions have a generalized, symmetric distribution on the extensor surfaces of the trunk and extremities. Localized PN exists, for example, in local dermatologic (leg venous insufficiency) and neuropathic (eg, brachioradial pruritus at the arms) diseases. The central back is difficult for patients to reach with their hands, leaving them unable to scratch it. This untouched area of the skin usually resembles a butterfly shape and is thus aptly named the "butterfly sign"[1,9,27] (Fig. 1). PN is an intensely pruritic condition. Most of the affected patients report a combination of sensations rather than just only pruritus, ranging from warmth and cold to stinging, burning, and tingling. These sensations occur independent of the etiology.[4]

In addition to the sensorial and visually evident symptoms, PN is known to have a significant, negative influence on patients' quality of life owing to sleep disturbances, behavioral and adjustment disorders, social isolation, and psychological hardship.[28,29]

ETIOLOGIC FACTORS
Dermatoses

Several inflammatory dermatoses have been linked to PN, of which atopic eczema has been

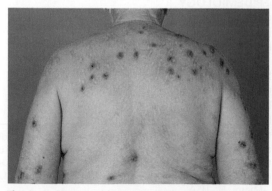

Fig. 1. A 77-year-old woman with prurigo nodularis owing to atopic predisposition with typical distribution of lesions, including the "butterfly sign" (no lesions on the center of the back).

identified as the most frequently occurring.[30] The vicious itch–scratch cycle that sustains PN occurs as a result of the dermatoses evolving in combination with itch. PN is thought to coexist with inflammatory dermatoses or persist after their treatment. Pruriginous atopic eczema is a term used to describe this association, because it echoes the synchronism and biological links between both conditions. Despite showing no signs of an active dermatosis, many patients with PN have an atopic background.

Although infrequent, pruritic cutaneous T-cell lymphoma, lichen planus, and dermatitis herpetiformis have the potential to cause PN.[4] PN lesions may indicate the initial clinical signs of an incipient bullous pemphigoid in some patients, especially the elderly.[31,32] Conducting a direct immunofluorescence examination in suspected cases of bullous pemphigoid in the elderly is recommended to establish a diagnosis.[33] Some patients have previous scabies leading to an itch–scratch cycle, the so-called nodular scabies. It is important to ensure the complete eradication of the scabies mites. Almost all patients who have atopy have in common a dry lichenified skin on top of the nodules, but also in between owing to the atopic predisposition, use of skin damaging measures, and/or as a consequence of scratching.

Most Common Systemic and Neurologic Diseases

It is estimated that 18% to 60% of patients with chronic renal failure are impacted by chronic itch.[34,35] More than one-half of these patients selected for a study on chronic pruritus as a result of chronic renal failure presented with PN.[36] Of patients on hemodialysis, 10% exhibited excoriations and scratched nodules typical to the clinical picture of PN in a representative, prospective, cross-sectional study on patients in dialysis units (GEHIS [German Epidemiological Hemodialysis Itch Study]).[37]

A connection between PN and diabetes mellitus has also been established.[38] PN lesions with nodules resembling Kyrle disease often occur in both chronic renal failure and diabetes mellitus (Fig. 2).[39,40] Kyrle disease was recently determined to be a variation of PN.[41] Interestingly, chronic pruritus owing to liver diseases was found to rarely cause PN.[42] PN frequently accompanies infections such as human immunodeficiency virus more often than other diseases.[43] Experts have correlated the severity of PN with decreased quantities of CD4 cells. A high human immunodeficiency virus prevalence may thus denote a high

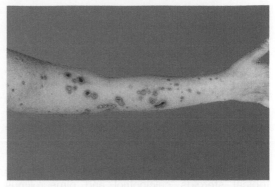

Fig. 2. Prurigo nodularis owing to diabetes mellitus type II in a 43-year-old patient resembling Kyrle disease.

PN prevalence. The symptoms of PN generally improve after treatment with antiretrovirals.[43]

PN can become localized owing to neuropathic diseases causing damage to cutaneous or extracutaneous nerves.[44] PN not only periodically arises owing to a postherpetic neuralgia,[45] but also in the context of several neuropathic forms of chronic pruritus, such as brachioradial pruritus localized mainly to the dermatome C5/C6.[46]

Psychiatric Disorders

PN can also develop as a result of psychogenic pruritus triggered by depression, anxiety, obsessive compulsive disorders, and tactile hallucinations,[47] and is a separate entity from skin picking disorder, a nonpruritic mental disorder that leads patients to perform body-focused repetitive behavior, such as scratching.[48] Skin picking disorder corresponds with mental disorders and/or pathologic behaviors, further emphasizing the need for identification of the underlying illness.[48]

TREATMENT OF PRURIGO NODULARIS

Therapies for PN generally aim to interrupt the vicious itch–scratch This therapeutic principle applies regardless of the cause for the chronic pruritus. An individual therapeutic plan must first be prepared that considers the patient's age, comorbidities, severity, and manifestation of their PN, as well as restrictions to the quality of life and expected side effects.[49] For better compliance and adherence, the various possibilities associated with the therapy, including its advantages and disadvantages, side effects, duration, possible use of off-label substances, and many therapeutic stages, should be explained individually. The treatment of PN usually extends over a prolonged period of time, which can be frustrating in cases of severe mental and physical stress and, occasionally, one too many treatment failures.[49] A good long-term management of the patient is thus required.

Owing to a lack of data from randomized controlled trials, PN remains difficult to treat. A multimodal treatment algorithm can be adopted for this purpose[49] (Fig. 3). A decrease in itching and the healing of PN lesions should be the main goals of a symptomatic therapy. Emollients are recommended as both a basis therapy and general therapeutic measure.

With regard to topical therapies for PN, the topical steroids calcipotriol and pimecrolimus have previously been analyzed in randomized controlled trials. All other substances have been described in CS. When compared with an antipruritic moisturizing cream (visual analog scale [VAS] of 0–10; 5.6 after use), betamethasone 0.1% cream was found to significantly reduce itch (VAS before, 8.8; VAS after, 3.9) and resulted in flattened nodules.[50] Further clinical improvement was noted after direct injection of triamcinolone acetonide into patients' nodules.[51] Topical steroids can conveniently be used in combination with an occlusive dressing to treat inflamed pruriginous lesions.[52] Topical calcineurin inhibitors may serve as a long-term treatment option. Pimecrolimus exhibits ameliorating effects on itch similar to those of hydrocortisone (VAS before pimecrolimus, 7.1; VAS after pimecrolimus, 4.4 [P<.001]; VAS after hydrocortisone. 4.5 [P<.001]) and has a marked impact on PN.[53] It was established that PN lesions were significantly decreased in patients treated with calcipotriol ointment, a vitamin D derivative, when compared with those with betamethasone valerate.[54] In another investigation, the skin's condition improved after the application of topical capsaicin, inhibiting localized, neuropathic forms of PN, thus resulting in improvements to the skin's condition.[55,56] Topical ketamine, used in combination with amitriptyline with and without lidocaine, is an additional method of treatment used mainly in the United States that targets the transient receptor potential channels, similar to capsaicin.[57,58]

Phototherapy, especially psoralen and ultraviolet (UV)A, UVA, and UVB light,[59] is a feasible viable therapeutic alternative for many patients, such as the elderly with multiple comorbidities and medications. Narrowband UVB therapy is, however, a

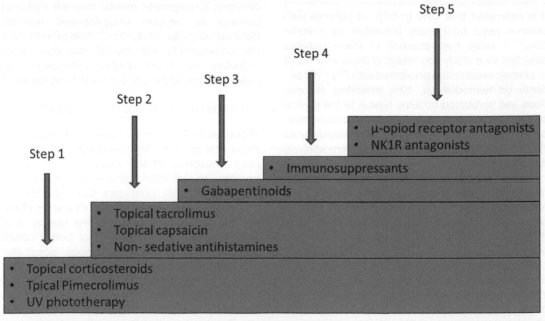

Fig. 3. Treatment algorithm for prurigo nodularis. NK1R, neurokinin-1 receptor; UV, ultraviolet. (*Data from* Ständer S, Zeidler C, Augustin M, et al. S2k guidelines for the diagnosis and treatment of chronic pruritus - update - short version. J Dtsch Dermatol Ges 2017;8:860–72; with permission.)

more current, effective option.[59] Patients treated with a combination of psoralen and UVA and a 308-nm excimer laser showed an accelerated healing.[59] Another treatment method, a modified Goeckermen regimen in which a daily, multistep broadband UVB treatment is performed and after which crude coal tar and topical steroids are applied to the skin under occlusion, has provided positive results[60]; however, the potentially carcinogenic nature of tar must be further investigated. For this reason, this modified regimen should be used with caution and offered only to selected patients.[61]

Owing to the increased quantities of mast cells detected in PN lesions, antihistamines are frequently used as treatments for PN. A high dose of a nonsedating antihistamine was combined, if needed, with a sedating antihistamine at nighttime, as described in a case series.[62] However, nowadays, sedating antihistamines are no longer recommended owing to side effects. Antihistamines and leukotriene inhibitors reduced the number of patients' PN lesions from between 10 and 290 (mean, 107.6) before treatment to between 0 and 154 after treatment (mean, 42.7).[63] These data, however, are based solely on individual reports and most experts concede that antihistamines are not a sufficient treatment method for PN.[64] There are currently insufficient data from systematic analyses and randomized controlled trials on the application of antihistamines for PN.

The introduction of the gabapentinoids gabapentin and pregabalin to patients with PN should be considered in patients with painful, neuropathic subqualities, and therapy-refractory to previous therapies. Gabapentinoids have proven to successfully treat chronic pruritus in randomized controlled trials.[65] Improvements of PN have thus far only been reported in case series.[66,67] Experts have yet to fully grasp its mechanisms of action, although it is suspected that stabilization of the spinal nerve membrane caused by calcium channel blockage, inhibition of glutamate synthesis, and the reinforcement of the GABA inhibitory mechanisms so that incoming signals are halted at the presynaptic membrane, are involved.[67] When prescribing gabapentinoids to the elderly or those with renal failure, it is necessary to consider the side effects profile and dosage adjustments.

μ-Opioid receptor antagonists such as naloxone (intravenous) and naltrexone (oral) have previously demonstrated efficacy for patients with PN in case series.[68] A randomized controlled trial for cholestatic pruritus documented a considerable decrease in itch intensity.[69] Of patients with PN of a dermatologic origin, 67.7% described improved symptoms in a case series, and 38% reported a complete healing of the PN.[70] Despite the efficacy of μ-opioid receptor antagonists, there are several side effects to consider that occur during the first few days of an oral treatment, including dizziness and vomiting. A polytherapy of κ-opioid receptor agonists and μ-opioid receptor antagonists (eg, butorphanol) may also have an antipruritic effect on PN.[71,72]

Paroxetine, amitryptiline, and mirtazapine are antidepressants that have demonstrated beneficial effects on patients with severe PN. Skin lesions caused by scratching were either partially or completely healed in patients participating in a 2-arm proof-of-concept study. This same patient group also reported a significantly decreased pruritus intensity.[73]

Immunosuppressants also comprise a viable therapeutic option for severe PN, although care must be taken to weigh their risk–benefit ratio. The success of immunosuppressive substances such as cyclosporine and methotrexate has been documented in case series.[74,75] It is vital to carefully monitor the blood pressure and other values, especially those of the kidneys, during immunosuppressive therapy. Thalidomide, a neurotoxic and teratogenic drug, has been described in several case series for PN.[76,77] Data from 280 patients with chronic pruritus, mostly with PN, were published in a recent review[78] that analyzed their treatment with thalidomide. It was found that, although the symptoms of PN and the itch intensity were reduced, the incidence rate of peripheral neuropathy was approximately 20% during the initial year of treatment.[79] As a result, thalidomide is considered a last choice in only the most severe cases of PN. Despite the success of its second-generation successor, lenalidomide, for treating pruritus and PN lesions in case reports, there is conflicting information regarding its neurotoxicity.[80]

A polytherapy of immunoglobins and methotrexate has also displayed an antipruritic effect for the treatment of PN related to atopic dermatitis.[81]

Novel Approaches

Increased levels of IL-31 and receptors for SP and opioids are, based on our current understanding of PN's pathomechanisms, currently the most promising targets in PN therapy.

The neurokinin-1 receptor antagonists aprepitant (German register: DRKS00005594) and serlopitant (VPD-737; ClinicalTrial.Gov: NCT02196324) have also been examined in recent randomized controlled trials on PN. The recent trial on serlopitant determined that the majority of the participating patients with PN had significantly reduced itch,[82] as was demonstrated in the previous care series for aprepitant.[23]

The efficacy of nalbuphine, a dual opioid receptor μ-antagonist/κ-agonist, is currently undergoing testing for PN treatment in the United States and Europe (NCT02174419) and seems to be promising. The application of nalbuphine for patients with uremic pruritus resulted in a decreased itch intensity in another recent randomized controlled trial.[83]

Another main aim of future trials on PN is to analyze the antipruritic effect of IL-31 blockage at the respective receptor. Nemolizumab, another substance, was confirmed to exhibit clinically meaningful improvements of this symptom in investigations on atopic dermatitis, a similar itch disease.[84,85]

SUMMARY

Based on neuronal sensitization processes, PN is closely intertwined with the vicious itch–scratch cycle. The proper management of PN will continue to present a therapeutic challenge as long as its pathophysiology remains unclear. Multiple ongoing randomized controlled trials conducted on novel targets, including the IL-31, neurokinin-1, and other various opioid receptors, provide hope for effective treatments for this stubborn, chronically itchy disease.

REFERENCES

1. Schedel F, Schurmann C, Metze D, et al. Prurigo. Clinical definition and classification. Hautarzt 2014; 65:684–90 [in German].
2. Pereira MP, Steinke S, Zeidler C, et al. European Academy of Dermatology and Venereology European Prurigo Project: expert consensus on the definition, classification and terminology of chronic prurigo. J Eur Acad Dermatol Venereol 2017. https://doi.org/10.1111/jdv.14570.
3. Tanaka M, Aiba S, Matsumura N, et al. Prurigo nodularis consists of two distinct forms: early-onset atopic and late-onset non-atopic. Dermatology 1995;190:269–76.
4. Iking A, Grundmann S, Chatzigeorgakidis E, et al. Prurigo as a symptom of atopic and non-atopic diseases: aetiological survey in a consecutive cohort of 108 patients. J Eur Acad Dermatol Venereol 2013; 27:550–7.
5. Mollanazar NK, Sethi M, Rodriguez RV, et al. Retrospective analysis of data from an itch center: integrating validated tools in the electronic health record. J Am Acad Dermatol 2016;75:842–4.

6. Schneider G, Driesch G, Heuft G, et al. Psychosomatic cofactors and psychiatric comorbidity in patients with chronic itch. Clin Exp Dermatol 2006;31: 762–7.
7. Amer A, Fischer H. Prurigo nodularis in a 9-year-old girl. Clin Pediatr (Phila) 2009;48:93–5.
8. Vachiramon V, Tey HL, Thompson AE, et al. Atopic dermatitis in African American children: addressing unmet needs of a common disease. Pediatr Dermatol 2012;29:395–402.
9. Vaidya DC, Schwartz RA. Prurigo nodularis: a benign dermatosis derived from a persistent pruritus. Acta Dermatovenerol Croat 2008;16:38–44.
10. Pautrier LM. Le neurone de la lichenification circonscrite nodulaire chronique (lichen ruber obtusus corne prurigo nodularis). Annales de Dermatologic Syph 1954;81(5):481–90.
11. Weigelt N, Metze D, Stander S. Prurigo nodularis: systematic analysis of 58 histological criteria in 136 patients. J Cutan Pathol 2010;37:578–86.
12. Schuhknecht B, Marziniak M, Wissel A, et al. Reduced intraepidermal nerve fibre density in lesional and nonlesional prurigo nodularis skin as a potential sign of subclinical cutaneous neuropathy. Br J Dermatol 2011;165:85–91.
13. Raap U, Ikoma A, Kapp A. Neurophysiology of pruritus. Hautarzt 2006;57:379–80, 382–4. [in German].
14. Groneberg DA, Serowka F, Peckenschneider N, et al. Gene expression and regulation of nerve growth factor in atopic dermatitis mast cells and the human mast cell line-1. J Neuroimmunol 2005; 161:87–92.
15. Johansson O, Liang Y, Emtestam L. Increased nerve growth factor- and tyrosine kinase A-like immunoreactivities in prurigo nodularis skin – an exploration of the cause of neurohyperplasia. Arch Dermatol Res 2002;293:614–9.
16. Liang Y, Marcusson JA, Jacobi HH, et al. Histamine-containing mast cells and their relationship to NGFr-immunoreactive nerves in prurigo nodularis: a reappraisal. J Cutan Pathol 1998;25:189–98.
17. Sonkoly E, Muller A, Lauerma AI, et al. IL-31: a new link between T cells and pruritus in atopic skin inflammation. J Allergy Clin Immunol 2006;117: 411–7.
18. Arai I, Tsuji M, Takeda H, et al. A single dose of interleukin-31 (IL-31) causes continuous itch-associated scratching behaviour in mice. Exp Dermatol 2013;22:669–71.
19. Raap U, Wichmann K, Bruder M, et al. Correlation of IL-31 serum levels with severity of atopic dermatitis. J Allergy Clin Immunol 2008;122:421–3.
20. Cevikbas F, Wang X, Akiyama T, et al. A sensory neuron-expressed IL-31 receptor mediates T helper cell-dependent itch: involvement of TRPV1 and TRPA1. J Allergy Clin Immunol 2014;133(2):448–60.

21. Almeida TA, Rojo J, Nieto PM, et al. Tachykinins and tachykinin receptors: structure and activity relationships [review]. Curr Med Chem 2004;11(15): 2045–81.

22. Haas S, Capellino S, Phan NQ, et al. Low density of sympathetic nerve fibers relative to substance P-positive nerve fibers in lesional skin of chronic pruritus and prurigo nodularis. J Dermatol Sci 2010;58: 193–7.

23. Stander S, Siepmann D, Herrgott I, et al. Targeting the neurokinin receptor 1 with aprepitant: a novel antipruritic strategy. PLoS One 2010;5: e10968.

24. Liang Y, Jacobi HH, Reimert CM, et al. CGRP-immunoreactive nerves in prurigo nodularis–an exploration of neurogenic inflammation. J Cutan Pathol 2000;27:359–66.

25. Bobko S, Zeidler C, Osada N, et al. Intraepidermal nerve fibre density is decreased in lesional and inter-lesional prurigo nodularis and reconstitutes on healing of lesions. Acta Derm Venereol 2016;96: 404–6.

26. Pereira MP, Pogatzki-Zahn E, Snels C, et al. There is no functional small-fiber neuropathy in prurigo nodularis despite neuroanatomical alterations. Exp Dermatol 2017;26(10):969–71.

27. Schedel F, Schürmann C, Augustin M, et al. Prurigo nodularis: introduction of a re-defined classification and Prurigo Activity Score (PAS). Acta Derm Venereol 2013;93:610.

28. Weisshaar E, Szepietowski JC, Darsow U, et al. European guideline on chronic pruritus. Acta Derm Venereol 2012;92:563–81.

29. Tessari G, Dalle Vedove C, Loschiavo C, et al. The impact of pruritus on the quality of life of patients undergoing dialysis: a single centre cohort study. J Nephrol 2009;22:241–8.

30. Pugliarello S, Cozzi A, Gisondi P, et al. Phenotypes of atopic dermatitis. J Dtsch Dermatol Ges 2011;9: 12–20.

31. Al-Salhi W, Alharithy R. Pemphigoid nodularis. J Cutan Med Surg 2015;19:153–5.

32. Cliff S, Holden CA. Pemphigoid nodularis: a report of three cases and review of the literature. Br J Dermatol 1997;136:398–401.

33. Feliciani C, Joly P, Jonkman MF, et al. Management of bullous pemphigoid: the European Dermatology Forum Consensus in collaboration with the European Academy of Dermatology and Venereology. Br J Dermatol 2015;172:867–77.

34. Solak B, Acikgoz SB, Sipahi S, et al. Epidemiology and determinants of pruritus in pre-dialysis chronic kidney disease patients. Int Urol Nephrol 2016;48: 585–91.

35. Bohme T, Heitkemper T, Mettang T, et al. Clinical features and prurigo nodularis in nephrogenic pruritus. Hautarzt 2014;65:714–20 [in German].

36. Hayani K, Weiss M, Weisshaar E. Clinical findings and provision of care in haemodialysis patients with chronic itch: new results from the German Epidemiological Haemodialysis Itch Study. Acta Derm Venereol 2016;96:361–6.

37. Tseng HW, Ger LP, Liang CK, et al. High prevalence of cutaneous manifestations in the elderly with diabetes mellitus: an institution-based cross-sectional study in Taiwan. J Eur Acad Dermatol Venereol 2015;29:1631–5.

38. White CR Jr, Heskel NS, Pokorny DJ. Perforating folliculitis of hemodialysis. Am J Dermatopathol 1982;4:109–16.

39. Hurwitz RM, Melton ME, Creech FT 3rd, et al. Perforating folliculitis in association with hemodialysis. Am J Dermatopathol 1982;4:101–8.

40. Kestner RI, Stander S, Osada N, et al. Acquired reactive perforating dermatosis is a variant of prurigo nodularis. Acta Derm Venereol 2017;97: 249–54.

41. Mettang T, Vonend A, Raap U. Prurigo nodularis: its association with dermatoses and systemic disorders. Hautarzt 2014;65:697–703 [in German].

42. Magand F, Nacher M, Cazorla C, et al. Predictive values of prurigo nodularis and herpes zoster for HIV infection and immunosuppression requiring HAART in French Guiana. Trans R Soc Trop Med Hyg 2011;105:401–4.

43. Ouattara I, Eholie SP, Aoussi E, et al. Can antiretroviral treatment eradicate Prurigo nodularis in HIV infected patients? Med Mal Infect 2009;39:415–6 [in French].

44. Stumpf A, Stander S. Neuropathic itch: diagnosis and management. Dermatol Ther 2013;26:104–9.

45. De D, Dogra S, Kanwar AJ. Prurigo nodularis in healed herpes zoster scar: an isotopic response. J Eur Acad Dermatol Venereol 2007;21:711–2.

46. Mirzoyev SA, Davis MD. Brachioradial pruritus: Mayo Clinic experience over the past decade. Br J Dermatol 2013;169:1007–15.

47. Stander S, Weisshaar E, Mettang T, et al. Clinical classification of itch: a position paper of the international forum for the study of itch. Acta Derm Venereol 2007;87:291–4.

48. Gieler U, Consoli SG, Tomas-Aragones L, et al. Self-inflicted lesions in dermatology: terminology and classification–a position paper from the European Society for Dermatology and Psychiatry (ESDaP). Acta Derm Venereol 2013;93:4–12.

49. Ständer S, Zeidler C, Augustin M, et al. S2k guidelines for the diagnosis and treatment of chronic pruritus - update - short version. J Dtsch Dermatol Ges 2017 Aug;15(8):860–72.

50. Saraceno R, Chiricozzi A, Nistico SP, et al. An occlusive dressing containing betamethasone valerate 0.1% for the treatment of prurigo nodularis. J Dermatolog Treat 2010;21:363–6.

51. Richards RN. Update on intralesional steroid: focus on dermatoses. J Cutan Med Surg 2010;14:19–23.
52. Wallengren J. Prurigo: diagnosis and management. Am J Clin Dermatol 2004;5:85–95.
53. Siepmann D, Lotts T, Blome C, et al. Evaluation of the antipruritic effects of topical pimecrolimus in non-atopic prurigo nodularis: results of a randomized, hydrocortisone-controlled, double-blind phase II trial. Dermatology 2013;227:353–60.
54. Wong SS, Goh CL. Double-blind, right/left comparison of calcipotriol ointment and betamethasone ointment in the treatment of prurigo nodularis. Arch Dermatol 2000;136:807–8.
55. Stander S, Luger T, Metze D. Treatment of prurigo nodularis with topical capsaicin. J Am Acad Dermatol 2001;44:471–8.
56. Stander S, Moormann C, Schumacher M, et al. Expression of vanilloid receptor subtype 1 in cutaneous sensory nerve fibers, mast cells, and epithelial cells of appendage structures. Exp Dermatol 2004;13:129–39.
57. Griffin JR, Davis MD. Amitriptyline/ketamine as therapy for neuropathic pruritus and pain secondary to herpes zoster. J Drugs Dermatol 2015;14:115–8.
58. Lee HG, Grossman SK, Valdes-Rodriguez R, et al. Topical ketamine-amitriptyline-lidocaine for chronic pruritus: a retrospective study assessing efficacy and tolerability. J Am Acad Dermatol 2017;76(4):760–1.
59. Hammes S, Hermann J, Roos S, et al. UVB 308-nm excimer light and bath PUVA: combination therapy is very effective in the treatment of prurigo nodularis. J Eur Acad Dermatol Venereol 2011;25:799–803.
60. Sorenson E, Levin E, Koo J, et al. Successful use of a modified Goeckerman regimen in the treatment of generalized prurigo nodularis. J Am Acad Dermatol 2015;72:e40–42.
61. Paghdal KV, Schwartz RA. Topical tar: back to the future. J Eur Acad Dermatol Venereol 2009;61:294–302.
62. Schulz S, Metz M, Siepmann D, et al. Antipruritic efficacy of a high-dosage antihistamine therapy. Results of a retrospectively analysed case series. Hautarzt 2009;60:564–8 [in German].
63. Shintani T, Ohata C, Koga H, et al. Combination therapy of fexofenadine and montelukast is effective in prurigo nodularis and pemphigoid nodularis. Dermatol Ther 2014;27:135–9.
64. Gunal AI, Ozalp G, Yoldas TK, et al. Gabapentin therapy for pruritus in haemodialysis patients: a randomized, placebo-controlled, double-blind trial. Nephrol Dial Transplant 2004;19:3137–9.
65. Gencoglan G, Inanir I, Gunduz K. Therapeutic hotline: treatment of prurigo nodularis and lichen simplex chronicus with gabapentin. Dermatol Ther 2010;23:194–8.
66. Mazza M, Guerriero G, Marano G, et al. Treatment of prurigo nodularis with pregabalin. J Clin Pharm Ther 2013;38:16–8.
67. Scheinfeld N. The role of gabapentin in treating diseases with cutaneous manifestations and pain. Int J Dermatol 2003;42:491–5.
68. Phan NQ, Lotts T, Antal A, et al. Systemic kappa opioid receptor agonists in the treatment of chronic pruritus: a literature review. Acta Derm Venereol 2012;92:555–60.
69. Bergasa NV. The pruritus of cholestasis: facts. Hepatology 2015;61:2114.
70. Stander S, Bockenholt B, Schurmeyer-Horst F, et al. Treatment of chronic pruritus with the selective serotonin re-uptake inhibitors paroxetine and fluvoxamine: results of an open-labelled, two-arm proof-of-concept study. Acta Derm Venereol 2009;89:45–51.
71. Dawn AG, Yosipovitch G. Butorphanol for treatment of intractable pruritus. J Am Acad Dermatol 2006;54:527–31.
72. Papoiu ADP, Kraft RA, Coghill RC, et al. Butorphanol suppression of histamine itch is mediated by nucleus accumbens and septal nuclei: a pharmacological fMRI study. J Invest Dermatol 2015;135(2):560–8.
73. Brasileiro LE, Barreto DP, Nunes EA. Psychotropics in different causes of itch: systematic review with controlled studies. An Bras Dermatol 2016;91(6):791–8.
74. Siepmann D, Luger TA, Stander S. Antipruritic effect of cyclosporine microemulsion in prurigo nodularis: results of a case series. J Dtsch Dermatol Ges 2008;6:941–6.
75. Spring P, Gschwind I, Gilliet M. Prurigo nodularis: retrospective study of 13 cases managed with methotrexate. Clin Exp Dermatol 2014;39:468–73.
76. Andersen TP, Fogh K. Thalidomide in 42 patients with prurigo nodularis Hyde. Dermatology 2011;223:107–12.
77. Taefehnorooz H, Truchetet F, Barbaud A, et al. Efficacy of thalidomide in the treatment of prurigo nodularis. Acta Derm Venereol 2011;91:344–5.
78. Sharma D, Kwatra SG. Thalidomide for the treatment of chronic refractory pruritus. J Am Acad Dermatol 2016;74:363–9.
79. Liu H, Gaspari AA, Schleichert R. Use of lenalidomide in treating refractory prurigo nodularis. J Drugs Dermatol 2013;12:360–1.
80. Kanavy H, Bahner J, Korman NJ. Treatment of refractory prurigo nodularis with lenalidomide. Arch Dermatol 2012;148:794–6.
81. Feldmeyer L, Werner S, Kamarashev J, et al. Atopic prurigo nodularis responds to intravenous immunoglobulins. Br J Dermatol 2012;166:461–2.
82. Ständer S, Kwon P, Luger TA. Randomized, double-blind, placebo-controlled, study of the neurokinin-1 receptor (NK1-R) antagonist serlopitant in subjects with prurigo nodularis (PN). Annual Meeting of the

American Association of Dermatology 2017). Orlando, March 3–7, 2017.

83. Hawi A, Alcorn H Jr, Berg J, et al. Pharmacokinetics of nalbuphine hydrochloride extended release tablets in hemodialysis patients with exploratory effect on pruritus. BMC Nephrol 2015;16:47.

84. Ruzicka T, Hanifin JM, Furue M, et al. Anti-interleukin-31 receptor A antibody for atopic dermatitis. N Engl J Med 2017;376:826–35.

85. Schneider LC. Ditching the itch with anti-type 2 cytokine therapies for atopic dermatitis. N Engl J Med 2017;376:878–9.

Chronic Pruritus in the Geriatric Population

Taige Cao, MD[a], Hong Liang Tey, MD[a,b],*, Gil Yosipovitch, MD[c]

KEYWORDS

- Pruritus • Geriatrics • Therapeutics • Diagnosis • Classification

KEY POINTS

- Chronic pruritus in the geriatric population is defined by pruritus that persists for more than 6 weeks experienced by people 65 year old and above.
- Aging is associated with pathologic changes is the epidermal barrier, immune system, and the nervous system that predispose the elderly to itch.
- In our approach to the clinical problem, we dichotomize pruritus based on its pathogenesis, either histaminergic or predominantly nonhistaminergic.
- Topical treatments are generally safe for the elderly population; systemic treatments are chosen depending on the condition with consideration of comorbid diseases and drug interactions.
- Numerous new medications are currently undergoing clinical trials and they are anticipated to enter the clinics in the near future.

INTRODUCTION

Chronic pruritus in the geriatric population, as defined by pruritus that persists for more than 6 weeks experienced by people 65 years old and above, is an increasing health care problem.[1] Medical advances, decreasing fertility rates, and longer life expectancies have given rise to a rapidly aging population, especially in developed countries. In 2017, there are an estimated 962 million people aged 60 or over in the world, comprising 13% of the global population. The population aged 60 or above is growing at a rate of about 3% per year. By 2050, all regions of the world except Africa will have nearly one-quarter or more of their populations at ages 60 and above. The number of older persons in the world is projected to be 1.4 billion in 2030 and 2.1 billion in 2050.[2] By then, geriatric conditions will impose the greatest strain on global health.

It is believed that the incidence of pruritus increases with age; however, there is a dearth of well-designed epidemiologic research to establish this. Depending on region and sample size, the prevalence of itch in the elderly was estimated to be between 11.5% and 41.0%.[3] A working population survey found that the prevalence of current chronic pruritus increased with age from 12.3% (16–30 years) to 20.3% (61–70 years).[4] A cross-sectional study of 302 geriatric patients in the Hispanic population in Mexico demonstrated the prevalence of chronic itch was 25%.[5] In another study of 68 noninstitutionalized persons, two-thirds of the group and 83% of octogenarians reported medical concerns regarding their skin, with pruritus being the most frequent complaint.[6] In a study conducted in Thailand involving 149 elderly patients, pruritic diseases were the most commonly reported disease (41%), of which xerosis (synonymous with senescent itch) was the most frequent (38.9%).[7]

Disclosure: The authors have nothing to disclose.
[a] National Skin Centre, 1 Mandalay Road, Singapore 308205, Singapore; [b] Lee Kong Chian School of Medicine, Nanyang Technological University, 11 Mandalay Road, Singapore 308232, Singapore; [c] Department of Dermatology and Cutaneous Surgery, Itch Center Miller School of Medicine, 1295 NW 14th Street, University of Miami Hospital South Building Suites K-M, Miami, FL 33125, USA
* Corresponding author. National Skin Centre, 1 Mandalay Road, Singapore 308205, Singapore.
E-mail address: teyhongliang111@yahoo.com

Dermatol Clin 36 (2018) 199–211
https://doi.org/10.1016/j.det.2018.02.004

derm.theclinics.com

The consequences of chronic pruritus are especially significant in the elderly population, which include a decreased quality of life, diminished mental health, and an impact on the health care economy. A recent German study by Makrantonaki and collegues[8] on 110 hospitalized geriatric patients revealed that pruritus showed a positive correlation with the duration of hospitalization and a negative correlation with the Barthel index and Tinetti score on the day of discharge. The latter indicates that pruritus has a significant impact on the physical condition and on the static and dynamic balance abilities of the elderly with multiple morbidities, respectively.[8] Insomnia and depression can result, and this condition is especially worse in the elderly with interrupted sleep.[9] In addition, pruritus can be aggravated by the complex psychosocial factors that are often present in the elderly.[10]

PATHOPHYSIOLOGY OF ITCH IN THE ELDERLY

Aging is associated with pathologic changes is the epidermal barrier, immune system, and nervous system, which predisposes the elderly to itch.

Epidermal Barrier

The epidermal barrier of the skin deteriorates with aging. The epidermal barrier is formed in the stratum corneum with corneal cells and intercellular lipids, forming a watertight configuration.[11] Xerosis of aging skin is not only caused by deficient sebum production, but also by a complex dysfunction of the stratum corneum. With aging, there are decreased skin surface lipids, increased transepidermal water loss, and decreased corneal hydration, which ultimately contributes to xerosis.[12] Aquaphorin-3 (AQP3), a membrane channel, allows the passage of glycerol and water. AQP3 gene expression was found to be significantly reduced in the skin of people aged 60 years and over.[13] A reduction of facilitated water permeability and glycerol transport translates to a decrease in epidermal and stratum corneum hydration and glycerol content, leading to xerosis. Sweat and sebum production are also reduced and barrier repair is diminished.[14,15] Elderly patients with pruritus are found to have clinically drier skin than age- and sex-matched control subjects. Xerosis may be causally implicated in up to 38% of generalized pruritus.[7] This finding is further supported by another study demonstrating that, although 69% of patients with itch presented with xerosis, only 18% of patients without itch presented with xerosis ($P<.001$).[5]

The decrease in skin surface lipids has been attributed to the increase in epidermal surface pH, which leads to reduced activity of lipid-forming enzymes and production of ceramide in the stratum corneum.[16] The decrease in the lipid formation capacity and fluid loss affect the epidermal barrier function and could contribute to pruritus of advanced aging. A study revealed that intracorneal cohesion is increased in pruritus of advanced aging, similar to that observed in dermatoses such as psoriasis, ichthyosis, and atopic eczema.[17] This feature predisposes the elderly to the development of other skin conditions, such as contact dermatitis.

Immune System

The age-associated alteration in systemic immunity with aging is referred to as immunosenescence. It is characterized by both a decrease in cell-mediated immune function and humoral immune responses.[18] Immunosenescence consists of defects within the innate immune system with a pathologic shift toward proinflammatory activity with an allergic phenotype. This dysregulation is hallmarked by a change toward type 2 dominance (Th2), with chronically increased levels of interleukin-6 and tumor necrosis factor-α.[19] It has been proposed that, during the aging process, there is a thymic involution with a loss of naive T cells, a decrease in T-cell regeneration, and a decrease in T-cell receptors. Impaired T-cell regulatory function leads to the change to Th2 dominance. Th2 dominance, in turn, may possibly predispose elderly individuals to allergic and mast cell disorders,[20] which in turn result in itch. In a recent report of 4 patients with chronic idiopathic pruritus, there was a decrease in serum immunoglobulin (Ig)G level, but not IgA or IgM levels. It has been suggested that the B cell defect could be considered a form of common variable immunodeficiency, acquired as a consequence of the aging process.[21]

It has also been proposed that there can be an autoimmune component to the pruritus of advanced aging. Aging is associated with a loss of self-tolerance against cutaneous autoantigens.[22] Macrophages are affected by aging, resulting in a compromise of the inductive phase of the immune response and phagocytic capabilities.[23] An example is bullous pemphigoid, in which patients can have generalized itch for years without blistering. Pruritus may be the consequence of antibodies developing against the basement membrane zone antigens.[24]

Nervous System

Aging also affects the nervous system and predisposes one to pruritus. Although no significant decrement in intraepidermal nerve fiber density with age is observed,[25] it is hypothesized that a subclinical neuropathy secondary to degeneration is present in elderly with pruritus.[26,27] There is a decrease in the itch threshold to stimuli; a deficiency in hydration may also be accountable in this reduction, because emollients improve the accuracy of sensory perception in elderly patients.

Age-related involution of the brain and multiple subclinical cerebral infarcts may also interrupt the pruritus pathway ,which goes through the thalamus and internal capsule and terminates in the sensory cortex.[28,29] These patients often complain of both itching and additional forms of dysesthesia (numbness, burning, or tingling sensations) and present with secondary skin changes from scratching, namely, lichen simplex chronicus, prurigo nodularis, and secondary cutaneous amyloidosis (**Fig. 1**). The typical topical antiinflammatory agents are ineffective, and some cases respond only to application of ice.[30]

APPROACH TO CHRONIC PRURITUS IN THE GERIATRIC POPULATION

Pruritus in the elderly has many causes. It can occur by itself or in association with primary skin disorders (eg, xerosis, atopic dermatitis, and scabies), systemic disorders (eg, chronic renal failure and liver diseases), neurologic disorders (eg, notalgia paraesthetica and brachioradial pruritus), psychogenic disorders, adverse drug reactions or a combination of these disorders.[31] In our approach to the clinical problem, we dichotomize pruritus based on its pathogenesis—histaminergic versus predominantly nonhistaminergic itch, such that suitable treatments can be instituted accordingly.

HISTAMINERGIC ITCH
Chronic Urticaria

Chronic urticaria is defined by the presence of recurrent urticaria, with or without angioedema,

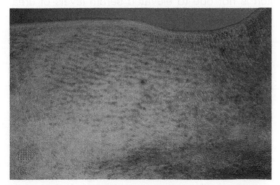

Fig. 1. Macular amyloidosis secondary to eczema.

for a period of 6 weeks or longer.[32] The pruritus in chronic urticaria is often described as a stinging, tickling, or burning that is often worse at night and may be triggered by ambient heat and sweating. An increase in itch intensity has been associated with stress.[33] Although chronic urticaria has a peak incidence in the 20- to 40-year age category,[34] in a retrospective investigation conducted on a large cohort of patients with chronic urticaria from the National Health Insurance Research Database of Taiwan, Chen and colleagues[35] found that one-quarter of the patients were in the age range of 60 to 79 years and 3.4% were 80 years and older. Notably, patients greater than 40 years of age had a prolonged duration of disease. A study performed by Magen and collaborators[36] on 1598 adults suffering from chronic spontaneous urticaria found that 9.4% were elderly.

Various authors have emphasized the role of drug-induced urticaria in the geriatric population.[37] Although international guidelines do not recommend a specific workup for elderly populations, urticaria secondary to a systemic drug (especially aspirin and angiotensin-converting enzyme inhibitors) or topical agents should be excluded, because polypharmacy and the use of topical medicaments are common in the elderly. Systemic diseases may also induce urticaria more commonly in the elderly. A recent study based on Mayo Clinic's electronic database revealed that patients presenting a new diagnosis of chronic urticaria at older ages were more likely to have underlying monoclonal gammopathy of undetermined significance.

PAROXYSMAL HISTAMINERGIC ITCH

In our itch clinic, we receive many referrals from dermatologists for patients presenting with severe itch affecting different parts of the body and are unresponsive to typical treatment with antihistamines. These patients are typically adults and the elderly. There are no associated primary skin lesions that can be detected, and physicians witness the absence of rash when the patients are actively itching. No urticarial rashes or dermographism can be elicited from the history and physical testing, respectively. The itch is typically intense. We term this condition descriptively, as paroxysmal histaminergic itch. This presentation could be a part of a mast cell activation syndrome, but other symptoms and signs are typically absent. Regular treatment with antihistamines with timely administration before the usual timings of itch occurrence often enables control of the symptoms. Of note, the antihistamine selected should have a long enough duration of action to cover the period of itching. Recognition of this condition is essential to providing expedient alleviation of this debilitating condition. In contrast, secondary causes, such as a drug cause, need to be excluded first. A careful history and physical examination are also necessary to check for an underlying paraneoplastic cause, especially in persistent cases. In refractory cases, immunosuppressant agents can be useful.

PREDOMINANT NONHISTAMINERGIC ITCH
Asteatotic Eczema

Asteatotic eczema is characterized by pruritic, dry, and scaly fissured skin. It commonly occurs on the shins of elderly patients and may progress to the thighs, trunk, and upper extremities. It usually spares the face, neck, palms, and soles. Both endogenous and exogenous causes contribute to dry skin. The most common cause is aging. Other predisposing and aggravating factors include a dry climate with low humidity, excessive exposure to water and soap, ichthyosis vulgaris, venous insufficiency, renal failure, and AIDS. Itching and stinging sensations result from xerosis. Subsequent inflammation occurs as a result of the impaired skin barrier and this is further perpetrated by scratching, rubbing, and the application of irritative substances.

Scabies

Scabies is a parasitic infestation caused by the mite *Sarcoptesscabiei* (var. *hominis*). The estimated prevalence ranges widely between populations from 0.2% to 71.0%, with as many as 100 million people affected worldwide.[38] Scabies is an extremely itchy condition more commonly found in residents of nursing homes and geriatric wards. The pruritus is the result of a delayed type IV hypersensitivity reaction to the mite, mite feces, and mite eggs.[39] To differentiate scabies infection from eczema, one clue is the presence of crusting along skin folds. Commonly in scabies infection, the hands, and palmar and wrist creases are involved, in addition to the finger and toe webs. The neck, temples, forehead, and scalp may be infested in geriatric patients. Elderly patients who present with generalized exfoliative dermatitis should be checked carefully for features of scabies infection, because scabies is not an infrequent cause of generalized exfoliative dermatitis in this group of patients. In elderly patients, misdiagnosis typically leads to use of topical steroids, with further delay in proper diagnosis and treatment. For further information, see Arnaud Jannic and colleagues' article, "Scabies Itch," in this issue.

BULLOUS PEMPHIGOID

Bullous pemphigoid is an autoimmune, subepidermal blistering disease that more commonly presents in people over 80 years of age, and mostly affects people over 50 years of age.[40–42] It may start with pruritus in the prodromal stage, while blisters develop weeks or months later.[43] The initial skin lesions may consist of erythematous, excoriated papules or nodules and urticarial or eczematous plaques.

Sometimes, patients have been reported to manifest with itch combined with immunopathologic findings compatible with bullous pemphigoid, but without primary skin lesions or blisters, despite being followed for several months or even years.[44] According to the definitions from an international expert panel, pruritus is considered a sufficient symptom for the diagnosis of bullous pemphigoid if the immunologic criteria are met.[43] In a Swiss study population, 20% of 160 patients diagnosed with bullous pemphigoid did not have blisters. In this study, most of these patients were older than 70 years, with a follow-up of 4 months to 6 years.[45] In view of this finding, early bullous pemphigoid should be considered in elderly patients without apparent blisters. Screening investigation of serum indirect immunofluorescence can be performed, because it provides the greatest sensitivity (>90%) among the immunologic investigations for bullous pemphigoid.[46]

Systemic Diseases

Numerous systemic conditions have been related to chronic itch in the elderly. Systemic conditions may cause itch with or without the presence of a rash.

Renal pruritus

Itch associated with end-stage chronic kidney disease may be referred to as renal pruritus or uremic pruritus. Despite the name of uremic pruritus, the itch is not due to elevated serum levels of urea. Renal pruritus is most commonly described as a daily or near-daily occurrence of itch that spans large bilaterally symmetric body areas, without an associated primary skin lesion. Renal pruritus can vary from a generalized itch to a localized itch affecting the back, face, and arms. The prevalence of renal pruritus in geriatric patients has not been assessed. However, it is well known that end-stage renal failure is becoming a geriatric problem. Among incident patients, those older than age 75 years outnumber those age 65 to 74 years and have the highest incident growth rate.[30] Contributing factors include an increased prevalence of diabetes and hypertension, improved life expectancy, and increased availability of dialysis therapy to the elderly. High permeability dialysis may possibly improve pruritic symptoms in elderly patients[47]; however, renal pruritus still affects up to 42% of patients on hemodialysis.[48]

Renal pruritus intensity is associated with multiple health-related quality-of-life outcomes, such as sleep quality, mood, and social function, and is associated independently with mortality. The pathophysiology of renal pruritus is not fully understood and likely is multifactorial. Subclinical or overt uremic neuropathy, skin or nerve inflammation in the context of kidney failure–associated chronic systemic inflammation, or an increase in activity of μ-opioid receptors owing to kidney failure have all been implicated.[49,50] For further details, refer to Radomir Reszke and Jacek C. Szepietowski's article, "End-Stage Renal Disease Chronic Itch and Its Management," in this issue.

Chronic liver disease and cholestasis-associated pruritus

The peak age range of complications occurring in chronic liver disease, namely cirrhosis, liver failure, and hepatocellular carcinoma, is 65 to 74 years and pruritus is one of the symptoms encountered in these patients.[51] Itching is a presenting symptom in 25% of those with jaundice from biliary obstruction or other causes, such as cirrhosis, pancreatic cancer, or hepatitis.[52]

Several lines of evidence have suggested the mechanisms by which pruritus is induced in cholestatic conditions. First, accumulated bile salts are thought to act as pruritogens.[53] Second, endogenous opioid levels have been reported increased in cholestatic patients.[54,55] The activation of μ-opioid receptors induces pruritus, with μ-opioid receptor antagonists showing antipruritic effects in patients with chronic cholestasis.[56] More recent evidence has implicated autotaxin and lysophosphatidic acid as potential mediators of cholestatic pruritus.[57] In severe cases, liver transplantation may be the only treatment capable of fully reliving itch in the context of chronic liver disease. However, transplantations in frail old people and in elderly people with very poor liver function are associated with increased morbidity and limited survival. For additional information, please see Miriam M. Düll and Andreas E. Kremer's article, "Management of Chronic Hepatic Itch," in this issue.

Paraneoplastic itch

The prevalence of malignancies has increased with increasing life expectancy worldwide. Chronic itch could be a presenting sign of malignancy. The intensity and extent of pruritus do not correlate with the extent of tumor involvement. Pruritus of lymphoma is the common prototype of paraneoplastic itch and can precede other clinical signs by weeks and months.[58] Paraneoplastic pruritus has also been associated with solid tumors. Therefore, persistent and unexplained pruritus that are resistant to common treatments should alert the physician to consider screening for an underlying malignancy. Generalized pruritus has been described in rare cases of Waldenström macroglobulinemia and as a preceding sign in patients with multiple myeloma, but there are no data on its prevalence.[59,60]

A proposed hypothesis on the pathogenesis of pruritus in malignant condition includes chemical release by necrotic tumor cells into the blood circulation, the production of chemical mediators by tumor cells, allergic reaction to tumor-specific antigens, increased proteolytic activity, and histamine release.

Neuropathic Itch

Neuropathic itch has a greater propensity to occur in the elderly population and it behooves health care providers to have a better understanding of the common causes of neuropathic itch. One common cause of neuropathic itch is postherpetic neuralgia. The incidence of acute herpes zoster and the complication of postherpetic neuralgia is higher in the elderly owing to an impaired immune system.[61] Between 30% and 58% of patients with postherpetic neuralgia experience pruritus at the site of herpes zoster.[62] Symptoms commonly occur when eruption occurs on the head, face, or neck.

Another classic example of neuropathic itch is notalgia paraesthetica (**Fig. 2**). Although patients

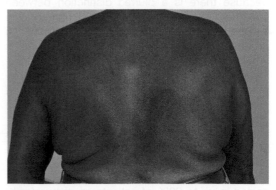

Fig. 2. Notalgia paraesthetica, a chronic sensory neuropathy characterized by pruritus of the upper to middle back associated with hyperpigmentation of the affected area.

as young as 21 years old have been reported, it is mainly a disease of the middle-aged and elderly.[63] Patients usually reports unilateral pruritus involving the skin medial to the scapular boarder on the mid or upper back. Cutaneous changes secondary scratching such as hyperpigmentation can be observed. In chronic cases, secondary amyloid deposition may be seen. The proposed etiology is that there is nerve entrapment of the dorsal rami of spinal nerves that arise from T2 to T6 when they run a long course up through the thick muscles of the back. A similar condition owing to nerve injury—brachioradial pruritus—is characterized by itch, burning, stinging, and tingling sensation in the areas of skin on either or both arms.[64] Most commonly affected area is the mid arm, but the forearms and upper extensor arms can also be affected. Nerve damage can be radiculopathy at the cervical spine or neuropathy of a cutaneous branch of the brachial nerves. See Jordan Daniel Rosen and colleagues' article, "Diagnosis and Management of Neuropathic Itch," in this issue, for further details.

Drug-Related Itch

Many systemic and topical drugs can cause pruritus and polypharmacy is a prevalent problem in the elderly patients. A large epidemiologic study from the 1980s showed that, among hospitalized patients, pruritus without concomitant skin lesions accounted for approximately 5% of adverse reactions after drug intake.[65] Another study of 200 patients with drug reactions revealed that 12.5% showed pruritus without skin lesions.[66] Specifically for the elderly population, a large Turkish study on 4099 geriatric patients greater than 65 years old estimated the prevalence of drug-related pruritus to be 1.4%.[67] However, there are difficulties in determining the exact prevalence because there is a blurred distinction between pure drug-induced pruritus without primary skin lesions and symptomatic pruritus accompanying drug-induced urticaria or lichenoid eruptions. It is also difficult to differentiate between drug-induced pruritus and pruritus caused by the primary disease, especially in cases of underlying malignancy, such as lymphoma treated with chemotherapeutic agents.

Notably, new targeted chemotherapies, such as epidermal growth factor receptor inhibitors and novel antimelanoma drugs, have the significant adverse effect of pruritus.[68] Pruritus has been reported in up to 29% of patients on vemurafenib, a B-Raf inhibitor used in the treatment of melanoma.[69] Another antimelanoma drug, ipilimumab, which is a human monoclonal antibody (IgG1)

against CTLA-4, causes pruritus in 31% of patients.[70] The incidence rates of all-grade and high-grade pruritus for patients treated with the epidermal growth factor receptor inhibitors cetuximab, erlotinib, and panitumumab were 31% and 2%, respectively. The highest incidence rate of pruritus is seen in patients treated with panitumumab, followed by cetuximab and erlotinib.[68] See Jennifer Wu and Mario E. Lacouture's article, "Pruritus Associated with Targeted Anticancer Therapies and Their Management," in this issue, for further details.

The main contributors to drug-induced itch in the elderly from a large case-control study including cardiac (diuretics, angiotensin-converting enzyme inhibitors, calcium channel blockers, lipid-lowering drugs), salicylic, and chemotherapeutic agents.[71] The pathogenesis of drug-induced pruritus ranges widely, which includes drug-induced skin eruptions, cholestatic liver injury, phototoxicity, xerosis, drug and/or drug metabolite deposition in the skin, and neuropathy.

MANAGEMENT
Topical Agents

Topical therapies are particularly appropriate in the elderly population because comorbidities and polypharmacy are common and there is a corresponding high risk of side effects and drug interactions. Topical therapies can provide broad-based itch relief for different types of itch and serve as adjuvant to systemic medications.

Emollients

By coating the skin with lipids, emollients counteract the epidermal barrier dysfunction present in asteatotic eczema and create an effective barrier that prevents the movement of water out of the skin. Also, they contain humectants to retain water, which moisturizes the skin. Emollients are steroid-sparing agents, because their use reduces the requirement for topical corticosteroids.[72] This factor is especially relevant for geriatric patients, who are prone to senile purpura owing to a significant decrease in collagen and elastin fibers in the dermis and vasculature in old age. In addition to reducing collagen and glycosaminoglycan synthesis, topical steroids can impair the immune response, which may result in infection subsequent to sustaining broken skin.

Menthol

One notable example of topical antipruritic therapeutics is menthol. Menthol activates TRPM8, a nonselective cation channel. The cold signaling inhibits experimental and disease-related pruritus. It is assumed that the itch relief results from activation of cutaneous Aδ fibers and spinal B5-I inhibitory interneurons, which produces a stable antipruritic effect without tachyphylaxis.[73] The main advantage of menthol is that it is applicable for various types of itch originating from the skin and has a favorable risk–benefit profile. However, its use is limited by its short duration of itch relief and repeated application is required.

Menthol-based moisturizing creams, such as one containing ceramides, serve to inhibit itch and restore skin barrier function concurrently.[74] This property is particularly useful for itch associated with asteatosis, which commonly occurs in the elderly.

Capsaicin and topical calcineurin inhibitors

Capsaicin is a substance derived from chili peppers that has been used for the treatment of pruritus. The mechanism of action for capsaicin involves its ability to activate transient release potential vanilloid-1, an ion channel in cutaneous nerve fibers. Activation of transient release potential vanilloid-1 stimulates neurons to release and eventually deplete certain neuropeptides, including substance P.[75] Substance P can cause vasodilation and release histamine from mast cell. By depleting these neuropeptides, the transmission of pruritus by nerve fibers is inhibited.

Capsaicin has been reported to treat neuropathic disorders (nostalgia paresthetica and brachioradial pruritus),[76] aquagenic pruritus, and pruritus associated with chronic renal disease.[77] In contrast, no therapeutic benefit has been seen in atopic dermatitis.

In addition to having antiinflammatory effects, topical calcineurin inhibitors have antipruritic effects and they seem to work in a similar mechanism as capsaicin through activation of transient release potential vanilloid-1.[78] Topical calcineurin inhibitors have been successfully used in treating itch in patients with pruritic inflammatory diseases (atopic dermatitis,[79] lichen simplex chronicus,[80] lichen sclerosus, and chronic graft-versus-host disease) and neuropathic itch (nostalgia paraesthetica[81] and meralgiaparesthetica[82]).

Topical anesthetics

Topical anesthetics, such as pramoxine and polidocanol, have been used as ingredients in topical preparations for their antipruritic effects. A pramoxine1% topical therapy was found to be more effective than control lotion in the management of uremic pruritus.[83] An open-label study of 5% urea and 3% polidocanol demonstrated a significant reduction of pruritus in patients with atopic dermatitis, contact dermatitis, and psoriasis.[84] In

a recent retrospective study by Lee and colleagues,[85] the combination of topical ketamine–amitriptyline–lidocaine is effective as a single or adjuvant therapy when treating various pruritic conditions, and is especially useful in neuropathic itch and prurigo nodularis. Its proposed mechanism of action is aimed at reducing hypersensitivity of peripheral nerve fibers through blockade of N-methyl-D-aspartate receptor and sodium channels.

Topical phosphodiesterase 4 inhibitor

Topical steroids are commonly used for itch in inflammation but have many side effects for frail skin. Crisaborole topical ointment, 2% is a benzoxaborole, nonsteroidal, topical, antiinflammatory phosphodiesterase 4 inhibitor that has recently been approved by the US Food and Drug Administration to treat mild to moderate atopic dermatitis. Phosphodiesterase 4 is present in a variety of inflammatory cells, including mast cells, eosinophils, neutrophils, and macrophages. By inhibiting phosphodiesterase 4 and thus increasing levels of cyclic adenosine monophosphate, crisaborole controls inflammation. Its use has been shown to improve severity and itch in atopic dermatitis.[86]

SYSTEMIC MEDICATIONS
Histaminergic Itch

Antihistamines

In the treatment of histaminergic itch, the regular use of antihistamines should be advocated, because many patients use them on an as-needed basis. Patients should preemptively take the medications regularly. For example, if itch often occurs at night, the patient can take the medication at dinner regularly before the onset of itch. Often a higher off-label dose of antihistamine is required to adequately control the symptoms.

Both older, first-generation H1 antihistamines (eg, chlorpheniramine, hydroxyzine) and newer, second-generation H1 antihistamines (eg, cetirizine, loratadine, levocetirizine, desloratadine, fexofenadine) can be used. However, second-generation agents are preferred in the geriatric population.[87] First-generation antihistamines are lipophilic and readily cross the blood–brain barrier, causing sedating and anticholinergic side effects that may be dose limiting in some patients. Significant sedation and impairment of performance (eg, fine motor skills, driving skills, and reaction times) occur in more than 20% of patients.[88] Anticholinergic side effects include dry mouth, diplopia, blurred vision, urinary retention, and vaginal dryness.[89] These effects are especially pronounced in geriatric patients and, therefore, they have been prominently mentioned in the Beers List, a list of potentially inappropriate medications to be avoided in older adults.[90]

Second-generation antihistamines are minimally sedating, and have low incidences of anticholinergic effects that often complicate use of first-generation agents. They have few significant drug–drug interactions, and require less frequent dosing compared with first-generation agents. Comparing the efficacy of these agents, no clear superiority has been demonstrated among trials.[91]

In choosing a suitable antihistamine, consideration of comorbidities, which are common in the elderly population, is important. For example, cetirizine is excreted in the urine (70%; 50% as unchanged drug). Therefore, in patients with chronic kidney disease, dose reduction is required. Notably, levocetirizine is nondialyzable and its use is contraindicated in patients on hemodialysis. Also, in patients with liver dysfunction, the half-life of cetirizine is increased to from 9 to 14 hours; therefore, a dose adjustment may be necessary. In contrast, antihistamines such as bilastine are excreted mainly in the feces and a dose adjustment is not required.[92] If histaminergic itch is not well-controlled with the recommended dosage, the dose of antihistamines can be increase up to 4-fold of the recommended dosage in elderly patients with normal liver and kidney function.[93]

Another consideration in choosing a suitable antihistamine is its duration of action. In the geriatric population, where the polypharmacy is prevalent, a longer duration of action will allow less frequent dosing and provide a more convenient dosing regimen. Wheal and erythema inhibition by various antihistamines has been characterized by Simons and Simons.[92] For example, cetirizine has a short time to action of 0.7 hour and a prolonged duration of action of more than 24 hours. This is a superior choice as compared with acrivastine, which has a short duration of action of 8 hours.

Predominant Nonhistaminergic Itch

GABAergic drugs

GABAergic drugs, namely gabapentin and pregabalin, are effective in neuropathic itch and intractable itch from chronic renal and hepatic disease. A low dose is effective for itch typically, rather than the dosages recommended in the package insert. In the elderly, it is advisable to slowly titrate the dosage up because drowsiness and nausea are prominent side effects. Renal adjustment in the dosage is required for patients with chronic kidney disease according to the estimated

glomerular filtration rate. For patients on hemodialysis, 100 to 300 mg of oral gabapentin administered after each hemodialysis session was an effective and safe regimen for renal pruritus.[94,95] In acute herpes zoster, use of gabapentin can be considered to prophylactically prevent postherpetic neuralgia. Of note, patients with postherpetic neuralgia often experience itch in addition to pain and, in some patients, itch in a dermatomal distribution is the sole complaint.[96,97] The major risk factors for postherpetic neuralgia are older age, greater acute pain, and greater rash severity.

Antidepressants

Antidepressants have been used to reduce generalized pruritus of various types, including but not limited to psychogenic itch. Selective serotonin reuptake inhibitors (SSRIs; eg, paroxetine, sertraline, fluvoxamine, and fluoxetine) have demonstrated efficacy in pruritus in small studies.[98] One small randomized trial showed a modest antipruritic effect of paroxetine, as compared with placebo.[99] A small double-blind trial demonstrated the efficacy of sertraline (at a daily dose of 100 mg) for cholestatic itch.[100] However, among the SSRIs, fluoxetine is generally not recommended for use in the elderly because of its long half-life and prolonged side effects.[101] Paroxetine is also typically not recommended for use in the elderly because it has the greatest anticholinergic effect of all the SSRIs.[102] In addition, fluoxetine, paroxetine, and fluvoxamine have higher risks of drug–drug interactions. SSRIs considered to have the best safety profile in the elderly are citalopram, escitalopram, and sertraline.[103]

Case reports have also suggested that the oral noradrenergic and specific serotonergic antidepressant with H1 antihistaminic properties, mirtazapine (at a daily dose of 15 mg) may relieve nocturnal itch of various types, including cancer-related itching.[104] Improvement in intractable itch has been reported in a case series of patients with cutaneous T-cell lymphoma who were treated with a combination of low-dose mirtazapine and gabapentin or pregabalin.[105] Also, mirtazapine is considered to have a good safety profile in terms of drug–drug interactions.

Tricyclic antidepressants, such as amitriptyline, are also occasionally used at low dose to treat chronic pruritus (eg, neuropathic or psychogenic forms), although these agents have not been studied for this use in randomized trials.[106]

Opioid receptor agonists

Activation of kappa-opioid receptors in the central nervous system may inhibit itch. According to anecdotal reports, butorphanol, a kappa-opioid agonist and a mu-opioid antagonist that is administered intranasally and has been approved by the US Food and Drug Administration for the treatment of migraine, can reduce intractable itch associated with non-Hodgkin's lymphoma, cholestasis, and opioid use.[107]

Immunosuppressants

Immunosuppressants such as methotrexate, cyclosporine, azathioprine, and mycophenolate mofetil have been used for inflammatory pruritic skin diseases.[108,109] In the elderly population in which there is a higher prevalence of comorbidities, the immunosuppressant to be used should be carefully selected. Apremilast, an oral phosphodiesterase-4 inhibitor and an immunomodulatory imide drug, was shown to have an antipruritic effect in psoriasis. Given the favorable safety profile and the low risk of drug interactions, apremilast seems to be an appropriate agent for elderly patients.[110]

Potential Treatments on the Horizon

Novel medications that target specific pruritic cytokines and neurotrophins are undergoing clinical trials. Efficacy and safety results so far have been promising. Dupilumab, a monoclonal antibody that targets interleukin-4 and interleukin-13, has been shown to effectively reduce pruritus in patients with moderate to severe atopic dermatitis and has been launched in the United States and Europe.[111] Monoclonal antibodies targeting the pruritic interleukin-31 cytokine, nemolizumab have shown quantitative reduction in pruritus in a phase II trial.[112]

Substance P is a neuropeptide and an important mediator of proinflammatory mechanisms in the skin. It binds to the neurokinin-1 receptor, which is abundantly expressed in the skin and central nervous system. Neurokinin-1 antagonists were shown to have a significant antipruritic effect in acute and chronic pruritus in case reports and series, including in the treatment of drug-induced pruritus, paraneoplastic pruritus, prurigo nodularis, cutaneous T-cell lymphoma, and brachioradial pruritus.[113] Neurokinin-1 antagonists have so far shown a favorable safety profile and, therefore, may be a suitable agent for use in elderly patients.

Selective opioid receptor agonists target kappa-opioid and/or mu-opioid receptors on neurons to inhibit itch without activating other opioid receptors linked to classic opioid side effects, such as respiratory depression, constipation, and addiction. One such agent is nalfurafine, an oral kappa-opioid receptor agonist marketed in Japan for treatment of uremic pruritus in patients with chronic kidney disease undergoing hemodialysis and for refractory pruritus in chronic liver disease.[114] The drug is in phase II studies in the United States. Asimadoline, a highly selective, peripherally directed kappa-opioid agonist is undergoing clinical trial in adults with atopic dermatitis.[115]

PALLIATIVE CARE

End-of-life care is one of the main issues of the geriatric population. Patients in palliative care suffer from pruritus owing to various underlying causes and targeted treatment is recommended. In a Cochrane review published in June 2016, 50 studies that tested 39 different drugs in 1916 patients in palliative care with itch are included.[116] Possibly useful treatments included gabapentin, nalfurafine (a kappa-opioid receptor agonist only used in Japan), cromolyn sodium for itch associated with chronic kidney disease, rifampicin, and flumecinol for itch associated with liver problems. Paroxetine may be useful for patients in palliative care whatever the cause of the itching, although evidence was only available from 1 study.

Some patients in palliative care may receive prolonged administration of opioids for chronic pain. Pruritus is observed in 2% to 10% of patients on opioid medications.[117] The exact mechanism underlying opioid-induced pruritus is uncertain. Morphine is reported to cause histamine release from mast cells, whereas other opioids (namely, fentanyl, sufentanil, and oxymorphone) are less likely to produce histamine release. Therefore, switching from morphine to fentanyl or other opioids is a possible choice.[118] However, the role of histamine in opioid-induced pruritus remains controversial, and antihistamines demonstrate varying degrees of success.

There is increasing evidence that opioid-induced pruritus is mediated through central mu-opioid receptors. Low doses of opioid antagonists (eg, nalmefene 10–25 µg given intravenously, nalbuphine 1–5 mg given intravenously or intramuscularly) are effective for the treatment of pruritus in patients with noncancer pain receiving short-term opioids in the postoperative setting, without reversal of opioid analgesia.[119] However, the long-term use of opioid antagonists in patients with cancer pain who are experiencing prolonged opioid-induced pruritus has not been investigated.[120]

SUMMARY

Itch in the geriatric population is a prevalent and growing problem in the aging society. The pathophysiologic predisposition factors are abnormalities of the epidermal barrier, and the immune and nervous systems. Causes of pruritus are varied, but can be broadly dichotomized into histaminergic and nonhistaminergic pruritus to aid in the treatment of this condition. Topical treatments are safe for both types of itch, but relief is often temporary. For systemic treatment of histaminergic itch, the use of second-generation antihistamines is preferred. For nonhistaminergic itch, treatment varies in accordance with the associated disease. Although treatment options for nonhistaminergic itch are limited, much progress has been made in identifying itch-selective mediators over the last decade. Numerous new biologics and molecules are currently undergoing clinical trials and they are anticipated to enter the clinics in the near future.

REFERENCES

1. Orimo H, Ito H, Suzuki T, et al. Reviewing the definition of "elderly." Geriatr Gerontol Int 2006;6(3): 149–58.
2. Key findings & advance tables, World population prospects 2017 Revision, United Nations. Available at: https://esa.un.org/unpd/wpp/Publications/Files/WPP2017_KeyFindings.pdf. Accessed September 27, 2017.
3. Weisshaar E, Dalgard F. Epidemiology of itch: adding to the burden of skin morbidity. Acta Derm Venereol 2009;89(4):339–50.
4. Ständer S, Schäfer I, Phan NQ, et al. Prevalence of chronic pruritus in Germany: results of a cross-sectional study in a sample working population of 11,730. Dermatology 2010;221(3):229–35.
5. Valdes-Rodriguez R, Mollanazar NK, González-Muro J, et al. Itch prevalence and characteristics in a Hispanic geriatric population: a comprehensive study using a standardized itch questionnaire. Acta Derm Venereol 2015;95(4):417–21.
6. Beauregard S, Gilchrest BA. A survey of skin problems and skin care regimens in the elderly. Arch Dermatol 1987;123(12):1638–43.
7. Thaipisuttikul Y. Pruritic skin diseases in the elderly. J Dermatol 1998;25(3):153–7.
8. Makrantonaki E, Steinhagen-Thiessen E, Nieczaj R, et al. Prevalence of skin diseases in hospitalized geriatric patients: association with gender, duration of hospitalization and geriatric assessment. Z Gerontol Geriatr 2017;50(6):524–31.
9. Kini SP, DeLong LK, Veledar E, et al. The impact of pruritus on quality of life: the skin equivalent of pain. Arch Dermatol 2011;147(10):1153–6.
10. Tey HL, Wallengren J, Yosipovitch G. Psychosomatic factors in pruritus. Clin Dermatol 2013; 31(1):31–40.
11. Rawlings AV, Harding CR. Moisturization and skin barrier function. Dermatol Ther 2004;17(s1):43–8.
12. Yong AA, Cao T, Tan V, et al. Skin physiology in pruritus of advanced ageing. J Eur Acad Dermatol Venereol 2016;30(3):549–50.
13. Li J, Tang H, Hu X, et al. Aquaporin-3 gene and protein expression in sun-protected human skin decreases with skin ageing. Australas J Dermatol 2010;51(2):106–12.
14. Patel T, Yosipovitch G. The management of chronic pruritus in the elderly. Skin Ther Lett 2010;15(8):5–9.
15. Waller JM, Maibach HI. Age and skin structure and function, a quantitative approach (I): blood flow, pH, thickness, and ultrasound echogenicity. Skin Res Technol 2005;11(4):221–35.
16. Luebberding S, Krueger N, Kerscher M. Age-related changes in skin barrier function - quantitative evaluation of 150 female subjects. Int J Cosmet Sci 2013;35(2):183–90.
17. Long CC, Marks R. Stratum corneum changes in patients with senile pruritus. J Am Acad Dermatol 1992;27(4):560–4.
18. Candore G, Caruso C, Jirillo E, et al. Low grade inflammation as a common pathogenetic denominator in age-related diseases: novel drug targets for anti-ageing strategies and successful ageing achievement. Curr Pharm Des 2010;16(6): 584–96.
19. Franceschi C, Capri M, Monti D, et al. Inflammaging and anti-inflammaging: a systemic perspective on aging and longevity emerged from studies in humans. Mech Ageing Dev 2007; 128(1):92–105.
20. Lang PO, Mitchell WA, Lapenna A, et al. Immunological pathogenesis of main age-related diseases and frailty: role of immunosenescence. Eur Geriatr Med 2010;1(2):112–21.
21. Xu AZ, Tripathi SV, Kau AL, et al. Immune dysregulation underlies a subset of patients with chronic idiopathic pruritus. J Am Acad Dermatol 2016; 74(5):1017–20.
22. Goronzy JJ, Weyand CM. Immune aging and autoimmunity. Cell Mol Life Sci 2012;69(10):1615–23.
23. Agrawal A, Gupta S. Impact of aging on dendritic cell functions in humans. Ageing Res Rev 2011; 10(3):336–45.
24. Schmidt T, Sitaru C, Amber K, et al. BP180- and BP230-specific IgG autoantibodies in pruritic disorders of the elderly: a preclinical stage of bullous pemphigoid? Br J Dermatol 2014;171(2):212–9.
25. McArthur JC, Stocks EA, Hauer P, et al. Epidermal nerve fiber density: normative reference range and diagnostic efficiency. Arch Neurol 1998;55(12): 1513.
26. Hunter JA. Seventh age itch. BMJ 1985;291(6499): 842.
27. Nusbaum NJ. Aging and sensory senescence. South Med J 1999;92(3):267–75.

28. Bernhard JD. Phantom itch, pseudophantom itch, and senile pruritus. Int J Dermatol 1992;31(12): 856–7.

29. Jinks SL, Carstens E. Superficial dorsal horn neurons identified by intracutaneous histamine: chemonociceptive responses and modulation by morphine. J Neurophysiol 2000;84(2):616–27.

30. Berger TG, Steinhoff M. Pruritus in elderly patients–eruptions of senescence. Semin Cutan Med Surg 2011;30(2):113–7.

31. Ständer S, Weisshaar E, Mettang T, et al. Clinical classification of itch: a position paper of the International Forum for the Study of Itch. Acta Derm Venereol 2007;87(4):291–4.

32. Zuberbier T, Aberer W, Asero R, et al. The EAACI/GA(2) LEN/EDF/WAO Guideline for the definition, classification, diagnosis, and management of urticaria: the 2013 revision and update. Allergy 2014; 69(7):868–87.

33. Chung MC, Symons C, Gilliam J, et al. The relationship between posttraumatic stress disorder, psychiatric comorbidity, and personality traits among patients with chronic idiopathic urticaria. Compr Psychiatry 2010;51(1):55–63.

34. Moolani Y, Lynde C, Sussman G. Advances in understanding and managing chronic urticaria. F1000Research 2016;5:F1000 Faculty Rev-177.

35. Chen Y-J, Wu C-Y, Shen J-L, et al. Cancer risk in patients with chronic urticaria: a population-based cohort study. Arch Dermatol 2012;148(1):103–8.

36. Magen E, Mishal J, Schlesinger M. Clinical and laboratory features of chronic idiopathic urticaria in the elderly. Int J Dermatol 2013;52(11):1387–91.

37. Karakelides M, Monson KL, Volcheck GW, et al. Monoclonal gammopathies and malignancies in patients with chronic urticaria. Int J Dermatol 2006;45(9):1032–8.

38. Romani L, Steer AC, Whitfeld MJ, et al. Prevalence of scabies and impetigo worldwide: a systematic review. Lancet Infect Dis 2015;15(8):960–7.

39. Currie BJ, McCarthy JS. Permethrin and ivermectin for scabies. N Engl J Med 2010;362(8):717–25.

40. Brick KE, Weaver CH, Lohse CM, et al. Incidence of bullous pemphigoid and mortality of patients with bullous pemphigoid in Olmsted County, Minnesota, 1960 through 2009. J Am Acad Dermatol 2014;71(1):92–9.

41. Försti A-K, Jokelainen J, Timonen M, et al. Increasing incidence of bullous pemphigoid in Northern Finland: a retrospective database study in Oulu University Hospital. Br J Dermatol 2014; 171(5):1223–6.

42. Joly P, Baricault S, Sparsa A, et al. Incidence and mortality of bullous pemphigoid in France. J Invest Dermatol 2012;132(8):1998–2004.

43. Murrell DF, Daniel BS, Joly P, et al. Definitions and outcome measures for bullous pemphigoid:

44. Alonso-Llamazares J, Rogers RS, Oursler JR, et al. Bullous pemphigoid presenting as generalized pruritus: observations in six patients. Int J Dermatol 1998;37(7):508–14.

45. Di Zenzo G, Della Torre R, Zambruno G, et al. Bullous pemphigoid: from the clinic to the bench. Clin Dermatol 2012;30(1):3–16.

46. Yew YW, Tey HL. Sensitivities and utility of non-invasive serological tests in the diagnosis of bullous pemphigoid. Int J Dermatol 2016;55(9): e510–11.

47. Chen ZJ, Cao G, Tang WX, et al. A randomized controlled trial of high-permeability haemodialysis against conventional haemodialysis in the treatment of uraemic pruritus. Clin Exp Dermatol 2009; 34(6):679–83.

48. Pisoni RL, Wikström B, Elder SJ, et al. Pruritus in haemodialysis patients: international results from the Dialysis Outcomes and Practice Patterns Study (DOPPS). Nephrol Dial Transpl 2006; 21(12):3495–505.

49. Meyer TW, Hostetter TH. Uremia. N Engl J Med 2007;357(13):1316–25.

50. Mathur VS, Lindberg J, Germain M, et al. A longitudinal study of uremic pruritus in hemodialysis patients. Clin J Am Soc Nephrol 2010;5(8): 1410–9.

51. Setiawan VW, Stram DO, Porcel J, et al. Prevalence of chronic liver disease and cirrhosis by underlying cause in understudied ethnic groups: the multiethnic cohort. Hepatology 2016;64(6):1969–77.

52. Mela M, Mancuso A, Burroughs AK. Review article: pruritus in cholestatic and other liver diseases. Aliment Pharmacol Ther 2003;17(7):857–70.

53. Schoenfield LJ, Sjövall J, Perman E. Bile acids on the skin of patients with pruritic hepatobiliary disease. Nature 1967;213(5071):93–4.

54. Bergasa NV. Treatment of the pruritus of cholestasis. Curr Treat Options Gastroenterol 2004; 7(6):501–8.

55. Thornton JR, Losowsky MS. Plasma leucine enkephalin is increased in liver disease. Gut 1989;30(10):1392–5.

56. Thornton JR, Losowsky MS. Opioid peptides and primary biliary cirrhosis. BMJ 1988;297(6662): 1501–4.

57. Kremer AE, Martens JJWW, Kulik W, et al. Lysophosphatidic acid is a potential mediator of cholestatic pruritus. Gastroenterology 2010,139(3). 1008–18, 1018.e1.

58. Wang H, Yosipovitch G. New insights into the pathophysiology and treatment of chronic itch in patients with end-stage renal disease, chronic liver disease, and lymphoma. Int J Dermatol 2010; 49(1):1–11.

recommendations by an international panel of experts. J Am Acad Dermatol 2012;66(3):479–85.

59. Paredes-Suárez C, Fernández-Redondo V, Blanco MV, et al. Multiple myeloma with scleroderma-like changes. J Eur Acad Dermatol Venereol 2005;19(4):500–2.

60. Zelicovici Z, Lahav M, Cahane P. Pruritus as a presentation of myelomatosis. Br Med J 1977;2(6095):1154.

61. Glynn C, Crockford G, Gavaghan D, et al. Epidemiology of shingles. J R Soc Med 1990;83(10):617–9.

62. Oxman MN, Levin MJ, Johnson GR, et al. A vaccine to prevent herpes zoster and postherpetic neuralgia in older adults. N Engl J Med 2005;352(22):2271–84.

63. Huesmann T, Cunha PR, Osada N, et al. Notalgia paraesthetica: a descriptive two-cohort study of 65 patients from Brazil and Germany. Acta Derm Venereol 2012;92(5):535–40.

64. Pereira MP, Lüling H, Dieckhöfer A, et al. Brachioradial pruritus and notalgia paraesthetica: a comparative observational study of clinical presentation and morphological pathologies. Acta Derm Venereol 2018;98(1):82–8.

65. Bigby M, Jick S, Jick H, et al. Drug-induced cutaneous reactions. A report from the Boston Collaborative Drug Surveillance Program on 15,438 consecutive inpatients, 1975 to 1982. JAMA 1986;256(24):3358–63.

66. Raksha MP, Marfatia YS. Clinical study of cutaneous drug eruptions in 200 patients. Indian J Dermatol Venereol Leprol 2008;74(1):80.

67. Yalçin B, Tamer E, Toy GG, et al. The prevalence of skin diseases in the elderly: analysis of 4099 geriatric patients. Int J Dermatol 2006;45(6):672–6.

68. Fischer A, Rosen AC, Ensslin CJ, et al. Pruritus to anticancer agents targeting the EGFR, BRAF, and CTLA-4. Dermatol Ther 2013;26(2):135–48.

69. Rinderknecht JD, Goldinger SM, Rozati S, et al. RASopathic skin eruptions during vemurafenib therapy. PLoS One 2013;8(3):e58721.

70. Hodi FS, O'Day SJ, McDermott DF, et al. Improved survival with ipilimumab in patients with metastatic melanoma. N Engl J Med 2010;363(8):711–23.

71. Reich A, Ständer S, Szepietowski JC. Drug-induced pruritus: a review. Acta Derm Venereol 2009;89(3):236–44.

72. Pereira MP, Ständer S. Chronic pruritus: current and emerging treatment options. Drugs 2017;77(9):999–1007.

73. Peier AM, Moqrich A, Hergarden AC, et al. A TRP channel that senses cold stimuli and menthol. Cell 2002;108(5):705–15.

74. Tey H, Tay E, Tan W. Safety and anti-pruritic efficacy of a menthol-containing moisturizing cream. Skinmed 2017;15(6):437–9.

75. Knotkova H, Pappagallo M, Szallasi A. Capsaicin (TRPV1 agonist) therapy for pain relief: farewell or revival? Clin J Pain 2008;24(2):142–54.

76. Metz M, Krause K, Maurer M, et al. Treatment of notalgia paraesthetica with an 8% capsaicin patch. Br J Dermatol 2011;165(6):1359–61.

77. Papoiu ADP, Yosipovitch G. Topical capsaicin. The fire of a "hot" medicine is reignited. Expert Opin Pharmacother 2010;11(8):1359–71.

78. Pereira U, Boulais N, Lebonvallet N, et al. Mechanisms of the sensory effects of tacrolimus on the skin. Br J Dermatol 2010;163(1):70–7.

79. Fleischer AB, Boguniewicz M. An approach to pruritus in atopic dermatitis: a critical systematic review of the tacrolimus ointment literature. J Drugs Dermatol 2010;9(5):488–98.

80. Tan ES, Tan AS, Tey HL. Effective treatment of scrotal lichen simplex chronicus with 0.1% tacrolimus ointment: an observational study. J Eur Acad Dermatol Venereol 2015;29(7):1448–9.

81. Ochi H, Tan LX, Tey HL. Notalgia paresthetica: treatment with topical tacrolimus. J Eur Acad Dermatol Venereol 2016;30(3):452–4.

82. Grönhagen CM, Tey HL. Meralgia paresthetica successfully treated with topical 0.1% tacrolimus: a case report. Int J Dermatol 2016;55(1):e32–3.

83. Kircik LH. Efficacy and onset of action of hydrocortisone acetate 2.5% and pramoxine hydrochloride 1% lotion for the management of pruritus: results of a pilot study. J Clin Aesthet Dermatol 2011;4(2):48–50.

84. Freitag G, Höppner T. Results of a postmarketing drug monitoring survey with a polidocanol-urea preparation for dry, itching skin. Curr Med Res Opin 1997;13(9):529–37.

85. Lee HG, Grossman SK, Valdes-Rodriguez R, et al. Topical ketamine-amitriptyline-lidocaine for chronic pruritus: a retrospective study assessing efficacy and tolerability. J Am Acad Dermatol 2017;76(4):760–1.

86. Paller AS, Tom WL, Lebwohl MG, et al. Efficacy and safety of crisaborole ointment, a novel, nonsteroidal phosphodiesterase 4 (PDE4) inhibitor for the topical treatment of atopic dermatitis (AD) in children and adults. J Am Acad Dermatol 2016;75(3):494–503.e6.

87. Kalivas J, Breneman D, Tharp M, et al. Urticaria: clinical efficacy of cetirizine in comparison with hydroxyzine and placebo. J Allergy Clin Immunol 1990;86(6 Pt 2):1014–8.

88. Gray SL, Anderson ML, Dublin S, et al. Cumulative use of strong anticholinergics and incident dementia: a prospective cohort study. JAMA Intern Med 2015;175(3):401–7.

89. Grob J-J, Lachapelle J-M. Non-sedating antihistamines in the treatment of chronic idiopathic urticaria using patient-reported outcomes. Curr Med Res Opin 2008;24(8):2423–8.

90. By the American Geriatrics Society 2015 Beers Criteria Update Expert Panel. American Geriatrics

Society 2015 updated beers criteria for potentially inappropriate medication use in older adults. J Am Geriatr Soc 2015;63(11):2227–46.

91. Sharma M, Bennett C, Cohen SN, et al. H1-antihistamines for chronic spontaneous urticaria. Cochrane Database Syst Rev 2014;(11):CD006137.

92. Simons FE, Simons KJ. Clinical pharmacology of new histamine H1 receptor antagonists. Clin Pharmacokinet 1999;36(5):329–52.

93. Powell RJ, Du Toit GL, Siddique N, et al. BSACI guidelines for the management of chronic urticaria and angio-oedema. Clin Exp Allergy 2007;37(5): 631–50.

94. Gunal AI, Ozalp G, Yoldas TK, et al. Gabapentin therapy for pruritus in haemodialysis patients: a randomized, placebo-controlled, double-blind trial. Nephrol Dial Transpl 2004;19(12):3137–9.

95. Nofal E, Farag F, Nofal A, et al. Gabapentin: a promising therapy for uremic pruritus in hemodialysis patients: a randomized-controlled trial and review of literature. J Dermatol Treat 2016;27(6): 515–9.

96. Scheinfeld N. The role of gabapentin in treating diseases with cutaneous manifestations and pain. Int J Dermatol 2003;42(6):491–5.

97. Jagdeo J, Kroshinsky D. A case of post-herpetic itch resolved with gabapentin. J Drugs Dermatol 2011;10(1):85–8.

98. Ständer S, Böckenholt B, Schürmeyer-Horst F, et al. Treatment of chronic pruritus with the selective serotonin re-uptake inhibitors paroxetine and fluvoxamine: results of an open-labelled, two-arm proof-of-concept study. Acta Derm Venereol 2009;89(1):45–51.

99. Zylicz Z, Krajnik M, van Sorge AA, et al. Paroxetine in the treatment of severe non-dermatological pruritus: a randomized, controlled trial. J Pain Symptom Manage 2003;26(6):1105–12.

100. Mayo MJ, Handem I, Saldana S, et al. Sertraline as a first-line treatment for cholestatic pruritus. Hepatol Baltim Md 2007;45(3):666–74.

101. Barton C, Sklenicka J, Sayegh P, et al. Contraindicated medication use among patients in a memory disorders clinic. Am J Geriatr Pharmacother 2008; 6(3):147–52.

102. Bali V, Chatterjee S, Johnson ML, et al. Risk of mortality in elderly nursing home patients with depression using paroxetine. Pharmacotherapy 2017; 37(3):287–96.

103. Kok RM, Reynolds CF. Management of depression in older adults: a review. JAMA 2017;317(20): 2114–22.

104. Hundley JL, Yosipovitch G. Mirtazapine for reducing nocturnal itch in patients with chronic pruritus: a pilot study. J Am Acad Dermatol 2004; 50(6):889–91.

105. Demierre M-F, Taverna J. Mirtazapine and gabapentin for reducing pruritus in cutaneous T-cell lymphoma. J Am Acad Dermatol 2006;55(3):543–4.

106. Yosipovitch G, Samuel LS. Neuropathic and psychogenic itch. Dermatol Ther 2008;21(1):32–41.

107. Dawn AG, Yosipovitch G. Butorphanol for treatment of intractable pruritus. J Am Acad Dermatol 2006; 54(3):527–31.

108. Maley A, Swerlick RA. Azathioprine treatment of intractable pruritus: a retrospective review. J Am Acad Dermatol 2015;73(3):439–43.

109. Ko KC, Tominaga M, Kamata Y, et al. Possible antipruritic mechanism of cyclosporine A in atopic dermatitis. Acta Derm Venereol 2016; 96(5):624–9.

110. Sobell JM, Foley P, Toth D, et al. Effects of apremilast on pruritus and skin discomfort/pain correlate with improvements in quality of life in patients with moderate to severe plaque psoriasis. Acta Derm Venereol 2016;96(4):514–20.

111. Beck LA, Thaçi D, Hamilton JD, et al. Dupilumab treatment in adults with moderate-to-severe atopic dermatitis. N Engl J Med 2014;371(2):130–9.

112. Ruzicka T, Hanifin JM, Furue M, et al. Anti-interleukin-31 receptor A antibody for atopic dermatitis. N Engl J Med 2017;376(9):826–35.

113. Ständer S, Luger TA. NK-1 antagonists and itch. Handb Exp Pharmacol 2015;226:237–55.

114. Jaiswal D, Uzans D, Hayden J, et al. Targeting the opioid pathway for uremic pruritus: a systematic review and meta-analysis. Can J Kidney Health Dis 2016;3. 2054358116675345.

115. Tsukahara-Ohsumi Y, Tsuji F, Niwa M, et al. SA14867, a newly synthesized kappa-opioid receptor agonist with antinociceptive and antipruritic effects. Eur J Pharmacol 2010;647(1–3):62–7.

116. Siemens W, Xander C, Meerpohl JJ, et al. Pharmacological interventions for pruritus in adult palliative care patients. In: The Cochrane Collaboration, editor. Cochrane database of systematic reviews. Chichester (United Kingdom): John Wiley & Sons, Ltd; 2016.

117. Szarvas S, Harmon D, Murphy D. Neuraxial opioid induced pruritus: a review. J Clin Anesth 2003; 15(3):234–9.

118. Rogers E, Mehta S, Shengelia R, et al. Four strategies for managing opioid-induced side effects in older adults. Clin Geriatr 2013;21(4). Available at: https://www.ncbi.nlm.nih.gov/pmc/articles/PMC44 18642/. Accessed September 30, 2017.

119. Jannuzzi RG. Nalbuphine for treatment of opioid-induced pruritus: a systematic review of literature. Clin J Pain 2016;32(1):87–93.

120. Krajnik M, Zylicz Z. Understanding pruritus in systemic disease. J Pain Symptom Manage 2001; 21(2):151–68.

Diagnosis and Management of Neuropathic Itch

Jordan Daniel Rosen, BS[a,b], Anna Chiara Fostini, MD[a,b,c], Gil Yosipovitch, MD[a,b],*

KEYWORDS

• Itch • Pruritus • Neuropathic • Diagnosis • Treatment • Peripheral nerves

KEY POINTS

- Neuropathic pruritus is any injury or dysfunction along the afferent itch pathway that results in a sensation to scratch.
- Numerous neuropathic itch syndromes, affecting the peripheral and central nervous systems, exist and should be recognized by clinicians.
- Keys to diagnosis include obtaining a full clinical history and skin examination, imaging, and neurophysiologic studies.
- Treatment is challenging and requires tailoring therapies. The most common treatments are GABA-nergic anticonvulsant medications and topical anesthetics.

INTRODUCTION

Neuropathic pruritus, also known as neuropathic itch, is a form of nondermatologic chronic itch. When defined broadly, neuropathic pruritus refers to any injury or dysfunction along the afferent itch pathway that results in a sensation to scratch.[1] Neuropathic itch accounts for 8% to 19% of patients affected by chronic pruritus.[2,3] Furthermore, patients with chronic itch owing to neuropathic pruritus tend to have severe pruritus. A retrospective analysis of 597 patients with chronic pruritus investigated the intensity of itch of different origins and found neuropathic itch to be of severe intensity with a mean of 7.8 ± 1.8 on a numerical scale of 0 to 10.[3] Injury most commonly occurs within the peripheral nervous system, or, less commonly, within the central nervous system. Neuropathic itch can be distinguished from systemic forms of pruritus that occur in the absence of direct damage to the nervous system. Patients with chronic itch frequently suffer from depressed mood, interrupted slumber, strained interpersonal relationships, and an impaired quality of life.[4] Neuropathic itch can be challenging for clinicians to diagnose and manage because of the variety of clinical presentations and limited treatment options. Recent developments offer improved insight into the underlying pathophysiology, relevant clinical associations, and novel treatment options.

PATHOPHYSIOLOGY

Neuropathic itch may develop from a variety of etiologies, but the underlying pathophysiology has not been completely ascertained. It is understood

---

Disclosure Statement: The authors have nothing to disclose.

[a] Department of Dermatology and Cutaneous Surgery, University of Miami Miller School of Medicine, 1475 Northwest 12th Avenue, Miami, FL 33136, USA; [b] Miami Itch Center, University of Miami Miller School of Medicine, 1475 Northwest 12th Avenue, Miami, FL 33136, USA; [c] Department of Medicine, Section of Dermatology, University of Verona, 37126 Verona, Italy

* Corresponding author. 1600 Northwest 10th Avenue, Rosenstiel Medical Science Building, Room 2023A, Miami, FL 33136.

E-mail address: Gyosipovitch@med.miami.edu

Dermatol Clin 36 (2018) 213–224
https://doi.org/10.1016/j.det.2018.02.005
0733-8635/18/© 2018 Elsevier Inc. All rights reserved.

that damage to itch neurons or other cells involved in the itch circuitry causes neuropathic itch. Given their vulnerability, damage to the peripheral nerves is more likely to cause neuropathic itch than central nervous system injury. In neuropathic itch, compression, trauma, and other modes of direct damage to peripheral nerve fibers characteristically results in a dermatomal distribution of pruritus. However, extensive damage or central lesions may cause pruritus that expands beyond or involves multiple dermatomes. Moreover, pruritus owing to compression is typically localized to the corresponding dermatome, whereas nerve fiber degeneration can present as either localized or generalized pruritus. The location of the insult and the involvement of other neural pathways determine whether other symptoms, such as pain or autonomic changes, are also present. Allokinesis (itch evoked by light touch) and other forms of hypersensitivity result from peripheral and central sensitization of neurons, and are frequently associated with neuropathic itch. Although the changes in the underlying neural pathway that result in neuropathic pruritus are not known, the following mechanisms have been proposed: (1) disinhibition of inhibitory spinal interneurons, (2) overactivation of adjacent undamaged sensory nerves, (3) hyperexcitation of central itch neurons in the absence of ascending signaling, or (4) dysfunction of cortical somatosensory pathways. Recent findings have also implicated (5) alterations in neuronal ion channels as a possible mechanism.

PRINCIPLE DISEASE ENTITIES

There are multiple ways to group the various etiologies of neuropathic itch. In this article, neuropathic itch is categorized based on the location of the primary insult in the peripheral or central nervous system (Table 1).

Peripheral Nervous System

Postherpetic neuralgia
Shingles is a neurocutaneous condition caused by the reactivation of latent varicella zoster virus in somatic sensory ganglia. Nonspecific symptoms (ie, fever, malaise) may present before skin manifestations, and the skin manifestations are often followed by the onset of postherpetic neuralgia (PHN). PHN is classically characterized by allodynia, pain, and parasthesias. Studies in the last 2 decades have provided evidence to support the association of neuropathic itch with acute shingles and PHN. An epidemiologic study of 586 adults with shingles demonstrated that itch, usually mild or moderate, affected up to 58% of patients with

Table 1 Causes of neuropathic itch	
Peripheral Nervous System	Central Nervous System
Postherpetic neuralgia	Spinal cord disorders
Small fiber neuropathy	Syringomyelia
Diabetic neuropathic itch	Tumors
NaV1.7 mutations	Abscesses
Notalgia paresthetica	Transverse myelitis
Brachioradial pruritus	Neuromyelitis optica
Neuropathic anogenital pruritus	Brain disorders
Cheiralgia paresthetica	Stroke
Meralgia paresthetica	Multiple sclerosis
Suprascapular entrapment syndrome	Traumatic brain injury
Pudendal neuralgia	Abscesses
Scalp dysesthesia	Scrapie
Multilevel symmetric neuropathic pruritus	Creutzfeldt-Jakob disease
Prurigo nodularis	Trigeminal trophic syndrome
Dry eye itch	Uremic pruritus
Postburn itch	
Scar and keloid Itch	

acute shingles or PHN.[5] Postherpetic itch is more likely to occur after facial shingles than after truncal shingles.[5] The skin changes and sensory symptoms of PHN classically present in a single dermatome, but multiple adjacent dermatomes may also be involved. Risk factors for PHN include advanced age, immunosuppression, polyneuropathy, and herpes zoster ophthalmicus or oticus.[2] Treatment options include anticonvulsants such as carbamazepine and gabapentin; antidepressants such as amitriptyline, desipramine, fluoxetine, or paroxetine; and topical agents such as capsaicin or anesthetics.

Small fiber neuropathies and diabetic itch
Small fiber neuropathies (SFN) are diseases of thinly myelinated A-δ and unmyelinated C fibers. SFN are characterized by autonomic and sensory symptoms, such as burning, allodynia, hyperalgesia, itch, and excessive sweating. The major diagnostic criterion of SFN is the diminution of intraepidermal nerve fiber density (IENF).

Additional criteria include the signs and symptoms of SFN, the presence of normal sural nerve conduction, and/or altered quantitative sensory testing.[6] There are various etiologies of SFN, which may originate from metabolic, infectious, inflammatory, toxic, paraneoplastic, autoimmune, genetic, or idiopathic causes. A recent study of 41 patients affected by SFN found that 68% of subjects suffered from mild to severe neuropathic itch with an average intensity of 4.79 on a numeric scale from 0 to 10.[7] In this study, pruritus frequently occurred on a daily or near-daily basis, and most often occurred during the evening. The area of the body most commonly afflicted was the back (63%), followed by the foot (59%) and shin (56%).

Diabetes mellitus is one of the most common causes of SFN in developed countries. The prevalence of pruritus in diabetic subjects is significantly higher than in nondiabetic subjects (26.3% vs 14.6%). Furthermore, in diabetic patients, pruritus of unknown origin localized to the trunk occurs more frequently than in those without diabetes (11.3% vs 2.9%).[8] This form of pruritus was associated with other characteristics of diabetic polyneuropathy, including impaired blood pressure response in a head-up tilt test, numbness in the toes and soles, and Achilles tendon areflexia.[8] Neurotropic agents, such as gabapentin, may be useful in the treatment of this condition, although data are lacking.

Gain-of-function mutations in voltage-gated sodium channel

The voltage-gated sodium channel, NaV1.7, modulates cell excitability and ion channel functioning. NaV1.7 is widely expressed in the dorsal root ganglion and in sympathetic ganglion neurons and their small diameter axons. A novel clinical syndrome associated with the I739V variant of the SCN9A gene (which encodes NaV1.7) has been reported in 3 patients of the same family.[9] In this report, the syndromal findings are characterized by paroxysmal itch attacks (involving the shoulders, upper back, and upper limbs), followed by transient burning pain. The symptoms can be triggered by environmental factors such as warmth, hot drinks, or spicy food. Pruritus was also associated with impaired superficial sensations, such as hypoesthesia and hypoalgesia in the affected areas. Furthermore, biopsies from 2 of the 3 patients, demonstrated a significant decrease in IENF density, consistent with SFN. Together these findings suggest a neuropathic origin of itch. In these patients, the use of pregabalin reduced itch intensity and the frequency of pruritic episodes.[9]

Notalgia paresthetica

Notalgia parestethica is characterized by pruritus, in a circumscribed area of the back, especially over the medial scapular borders in the mid thoracic dermatomes. The classic physical examination finding is a hyperpigmented patch overlying the symptomatic area secondary to chronic scratching. Paresthesias are also often found in conjunction with pruritus. The changes leading to notalgia parestethica can be frequently attributed to radiculopathy of the primary dorsal rami of the spinal nerves. In one study, approximately 70% of patients with notalgia parestethica also had underlying vertebral column disease.[10] Damage to the peripheral nerves by musculoskeletal compression has been proposed as an alternative explanation.[11] Other associations with notalgia parestethica include trauma, diabetes mellitus, and multiple endocrine neoplasia syndrome type 2A. Therapy usually only provides symptomatic relief. Some benefits have been reported with capsaicin cream (0.075%–0.100%), 8% capsaicin patches, topical local anesthetics, oral medications such as gabapentin and antidepressants, and the injection of botulinum toxin type A.[2,12]

Brachioradial pruritus

Brachioradial pruritus is typically localized to a circumscribed area on the dorsolateral forearm along the C5/C6 dermatomes; however, it may spread to the shoulders, upper thorax or wrists. Brachioradial pruritus often occurs bilaterally and may be associated with tingling, burning, and stinging perceptions. Although brachioradial pruritus is typically localized, generalized pruritus has been described in some cases of brachioradial pruritus.[13,14] Factors leading to brachioradial pruritus include compression of the spinal cord or cervical radiculopathies, as seen in spinal stenosis. Brachioradial pruritus may worsen under exposure to ultraviolet light and warmth, and can be alleviated by cooling the area (also known as the ice-pack sign). Gabapentin has been described as one of the more effective treatments for brachioradial pruritus.[15] A recent comparison between treatment approaches in brachioradial pruritus in 49 patients showed meaningful reductions of itch with the antidepressants fluoxetine, amitriptyline, and doxepin.[16] Moreover, the comparison found that the most significant reductions in itch were associated with the highest itch intensities before treatment, and longer periods of therapy.[16] Brachioradial pruritus and notalgia parestethica may present similarly; however, there are distinctions that can aid in distinguishing the 2 diagnoses. A new study comparing different aspects of brachioradial pruritus and notalgia parestethica in 58 patients showed that patients with brachioradial pruritus reported stinging and burning more often than those with notalgia parestethica. The study found that IENF density decreased in the lesional skin of patients with brachioradial pruritus, but not in those with notalgia parestethica. In the brachioradial pruritus group, structural MRI abnormalities correlated more frequently with the localization of symptoms. Additionally, topical capsaicin was more efficacious in patients with brachioradial pruritus compared with those with notalgia parestethica.[17]

Neuropathic anogenital pruritus

Anogenital pruritus is defined as an itch localized to the anus, perianal, and/or genital skin. Whereas the origin remains unclear in some cases, anogenital pruritus without a primary rash should raise a high index of suspicion of neuropathic itch. In patients with anogenital pruritis of unknown origin, an underlying neuropathic disease process is often found. This supposition is supported by a study that found that 16 of 20 patients (80%) with anogenital pruritus of unknown origin had lumbosacral radiculopathy, representing nerve or nerve root compression.[18] This study reported positive patient outcomes with a steroid and lidocaine nerve block; however, the use of other treatments used to manage different forms of neuropathic itch are also effective in the treatment of neuropathic anogenital pruritus.

Other localized forms of neuropathic pruritus

Other localized neuropathic syndromes characterized by itch and pain have been reported. These syndromes include cheiralgia (hand) paresthetica, meralgia (lateral thigh) paresthetica, suprascapular entrapment syndrome, and pudendal neuralgia.

Scalp dysesthesia

Scalp dysesthesia occurs in the absence of a primary cutaneous disorder and presents with itching, burning, or stinging of the scalp. The symptoms may be localized or occur diffusely across the scalp. Women account for the vast majority of patients with scalp dysesthesia. Associations with psychiatric diseases, cervical spine diseases, and iatrogenic damage to peripheral nerves have been described.[19] In one study conducted on 15 female patients affected by scalp dysesthesia, 14 had abnormal cervical spine images. In particular, the most common radiographic abnormality was degenerative disk disease, which was present in 11 patients and occurred at C5 to C6 in 10 patients.[20] Diabetes mellitus has been recognized as a risk factor for chronic itch of the scalp in the geriatric population (odds ratio, 2.1; 95% confidence interval, 1.1–9.5; $P = .037$), and

this finding may correspond with the presence of SFN.[21] Oral and topical gabapentin, topical corticosteroids, antidepressants, and pregabalin have been used in treatment of scalp dysesthesia with varying degrees of success.[19,22]

Multilevel symmetric neuropathic pruritus

Multilevel symmetric neuropathic pruritus is characterized by generalized, symmetric, neuropathic pruritus and scratching lesions, which usually arise in patients in their 60s or older. The cause of multilevel symmetric neuropathic pruritus seems to be related to multilevel degenerative disc disease of the spine secondary to atherosclerosis and subsequent decreased blood flow to the intervertebral discs.[23] The use of low-dose gabapentin, sometimes in combination with mirtazapine, has shown promising results.[23]

Prurigo nodularis

Prurigo nodularis is a chronic, highly pruritic condition characterized by the presence of hyperkeratotic, excoriated, pruritic papules and nodules. The lesions are classically distributed symmetrically. Although contrasting data exist, findings in patients with prurigo nodularis and alterations in dermal and epidermal small diameter nerve fibers may suggest the presence of a SFN in some cases.[24] Hypoesthesia and paresthesia, as well as burning, tingling, and stinging sensations, may be present in patients with prurigo nodularis.[25] Randomized, controlled trials are scarce; however, some success has been shown with treatments such as topical steroids, ultraviolet phototherapy, anticonvulsants, cyclosporine, thalidomide, and aprepitant.[26]

Dry eye itch

Recent findings suggest that dry eye accompanied with chronic ocular pain and itch is of neuropathic origin.[27] Moreover, there is evidence that peripheral and central sensitization processes may be involved in generating and maintaining these ocular sensory symptoms.[28] Although data are lacking, high doses of gabapentin have showed efficacy in treating patients with symptoms of dryness and ocular pain who are not responsive to traditional therapies.[28]

Scars, postburn itch, and keloids

Postburn scars, postsurgery scars, hypertrophic scars and keloids can all cause long-lasting pruritus. In these conditions, the pruritus is often associated with burning or piercing sensations.[2] In those who sustain burn injuries, itch is present in about 87% of patients after 3 months, in 70% of patients after 1 year, and in 67% of patients after 2 years.[29] Neurophysiologic and pharmacologic evidence hints at a neuropathic mechanism of pruritus in patients with chronic burn injury associated with itch.[30]

Keloids are a form a pathologic scarring consisting of benign overgrowths of dense fibrous tissue that extends beyond the borders of the original wound. Symptoms of itch and pain are common in patients with keloids, and are present in 86% and 46% of patients, respectively.[31] Itch in keloids typically involves the border of the keloid, whereas pain is more commonly reported in the center of the keloid. The pruritus associated with keloids may be severe; in a recent study, the maximum reported intensity of itch experienced from a keloid was 7.7 on a numerical scale from 0 to 10.[31] Allodynia, allokinesis, and abnormal thermal and pain thresholds were also reported in patients. This constellation of symptoms may be due to neuropathic damage.[31] Treatment options for scar pruritus include gabapentin and pregabalin, as well as topical anesthetics.[2]

Central Nervous System

Spinal cord disorders

Different diseases of the spinal cord may cause itch, including syringomyelia, tumors (typically ependymomas and cavernous hemangiomas), abscesses, transverse myelitis, and neuromyelitis optica.[24,32,33] The location and distribution of itch depends on the site of the primary lesion. In a case series of 45 patients affected by neuromyelitis optica, 12 patients endorsed pruritus, 3 patients reported pruritus as the first symptom of a relapse, and 1 patient reported pruritus as the first symptom of the index episode.[32] Pathologic features of these entities, such as gliosis and hemosiderin, might provoke spontaneous activation of spinal itch neurons.[11]

Brain disorders

Any brain lesion affecting itch neurons can cause central neuropathic itch. Central neuropathic pruritus may be associated with central hypersensitization of nerve fibers, spontaneous firing of damaged nerves, and central neuronal deprivation of afferent input.[34,35] Stroke is the most common brain lesion associated with neuropathic itch. In particular, infarctions of the lateral medulla can cause Wallenberg's syndrome. Wallenberg's syndrome presents with itch, vertigo, nausea, dysphagia, dysarthria, ataxia, ipsilateral sensory loss of the face, and contralateral sensory loss of the trunk and extremities.[24] Less frequent lesions associated with neuropathic itch include multiple sclerosis, tumors within or near the brain, abscesses, and infections.[12] A case report of a patient with traumatic injury to the thalamic and prefrontal cortex described symptoms of generalized neuropathic itch.[36] Neuropathic itch is infrequently associated with prion diseases, such as scrapie and sporadic Creutzfeldt–Jakob disease; 6 of 31 patients with familial Creutzfeldt–Jakob disease reported pruritus.[37]

Trigeminal trophic syndrome is a condition in which abnormal sensations, particularly itching, burning, or stinging, lead to scratching. The associated cutaneous sensory loss in trigeminal trophic syndrome may permit scratching to continue to the point of self-injury. Unfortunately, trigeminal trophic syndrome often remains unrecognized by the physician. The most common causes of trigeminal trophic syndrome are cerebral vascular accidents, particularly stroke, and trigeminal nerve ablation, often in the context of treatment for trigeminal neuralgia.[19,38] Other less frequently described causes of trigeminal trophic syndrome are trauma, herpes zoster, multiple sclerosis, tumors, and abscesses.[38] Although any of the 3 branches of the trigeminal nerve can be involved, the maxillary branch (V2) is the most frequently affected. Treatment is challenging and includes the use of protective barrier, carbamazepine, diazepam, amitriptyline, and pimozide.[38]

Interestingly, a recent study demonstrated neuropathic changes in multiple gray matter regions of the brain in patients affected by uremic pruritus. This finding suggests that an underlying central neuropathy in patients with end-stage renal disease may specifically involve changes to structures involved in the cerebral processing of itch.[39]

CLINICAL EVALUATION OF THE PATIENT

A thorough history may provide critical information about the origin of pruritus in a patient. In particular, the characteristics of itch should be investigated in detail. Neuropathic itch syndromes may be suspected depending on the involved areas, the distribution of pruritus, the presence of dysesthetic symptoms, or the presence of comorbidities (eg, diabetes). For example, one should consider neuropathic origins of itch in patients with localized itch and a history of shingles, or radiculopathic itch and back pain in the context of a motor vehicle accident. The interview should always include a review of all current, and changes to, medications. The intensity of pruritus may be assessed by subjective scales, such as the visual analog scale or the numeric rating scale. A full dermatologic evaluation is fundamental to exclude inflammatory dermatosis as the primary cause of pruritus and to assess the presence of lesions secondary to scratching. Laboratory investigations with a complete blood count, erythrocyte sedimentation rate, thyroid, liver, and renal function tests are useful in excluding underlying systemic disease. Radiologic studies, specifically computed tomography or MRI, are used for detecting structural lesions that can impinge on cranial or spinal nerve roots. MRI is particularly useful in detecting the imaging abnormalities of brachioradial pruritus and notalgia paresthetica, and can be used to detect lesions of the brain and of the spinal cord. Neurophysiologic studies, specifically nerve conduction study and electromyography, are often used to document peripheral nerve damage. However, electromyography is insensitive in detecting SFN. In cases of SFN, the evaluation of IENF density can be used to confirm the diagnosis. The technique requires an immunofluorescence staining process of a skin sample with a primary antibody against the protein gene product 9.5. The IENF densities detected are then quantified according to international guidelines to determine their signifiance.[40] For example, an IENF density below the fifth percentile of the corresponding gender and age, in association with a suitable clinical history, suggests the presence of a SFN.[40] Additional testing in suspected cases of SFN may include thermal quantitative sensory testing, which can indicate possible sensory dysfunctions of C nerve fibers that transmit itch and pain and can serve as a quality marker of clinical improvement.[2]

TREATMENT

Neuropathic itch is a challenging condition for clinicians to manage. Although it would be ideal to target the source of the disease (eg, compressed spinal cord roots), thereby eliminating the corresponding sequelae, this strategy is rarely effective or practical. The majority of interventions are not curative. For patients with intractable pruritus, it is important to focus on symptomatic management and quality of life (**Fig. 1**). Commonly prescribed antipruritic medications, such as antihistamines and corticosteroids, have limited success in neuropathic pruritus. Alternate agents, such as oral gabapentin and topical capsaicin, tend to be the first-line agents in the management of neuropathic pruritus. However, the efficacy of pharmacologic treatments is largely based on clinician experience and case reports, and is not validated by controlled studies. In addition to medical treatments, patients may benefit from nonpharmacologic approaches and therapies. The consultation and coordination of care with other specialists and health care providers is critical given the comorbidities associated with the many conditions that cause neuropathic itch.

Topical Pharmacologic Treatments

Topical treatments can be applied in affected areas to achieve high local concentrations with

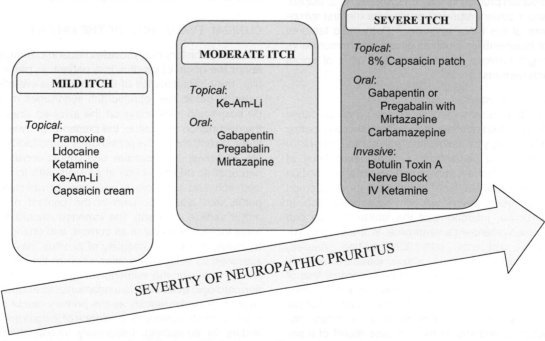

Fig. 1. Author's therapeutic ladder for neuropathic pruritus. IV, intravenous.

reduced risks of major adverse effects. During localized, less severe, or more acute forms of neuropathic itch, topical treatments may offer more rapid relief.

Capsaicin

Capsaicin, a metabolite found in chili peppers, is a commonly used topical treatment for neuropathic pruritus. Capsaicin activates the transient receptor potential cation channel, subfamily V-1 receptors found on C fibers, causing an intense depolarization. This results in the long-lasting desensitization of local nerve fibers and an improvement of pruritic symptoms. Capsaicin has shown success in treating the symptoms of PHN, notalgia paresthetica,[41] brachioradial pruritus,[42] and SFN.[14] Before achieving its antipruritic effects, the application of capsaicin is often followed by a hot or burning sensation that may be brief or last for several days. Patients are often very bothered by the burning sensation, but compliance may improve with the preapplication of a local anesthetic such as lidocaine[42] or a eutectic mixture of local anesthetic. The administration of nonprescription capsaicin (0.025%–0.100%) normally requires multiple applications to achieve a significant reduction in pruritus. We recommend higher concentrations of topical capsaicin, usually at 0.075% to 0.100%.[43] Furthermore, 8% capsaicin patches (NGX-4010) applied for 60 minutes may produce a greater and longer lasting antipruritic effect.[14,41,42,44] There is even a report of a single 8% capsaicin application abolishing neuropathic pruritus for more than a year.[41,42]

Anesthetics

The effectiveness of topical anesthetics in treating neuropathic pruritus varies among patients. However, the relatively low cost and minimal adverse effects make them worthwhile treatment modalities to explore. Some success has been reported with the application of the following topical anesthetics: eutectic mixture of local anesthetic, lidocaine, prilocaine, and pramoxine. A combination of topical 5% to 10% ketamine with 5 amitriptyline and 5% lidocaine (KeAmLi), which additionally targets ion channels, may improve itch in a variety of pruritic conditions, including neuropathic pruritus.[45] Ketamine can also be applied topically in combination with amitriptyline for treatment of brachioradial pruritus,[46] and mild relief of PHN and notalgia paresthetica.[47]

Topical calcineurin inhibitors

Topical calcineurin inhibitors are another low-risk option with variable efficacy in neuropathic itch. Topical tacrolimus applied to effected areas has shown some success in treating notalgia paresthetica,[48] trigeminal trophic syndrome,[49] and, in the authors' experience, anogenital itch. Similar to capsaicin, topical calcineurin inhibitors may cause a transient burning sensation. Topical application is not typically associated with the systemic immunosuppression that can occur with oral use of calcineurin inhibitors.

Menthol

Menthol, through activation of the TRPM-8 receptor, can elicit a cool sensation useful in the relief of itch. Although not commonly used in neuropathic pruritus, patients who report improvement of symptoms with cooling of the affected areas, such as those with brachioradial pruritus (ie, the ice-pack sign), may experience some relief using topical menthol up to 2%.

Other topical therapies

A variety of other topical therapies, such as gabapentin (10%–12%) and strontium hydrogel (Tricalm), may be effective in treating neuropathic pruritus.[20,50] In addition, topical acetylsalicylic acid (aspirin) can improve symptoms of neuropathic pain[51] and, in the author's experience, reduce pruritus in PHN and notalgia paresthetica.

Oral Pharmacologic Treatments

Many of the medications discussed in this section require higher doses to treat neuropathic itch compared with the recommended doses for use in other indications. When using systemic therapies for the treatment of neuropathic itch, it is important to use effective dosing to reach therapeutic levels. Generally, once a maximum therapeutic dose has been achieved, medications from a different class may be added to the regimen to achieve further reduction in itch.

Anticonvulsants

Gabapentinoids are a class of anticonvulsant medications that includes gabapentin (Neurontin) and pregabalin (Lyrica). These drugs are GABA-aminobutyric acid analogs that act by antagonizing the alpha-2-delta subunit of voltage-gated calcium channels. Gabapentin is approved by the UD Food and Drug Administration for the treatment of seizures and PHN,[52] and is effective in the treatment of neuropathic forms of itch, such as brachioradial pruritus, prurigo nodularis, and notalgia paresthetica.[53] There are promising case reports regarding the use of gabapentin in scalp dysesthesia,[20] pruritus associated with traumatic spinal cord injury,[54] and trigeminal trophic syndrome.[55] Gabapentin is typically dosed beginning at 300 to 600 mg at night, followed by an increase in dosage every 2 to 3 days as tolerated.[56] In our experience for neuropathic itch, doses as high as 3600 mg/d may be tolerable. Pregabalin has demonstrated success in the treatment of prurigo nodularis.[57] Pregabalin is dosed beginning with 50 mg twice daily and may be increased to a maximum total dose of 450 mg/d.[56] Despite similar mechanisms of action, a trial of pregabalin or gabapentin can be prescribed if a patient does not respond to the other agent. Sedative neurologic symptoms are the most common side effects of both gabapentin and pregabalin, but are generally well-tolerated by patients[57] and subside with continued treatment. Patients also often experience increased appetite, weight gain, constipation, and, less commonly, swelling of the lower legs. The kidneys eliminate both gabapentin and pregabalin, so drug levels must be followed closely in patients with impaired renal function.[58] Additionally, it is important to monitor for symptoms of withdrawal if either medication is discontinued abruptly.[59]

Although not as widely used as the gabapentinoids, 2 additional anticonvulsants, oxcarbazepine and carbamazepine, have been used in the treatment of neuropathic pruritus. In a small number of patients, oxcarbazepine has demonstrated some success in the treatment of notalgia paresthetica[60] and brachioradial pruritus.[61] Carbamazepine has been used to treat neuropathic itch in multiple sclerosis,[62] PHN, trigeminal trophic syndrome,[63] and brachioradial pruritus.[64] The pharmacodynamics of carbamazepine and oxcarbazepine are not entirely understood, but are believed to involve antagonism of voltage-gated sodium channels found on neurons.[65] Variations in the gene (SCN9A) encoding the voltage-gated sodium 1.7 receptor (NaV1.7) have been linked with a familial form of peripheral neuropathic itch.[66] Interestingly, monoclonal antibodies to NaV1.7 may be effective in the treatment of this type, as well as other forms of neuropathic itch.[67,68]

Antidepressants

Tricyclic antidepressants offer an additional therapeutic approach to neuropathic itch. Amitriptyline has been reported useful in the treatment of PHN itch, trigeminal trophic syndrome, notalgia paresthetica,[69] and brachioradial pruritus.[70] To minimize adverse effects, amitriptyline is typically given at night, beginning at a low dose of 5 to 10 mg, and then titrated upward. Patients may not experience benefits from the medications until 6 to 8 weeks of treatment.

Selective serotonin reuptake inhibitors and selective serotonin and norepinephrine inhibitors are used to treat certain types of pruritus. The selective serotonin and norepinephrine inhibitor, mirtazapine, can be used to treat neuropathic pain[71];

however, current research is lacking with regards to the use of selective serotonin reuptake inhibitors and selective serotonin and norepinephrine inhibitors in neuropathic itch. Treatment-resistant neuropathic pruritus may respond to a combination of gabapentin and mirtazapine because it reduces neural hypersensitization. Other antidepressants such as fluvoxamine and duloxetine[72] have also been reported to reduce pruritus.

Neurokinin-1 inhibitors

Neurokinin-1 (NK1) receptors are found throughout the body and the neural system. NK1 receptors bind the neuropeptide substance P. Substance P is involved in the transmission of pain and itch, and is suspected of playing a role in the pathogenesis of pruritic conditions. Aprepitant, an NK1 receptor inhibitor, is indicated for the treatment of chemotherapy-induced nausea and vomiting. Aprepitant has also demonstrated efficacy in the treatment of a variety of pruritic conditions, such as paraneoplastic itch[73] and prurigo nodularis.[74] In addition, a case report of a woman with brachioradial pruritus showed improvements in pruritus and pruritic lesions within 1 week of receiving 80 mg/d of aprepitant.[75] The adverse effects of aprepitant are typically well-tolerated by patients[76]; however, aprepitant is an inhibitor of CYP3A4 and can interact with other medications. Novel NK1 receptor inhibitors, such as serlopitant and tradipitant, have a higher affinity for brain NK1 receptors and are possibly more effective in treating neuropathic itch.

Opioids

Itch transmission is associated with activation of the mu-opioid receptor and antagonism of the kappa-opioid receptor. It has, therefore, been postulated that mu-opioid receptor antagonists and kappa-opioid receptor agonists may make for capable treatments of pruritus.[77] At night, 1 to 4 mg of intranasal butorphanol, an opioid with mixed activity, can reduce symptoms in patients with treatment-resistant chronic itch.[78] However, clinical evidence advocating for the use of opioid medications in patients with neuropathic itch is lacking.

Ketamine

Ketamine is an NMDA receptor antagonist that, when administered intravenously, can be used to treat neuropathic pain.[79] In the author's experience, patients with severe intractable neuropathic pruritus may also benefit from intravenous ketamine (0.5 mg/kg).

Oral lidocaine analogs

The use of the lidocaine analog, mexiletine, has been reported to improve cholestatic pruritus.[80]

Oral mexiletine can treat other pruritic conditions as well, and is a potential therapeutic option for the treatment of neuropathic itch.[81]

Future
Further exploration of the neuropathic itch pathway and development of pharmacologic agents targeting receptors, neurokinin 1 inhibitors, ion channels such as transient receptor potential channels (transient receptor potential cation channel, subfamily V), Mas-related G-protein coupled receptor, may yield future clinical applications.

Invasive Treatments

Botulinum toxin A
A small number of case series have suggested that injection of botulinum toxin A decreases pruritus in patients with notalgia paresthetica.[82,83] Treatment involves a series of injections of 1 to 5 U of botulinum toxin A at each of several points within the affected area, each point being located 1 to 2 cm apart. Botulinum toxin may decrease pruritus through the reduction of cholinergic transmission or release of substance P along itch pathways. The authors have had some success with this treatment; however, such benefits were not substantiated in a 20-patient double-blinded controlled study.[84] It is also speculated that botulinum toxin A may be useful in other forms of neuropathic itch, such as brachioradial pruritus.[85]

Interventional therapies
Interventional treatments, such as targeted nerve blocks or modulation of specific neural structures, provide alternative treatment strategies in selected patients with refractory neuropathic itch. There have been reported benefits with peripheral nerve stimulation in a case of notalgia paresthetica,[86] and with targeted nerve blocks in cases of post-herpetic itch[87] and notalgia paresthetica.[88] Additionally, a paravertebral injection of a mixture of triamcinolone acetonide and lidocaine has been reported to reduce pruritus in patients suffering from neuropathic anogenital pruritus.[18] Given the limited evidence and the inherent risks of surgery, neurosurgical decompression is rarely indicated. A less invasive, nonsurgical alternative is transcutaneous electrical nerve stimulation. Transcutaneous electrical nerve stimulation has been shown to partially relieve pruritus in those with localized notalgia paresthetica,[89] burn pruritus,[90] or brachioradial pruritus.[89,91] Potential future treatments for neuropathic itch may include transcranial direct current stimulation, repetitive transcranial magnetic stimulation, or epidural motor cortex stimulation.

Nonpharmacologic Treatments

Psychological interventions
Adopting a holistic approach to address the cognitive and emotional components of neuropathic itch may be considered. Although there are limited data on the psychological management of these patients, it may be useful as an additional therapy to control the itch–scratch cycle and improve quality of life. Cognitive behavior therapies include habit reversal training and relaxation training.[92] The goal of habit reversal training is to alter dysfunctional behavior by teaching patients to replace negative behaviors with neutral actions. This technique consists of awareness training, practicing a competing response whereby a patient replaces the dysfunctional behavior, and increasing motivation to better control scratching.[93] Habit reversal training has been shown to have positive effects on the treatment of some compulsive anxiety-related disorders and in the decrease of frequency of scratching in patients with itch-related dermatoses.[93] Relaxation training includes progressive muscle relaxation and autogenic training. Progressive muscle relaxation consists of exercises that determine the tension of certain muscle groups, followed by the subsequent relaxation of those muscles. Autogenic training is known to reduce stress and anxiety in different somatic diseases, and consists of asking subjects to concentrate mentally on certain body perceptions.[93] Biofield therapy with healing touch was reported to be effective in treating a patient affected by intractable central neuropathic itch.[36] Healing touch involves touching or placing one's hands above the body to facilitate healing. It has shown efficacy in reducing itch in patients with pain, as well as reducing stress, anxiety, and chronic pain in oncologic patients.[36,94–96]

Physical therapy and exercise
Strengthening and stretching exercises could be considered an adjunctive treatment in certain neuropathic itch conditions, especially those related to nerve impingement or compression. This intervention was applied in a case report of 2 individuals affected by notalgia paresthetica; the individuals both had a reduction in itch after the implementation of a muscle stretching and strengthening program.[97]

SUMMARY

Given the variety of presentations, extensive differential diagnoses, and limited number of definitive treatments, neuropathic itch is often difficult to diagnose and a challenge to treat. Management frequently requires trials with different treatments and the care of an interdisciplinary team of health care providers. Although neuropathic itch is often a debilitating and consuming condition for patients, awareness among clinicians and patients remains limited. It is important for future research to aid in validating the efficacy of current treatments and to continue to guide the development of novel therapeutic options.

REFERENCES

1. Yosipovitch G, Goodkin R, Wingard E, et al. Neuropathic pruritus. Itch: Basic Mech Ther 2004;27: 231–40.

2. Stumpf A, Ständer S. Neuropathic itch: diagnosis and management. Dermatol Ther 2013;26:104–9.

3. Mollanazar NK, Sethi M, Rodriguez RV, et al. Retrospective analysis of data from an itch center: integrating validated tools in the electronic health record. J Am Acad Dermatol 2016;75:842.

4. Kini SP, DeLong LK, Veledar E, et al. The impact of pruritus on quality of life: the skin equivalent of pain. Arch Dermatol 2011;147:1153–6.

5. Oaklander AL, Bowsher D, Galer B, et al. Herpes zoster itch: preliminary epidemiologic data. J Pain 2003;4:338–43.

6. Devigili G, Tugnoli V, Penza P, et al. The diagnostic criteria for small fibre neuropathy: from symptoms to neuropathology. Brain 2008;131:1912–25.

7. Brenaut E, Marcorelles P, Genestet S, et al. Pruritus: an underrecognized symptom of small-fiber neuropathies. J Am Acad Dermatol 2015;72:328–32.

8. Yamaoka H, Sasaki H, Yamasaki H, et al. Truncal pruritus of unknown origin may be a symptom of diabetic polyneuropathy. Diabetes Care 2010;33:150–5.

9. Devigili G, Eleopra R, Pierro T, et al. Paroxysmal itch caused by gain-of-function Na v 1.7 mutation. Pain 2014;155:1702–7.

10. Savk E, Savk SO. On brachioradial pruritus and notalgia paresthetica. J Am Acad Dermatol 2004;50: 800–1.

11. Dhand A, Aminoff MJ. The neurology of itch. Brain 2013;137:313–22.

12. Oaklander AL. Neuropathic itch. In: Carstens E, Akiyama T, editors. Itch: mechanism and treatment. Chapter 7. Boca Raton (FL): CRC Press/Taylor & Francis; 2014. p. 89–118.

13. Zeidler C, Lüling H, Dieckhöfer A, et al. Capsaicin 8% cutaneous patch: a promising treatment for brachioradial pruritus? Br J Dermatol 2015;172: 1669–71.

14. Kwatra SG, Stander S, Bernhard JD, et al. Brachioradial pruritus: a trigger for generalization of itch. J Am Acad Dermatol 2013;68:870–3.

15. Weisshaar E, Szepietowski JC, Darsow U, et al. European guideline on chronic pruritus. Acta Derm Venereol 2012;92:563–86.

16. Wachholz PA, Masuda PY, Pinto A, et al. Impact of drug therapy on brachioradial pruritus. An Bras Dermatol 2017;92:281–2.

17. Pereira MP, Luling H, Dieckhofer A, et al. Brachioradial pruritus and notalgia paraesthetica: a comparative observational study of clinical presentation and morphological pathologies. Acta Derm Venereol 2018;98(1):82–8.

18. Cohen AD, Vander T, Medvendovsky E, et al. Neuropathic scrotal pruritus: anogenital pruritus is a symptom of lumbosacral radiculopathy. J Am Acad Dermatol 2005;52:61–6.

19. Shumway NK, Cole E, Fernandez KH. Neurocutaneous disease: neurocutaneous dysesthesias. J Am Acad Dermatol 2016;74:215–28.

20. Thornsberry LA, English JC. Scalp dysesthesia related to cervical spine disease. JAMA Dermatol 2013;149:200–3.

21. Valdes-Rodriguez R, Mollanazar NK, González-Muro J, et al. Itch prevalence and characteristics in a Hispanic geriatric population: a comprehensive study using a standardized itch questionnaire. Acta Derm Venereol 2015;95:417–21.

22. Sarifakioglu E, Onur O. Women with scalp dysesthesia treated with pregabalin. Int J Dermatol 2013;52: 1417–8.

23. Ward RE, Veerula VL, Ezra N, et al. Multilevel symmetric neuropathic pruritus (MSNP) presenting as recalcitrant "generalized" pruritus. J Am Acad Dermatol 2016;75:774–81.

24. Misery L, Brenaut E, Le Garrec R, et al. Neuropathic pruritus. Nat Rev Neurol 2014;10:408–16.

25. Iking A, Grundmann S, Chatzigeorgakidis E, et al. Prurigo as a symptom of atopic and non-atopic diseases: aetiological survey in a consecutive cohort of 108 patients. J Eur Acad Dermatol Venereol 2013;27:550–7.

26. Fostini AC, Girolomoni G, Tessari G. Prurigo nodularis: an update on etiopathogenesis and therapy. J Dermatolog Treat 2013;24:458–62.

27. Crane AM, Feuer W, Felix ER, et al. Evidence of central sensitisation in those with dry eye symptoms and neuropathic-like ocular pain complaints: incomplete response to topical anaesthesia and generalised heightened sensitivity to evoked pain. Br J Ophthalmol 2017;101:1238–43.

28. Andersen HH, Yosipovitch G, Galor A. Neuropathic symptoms of the ocular surface: dryness, pain, and itch. Curr Opin Allergy Clin Immunol 2017;17: 373–81.

29. Vitale M, Fields-Blache C, Luterman A. Severe itching in the patient with burns. J Burn Care Rehabil 1990;12:330–3.

30. Goutos I. Neuropathic mechanisms in the pathophysiology of burns pruritus: redefining directions for therapy and research. J Burn Care Res 2013;34:82–93.

31. Lee S-S, Yosipovitch G, Chan Y-H, et al. Pruritus, pain, and small nerve fiber function in keloids: a

controlled study. J Am Acad Dermatol 2004;51: 1002–6.

32. Elsone L, Townsend T, Mutch K, et al. Neuropathic pruritus (itch) in neuromyelitis optica. Mult Scler J 2013;19:475–9.

33. Zhao S, Mutch K, Elsone L, et al. An unusual case of 'itchy paralysis': neuromyelitis optica presenting with severe neuropathic itch. Pract Neurol 2015;15: 149–51.

34. Yosipovitch G, Samuel LS. Neuropathic and psychogenic itch. Dermatol Ther 2008;21:32–41.

35. Binder A, Koroschetz J, Baron R. Disease mechanisms in neuropathic itch. Nature reviews. Neurology 2008;4:329.

36. Curtis AR, Tegeler C, Burdette J, et al. Holistic approach to treatment of intractable central neuropathic itch. J Am Acad Dermatol 2011;64:955–9.

37. Cohen OS, Chapman J, Lee H, et al. Pruritus in familial Creutzfeldt-Jakob disease: a common symptom associated with central nervous system pathology. J Neurol 2011;258(1):89–95.

38. Curtis AR, Oaklander AL, Johnson A, et al. Trigeminal Trophic Syndrome from stroke. Am J Clin Dermatol 2012;13:125–8.

39. Papoiu AD, Emerson NM, Patel TS, et al. Voxel-based morphometry and arterial spin labeling fMRI reveal neuropathic and neuroplastic features of brain processing of itch in end-stage renal disease. J Neurophysiol 2014;112:1729–38.

40. Lauria G, Bakkers M, Schmitz C, et al. Intraepidermal nerve fiber density at the distal leg: a worldwide normative reference study. J Peripher Nerv Syst 2010;15(3):202–7.

41. Andersen HH, Sand C, Elberling J. Considerable variability in the efficacy of 8% capsaicin topical patches in the treatment of chronic pruritus in 3 patients with notalgia paresthetica. Ann Dermatol 2016;28:86–9.

42. Misery L, Erfan N, Castela E, et al. Successful treatment of refractory neuropathic pruritus with capsaicin 8% patch: a bicentric retrospective study with long-term follow-up. Acta Derm Venereol 2015;95:864–5.

43. Papoiu AD, Yosipovitch G. Topical capsaicin. The fire of a 'hot' medicine is reignited. Expert Opin Pharmacother 2010;11:1359–71.

44. Andersen HH, Arendt-Nielsen L, Elberling J. Topical capsaicin 8% for the treatment of neuropathic itch conditions. Clin Exp Dermatol 2017;42:596–8.

45. Lee HG, Grossman SK, Valdes-Rodriguez R, et al. Topical ketamine-amitriptyline-lidocaine for chronic pruritus: a retrospective study assessing efficacy and tolerability. J Am Acad Dermatol 2017;76:760–1.

46. Poterucha TJ, Murphy SL, Davis MD, et al. Topical amitriptyline-ketamine for the treatment of brachioradial pruritus. JAMA Dermatol 2013;149:148–50.

47. Poterucha TJ, Murphy SL, Sandroni P, et al. Topical amitriptyline combined with topical ketamine for

the management of recalcitrant localized pruritus: a retrospective pilot study. J Am Acad Dermatol 2013;69:320–1.

48. Ochi H, Tan L, Tey H. Notalgia paresthetica: treatment with topical tacrolimus. J Eur Acad Dermatol Venereol 2016;30:452–4.

49. Nakamizo S, Miyachi Y, Kabashima K. Treatment of neuropathic itch possibly due to trigeminal trophic syndrome with 0.1% topical tacrolimus and gabapentin. Acta Derm Venereol 2010;90:654–5.

50. Papoiu AD, Valdes-Rodriguez R, Nattkemper LA, et al. A novel topical formulation containing strontium chloride significantly reduces the intensity and duration of cowhage-induced itch. Acta Derm Venereol 2013;93:520–4.

51. Kingery WS. A critical review of controlled clinical trials for peripheral neuropathic pain and complex regional pain syndromes. Pain 1997;73:123–39.

52. Neurontin(R) [package insert]. New York: Pfizer Inc; 2017.

53. Maciel AAW, Cunha PR, Laraia IO, et al. Efficacy of gabapentin in the improvement of pruritus and quality of life of patients with notalgia paresthetica. An Bras Dermatol 2014;89:570–5.

54. Crane DA, Jaffee KM, Kundu A. Intractable pruritus after traumatic spinal cord injury. J Spinal Cord Med 2009;32:436–9.

55. Sawada T, Asai J, Nomiyama T, et al. Trigeminal trophic syndrome: report of a case and review of the published work. J Dermatol 2014;41:525–8.

56. Leslie TA, Greaves MW, Yosipovitch G. Current topical and systemic therapies for itch. In: Cowen A, Yosipovitch G, editors. Pharmacology of itch. Handbook of experimental pharmacology, vol. 226. Berlin: Springer; 2015. p. 337–56.

57. Matsuda KM, Sharma D, Schonfeld AR, et al. Gabapentin and pregabalin for the treatment of chronic pruritus. J Am Acad Dermatol 2016;75:619–25.

58. Zand L, McKian KP, Qian Q. Gabapentin toxicity in patients with chronic kidney disease: a preventable cause of morbidity. Am J Med 2010;123:367–73.

59. Ehrchen J, Ständer S. Pregabalin in the treatment of chronic pruritus. J Am Acad Dermatol 2008;58: S36–7.

60. Şavka E, Bolukbasib O, Akyolb A, et al. Open pilot study on oxcarbazepine for the treatment of notalgia paresthetica. J Am Acad Dermatol 2001;45: 630–2.

61. Mataix J, Silvestre J, Climent J, et al. Brachioradial pruritus as a symptom of cervical radiculopathy. Actas Dermosifiliogr 2008;99:719–22 [in Spanish].

62. Yamamoto M, Yabuki S, Hayabara T, et al. Paroxysmal itching in multiple sclerosis: a report of three cases. J Neurol Neurosurg Psychiatry 1981;44:19–22.

63. Bhushan M, Parry E, Telfer N. Trigeminal trophic syndrome: successful treatment with carbamazepine. Br J Dermatol 1999;141:758–9.

64. Tait CP, Grigg E, Quirk CJ. Brachioradial pruritus and cervical spine manipulation. Australas J Dermatol 1998;39:168–70.

65. Ambrósio AF, Soares-da-Silva P, Carvalho CM, et al. Mechanisms of action of carbamazepine and its derivatives, oxcarbazepine, BIA 2-093, and BIA 2-024. Neurochem Res 2002;27:121–30.

66. Martinelli-Boneschi F, Colombi M, Castori M, et al. COL6A5 variants in familial neuropathic chronic itch. Brain 2017;140:555–67.

67. Lee J-H, Park C-K, Chen G, et al. A monoclonal antibody that targets a Na V 1.7 channel voltage sensor for pain and itch relief. Cell 2014;157:1393–404.

68. Kornecook TJ, Yin R, Altmann S, et al. Pharmacologic characterization of AMG8379, a potent and selective small molecule sulfonamide antagonist of the voltage-gated sodium channel NaV1. 7. J Pharmacol Exp Ther 2017;362:146–60.

69. Yeo B, Tey HL. Effective treatment of notalgia paresthetica with amitriptyline. J Dermatol 2013;40:505–6.

70. Barry R, Rogers S. Brachioradial pruritus–an enigmatic entity. Clin Exp Dermatol 2004;29:637–8.

71. Mattia C, Paoletti F, Coluzzi F, et al. New antidepressants in the treatment of neuropathic pain. A review. Minerva Anestesiol 2002;68:105–14.

72. Kouwenhoven TA, van de Kerkhof PCM, Kamsteeg M, et al. Use of oral antidepressants in patients with chronic pruritus: A systematic review. J Am Acad Dermatol 2017;77(6):1068–73.e7.

73. Ständer S, Luger TA. NK-1 antagonists and itch. In: Cowan A, Yosipovitch G, editors. Pharmacology of itch. Handbook of experimental pharmacology, vol. 226. Berlin: Springer; 2015. p. 237–55.

74. Ständer S, Siepmann D, Herrgott I, et al. Targeting the neurokinin receptor 1 with aprepitant: a novel antipruritic strategy. PLoS One 2010;5:e10968.

75. Ally MS, Gamba CS, Peng DH, et al. The use of aprepitant in brachioradial pruritus. JAMA Dermatol 2013;149:627–8.

76. Keller M, Montgomery S, Ball W, et al. Lack of efficacy of the substance P (neurokinin 1 receptor) antagonist aprepitant in the treatment of major depressive disorder. Biol Psychiatry 2006;59:216–23.

77. Tajiri K, Shimizu Y. Recent advances in the management of pruritus in chronic liver diseases. World J Gastroenterol 2017;23:3418.

78. Dawn AG, Yosipovitch G. Butorphanol for treatment of intractable pruritus. J Am Acad Dermatol 2006;54:527–31.

79. Maher DP, Chen L, Mao J. Intravenous ketamine infusions for neuropathic pain management: a promising therapy in need of optimization. Anesth Analg 2017;124:661–74.

80. Watson W. Intravenous lignocaine for relief of intractable itch. Lancet 1973;301:211.

81. Wood GJ, Akiyama T, Carstens E, et al. An insatiable itch. J Pain 2009;10:792–7.

82. Weinfeld PK. Successful treatment of notalgia paresthetica with botulinum toxin type A. Arch Dermatol 2007;143:980–2.

83. Wallengren J, Bartosik J. Botulinum toxin type A for neuropathic itch. Br J Dermatol 2010;163:424–6.

84. Maari C, Marchessault P, Bissonnette R. Treatment of notalgia paresthetica with botulinum toxin A: a double-blind randomized controlled trial. J Am Acad Dermatol 2014;70:1139–41.

85. Kavanagh G, Tidman M. Botulinum A toxin and brachioradial pruritus. Br J Dermatol 2012;166:1147.

86. Ricciardo B, Kumar S, O'callaghan J, et al. Peripheral nerve field stimulation for pruritus relief in a patient with notalgia paraesthetica. Australas J Dermatol 2010;51:56–9.

87. Yamanaka D, Kawano T, Shigematsu-Locatelli M, et al. Peripheral nerve block with a high concentration of tetracaine dissolved in bupivacaine for intractable post-herpetic itch: a case report. JA Clin Rep 2016;2:43.

88. Goulden V, Toomey P, Highet A. Successful treatment of notalgia paresthetica with a paravertebral local anesthetic block. J Am Acad Dermatol 1998;38:114–6.

89. Wallengren J, Sundler F. Cutaneous field stimulation in the treatment of severe itch. Arch Dermatol 2001;137:1323–5.

90. Hettrick HH, O'Brien K, Laznick H, et al. Effect of transcutaneous electrical nerve stimulation for the management of burn pruritus: a pilot study. J Burn Care Res 2004;25:236–40.

91. Şavk E, Şavk Ö, Şendur F. Transcutaneous electrical nerve stimulation offers partial relief in notalgia paresthetica patients with a relevant spinal pathology. J Dermatol 2007;34:315–9.

92. Tey HL, Wallengren J, Yosipovitch G. Psychosomatic factors in pruritus. Clin Dermatol 2013;31:31–40.

93. Schut C, Mollanazar NK, Kupfer J, et al. Psychological interventions in the treatment of chronic itch. Acta Derm Venereol 2016;96:157–63.

94. Wilkinson DS, Knox PL, Chatman JE, et al. The clinical effectiveness of healing touch. J Altern Complement Med 2002;8:33–47.

95. Danhauer SC, Tooze JA, Holder P, et al. Healing touch as a supportive intervention for adult acute leukemia patients: a pilot investigation of effects on distress and symptoms. J Soc Integr Oncol 2008;6:89.

96. Kemper KJ, Fletcher NB, Hamilton CA, et al. Impact of healing touch on pediatric oncology outpatients: pilot study. J Soc Integr Oncol 2009;7:12.

97. Fleischer AB, Meade TJ, Fleischer AB. Notalgia paresthetica: successful treatment with exercises. Acta Derm Venereol 2011;91:356–7.

Female Genital Itch

Jessica A. Savas, MD[a], Rita O. Pichardo, MD[b],*

KEYWORDS

- Vulvar pruritus • Vulvar itch • Anogenital pruritus • Vulvar dermatoses • Lichen simplex chronicus
- Atopic dermatitis • Lichen sclerosus • Lichen planus

KEY POINTS

- Female genital itch is a common presenting symptom of numerous conditions and thus requires a systematic approach to establish the correct diagnosis.
- Therapy should be initiated in a timely manner to avoid the prolongation of suffering and to prevent complications that may result in disfigurement and/or dysfunction.
- Long-term follow-up and a multidisciplinary approach are often required in this patient population.

INTRODUCTION

Vulvar pruritus is a common complaint among young girls and women presenting to primary care physicians, gynecologists, and dermatologists. Although the true prevalence of vulvar dermatoses is largely unknown, in one vulvar specialty clinic, pruritus of the anogenital region, was found to be the most common presenting symptom, reported by 70% of all male and female patients seen.[1,2] The potential causes of vulvar itch are vast and, more often than not, multifactorial. Although the etiopathogenesis of itch remains poorly understood, the mechanisms underlying vulvar itch are even less so. Vulvar pruritus is often complicated by several factors that are unique to the female anogenital anatomy. Among these factors, the complex innervation of genital skin, the presence of both stratified squamous and modified mucosal epithelia, as well as the introduction of various irritants via a direct connection to the urinary, reproductive, and digestive tracts feature most prominently.

Although pruritus in general has a profoundly negative impact on quality of life because of disruption in work and sleep, female genital itch further interferes with intimacy and sexual function, making it exceptionally distressing. Moreover, the great psychosocial stress caused by vulvar pruritus secondary to the sensitive nature of vulvar disease as well as the pervasive desire to scratch (a socially unacceptable public behavior) cannot be overstated.

Although vulvar pathologic condition may be broadly classified into inflammatory, environmental, neoplastic, and infectious causes, the primary focus of this article centers on the diagnosis and management of inflammatory vulvar dermatoses presenting with pruritus. The authors comment briefly on the more common infectious and neoplastic dermatoses as they pertain to potential differential diagnoses and also speak to their ability to coexist with or develop as a consequence of other primary inflammatory dermatoses.

General Vulvar History

The initial encounter with a patient presenting with a primary complaint of genital itch should include a detailed history guided by the intent of differentiating primary and secondary causes of pruritus. Symptom duration, severity, and aggravating and alleviating factors should be addressed first. Acute

Disclosure: The authors have nothing to disclose.
[a] Department of Dermatology, Wake Forest University School of Medicine, Winston-Salem, NC, USA;
[b] Department of Dermatology, Wake Forest University School of Medicine, 4618 Country Club Road, Winston-Salem, NC 27104, USA
* Corresponding author.
E-mail address: rpichard@wakehealth.edu

Dermatol Clin 36 (2018) 225–243
https://doi.org/10.1016/j.det.2018.02.006

onset of pruritus is often indicative of an infectious disease, although irritant or allergic contact dermatitis (ACD) may present acutely as well. Chronic pruritus, or itch lasting more than 6 weeks, is suggestive of an inflammatory, neoplastic, or hormone-mediated process.

Inquiry into secondary hygiene practices, including those that may have been implemented to alleviate the pruritus, associated odors, or presumed infection, is imperative. This will often reveal sources of external irritation, such as excessive washing, douching, and the application of feminine hygiene products that may be exacerbating or perpetuating the underlying process. Information regarding bowel and bladder control is also critical to obtain as incontinence of urine or feces as well as products used to manage these conditions, such as panty liners, Depends, and premoistened or premedicated wipes, are additional sources of irritants and allergens.

A thorough past dermatologic history should be gathered because this may reveal a known history of a relevant primary dermatosis affecting other cutaneous or mucosal sites, such as psoriasis, eczema, or lichen planus (LP). A reproductive history, including a history of urogenital malignancies, should be obtained. Clarification of menstrual or menopausal status is often helpful because many women may come with a diagnosis of atrophic vaginitis and may or may not be on estrogen therapy. Last, inquiry into whether sexual partners or other members of the household are experiencing similar symptoms may be useful because this may suggest infection or infestation.

Developing a questionnaire may be the most efficient way to collect all of the pertinent historical data. Patients can complete this before their evaluation so it can be referenced during the initial patient visit.

INFLAMMATORY
Atopic Dermatitis

Atopic dermatitis (AD) is a chronic, common noninfectious cause of vulvar itch that is often underdiagnosed by nondermatologists.[3]

Skin barrier dysfunction in vulvar skin is compounded by numerous other local factors, such as sweat, urine and/or feces, the use of irritating and/or allergenic products, hygiene practices, and certain lifestyle choices, such as repetitive friction from exercise and the use of tight-fitting clothing.

Diagnosis
Severe pruritus is the most common symptom of eczema and may be most pronounced at night. On physical examination, there is a broad spectrum of clinical presentation from poorly demarcated erythematous edematous plaques with vesicles (acute AD), erythematous patches, and plaques (subacute AD), to hyperpigmented lichenified plaques (chronic AD/lichen simplex chronicus [LSC]).

Lichen Simplex Chronicus

LSC is a descriptive term used in the setting of primary, localized, chronic scratching and rubbing of the vulva with no implication toward a specific cause.[4]

Although the actual cause of primary vulvar pruritus and the subsequent development of LSC remain unknown, several patients are ultimately identified as atopic, with either a personal or a family history of allergic rhinitis, hayfever, and/or asthma. It is important to note that LSC can and often will develop as a consequence of other pruritic inflammatory dermatoses of the vulva, namely irritant or ACD and lichen sclerosus (LS).

Regardless of the inciting incident, when itching prompts scratching or rubbing behavior, cutaneous nerve endings are further stimulated, triggering a stronger sensation of itch and thus leading to the "itch-scratch cycle" that is invariably identified in all cases of LSC.

Patients presenting with LSC will often report intermittent or incessant itch that is relieved, albeit temporarily, by scratching or rubbing behaviors. Identifying the presence of nighttime scratching is imperative when approaching treatment.

Environmental factors, such as excessive sweating or friction related to body habitus, exercise or tight-fitting clothing, the use of menstrual or incontinence pads, and the application of over-the-counter medications or other home remedies, may also contribute to perpetuating the itch-scratch cycle and should be addressed.

The importance of psychological factors cannot be overemphasized. Although many patients will not voluntarily offer that they are depressed or anxious, many can identify that their itching and subsequent scratching is exacerbated by stress.

On physical examination, LSC is characterized by ill-defined, erythematous, xerotic plaques with increased skin markings, or lichenification, and a variable degree of overlying scale. The most common site of involvement is the labia majora with occasional extension to the labia minora, mons pubis, or upper medial thighs (Fig. 1). The vagina is always spared.[5–8] Secondary excoriations are commonly encountered and can be differentiated from erosions or ulcers by their angulated appearance. Overlying serous and heme-crusting may be present and, depending on the degree, may indicate

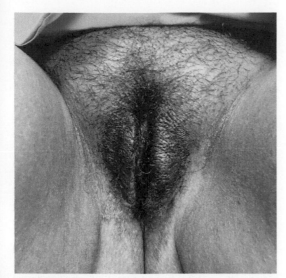

Fig. 1. Bilateral involvement of the labia majora with hyperpigmented lichenified plaques.

secondary infection. In longstanding lesions, melanocyte activation will lead to hyperpigmentation of the involved area and in severe or chronic cases prurigo nodule formation may occur.

A proper speculum examination and wet mount evaluation are important to rule out a concomitant vaginitis because this can frequently lead to chronic pruritus eventuating in the development of LSC.

Once the diagnosis of LSC has been established, the physician must determine whether the process is primary or secondary to an underlying disorder.

Although LSC is primarily a clinical diagnosis, if there is still question after initial treatment attempts or there remains a concern about an underlying inflammatory or neoplastic process, skin biopsy may be necessary.

Lichen Sclerosus et Atrophicus

Lichen sclerosus et atrophicus, or simply, lichen sclerosus, is a relatively common inflammatory disorder primarily affecting genital skin, and less frequently, extragenital skin. It may occur in men or women, but there appears to be a female preponderance. LS may affect women of all ages; however, peak incidence appears to be in postmenopausal women in the fifth and sixth decade. Young girls represent a minority of the patients presenting with LS.

The pathogenesis of LS has yet to be fully elucidated but is likely multifactorial with a role for both genetic and environmental factors.

Although the true prevalence of LS is unknown, one survey discovered that 1.7% of patients

presenting to a general gynecology practice were found to have LS.[9] A vulvar specialty clinic in England reported LS to be the most common disease evaluated and treated in their practice with 39% of their patients carrying the diagnosis.[10]

The vast majority of patients present because of severe, persistent vulvar pruritus, although rarely, LS may be asymptomatic. If pruritus leads to scratching, skin tears and erosions may develop because the skin is characteristically atrophic and fragile.

On genital examination, early lesions may be subtle, demonstrating only a thin, sharply demarcated rim of erythema that may or may not be slightly raised. Classically, well-marginated, hypopigmented, or white plaques primarily involving the vulva, perineum, and perianal skin are seen, producing the distinctive "figure-of-8" pattern. Additional findings that suggest a diagnosis of LS include the characteristic textural changes that accompany the white plaques. Wrinkling of the skin, likened to wet tissue paper, is the pathognomonic finding; however, smooth, shiny, white plaques and hyperkeratosis are other common features. Because of the severe pruritus, rubbing or scratching may result in a superimposed LSC with prominent epidermal thickening and lichenification. In approximately 75% of patients, the entire genital area is involved (vulva, perineum, and perianal).[11] The keratinized, hair-bearing labia majora is generally spared, and true vaginal involvement is uncommon.[12–16]

As lesions progress, hypopigmentation, sclerosis, and atrophy become more prominent and are often complicated by erosions, fissures and petechiae, or frank purpura (**Figs. 2** and **3**). In longstanding lesions, resorption of the clitoral hood, and fusion of the labia minora to the labia majora may occur, thus obscuring normal vaginal anatomy and leading to functional impairment. This can eventuate into complete loss of the labia minora and/or stenosis of the vaginal introitus, making intercourse impossible. Scarring risk appears to correlate directly with duration of disease and degree of hyperkeratosis.[11]

It is important to note that lesions of LS are sometimes associated with hyperpigmentation that can vary from ill-defined and patchy to strikingly irregular, dark brown or heterogeneously pigmented macules and patches resembling genital lentigines or atypical nevi.

Lichen Planus

LP is a T cell–mediated chronic inflammatory mucocutaneous disorder that may involve the skin, oral, or genital mucosa. There are numerous

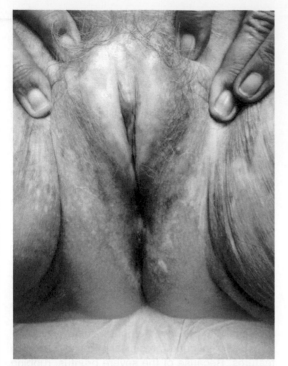

Fig. 2. Atrophy and hypopigmentation involving the labia and perineum with resorption of the labia minora.

clinical variants of LP with 3 subtypes most commonly affecting genital skin. These include papulosquamous, hypertrophic, and erosive with erosive being the most common subtype affecting the vulvovaginal area. Although the true incidence

of vulvar LP remains unknown, recent studies suggest that genital involvement occurs in 25% to 57% of women with oral LP.[17,18] LP is primarily a disease of women between the ages of 40 and 60, although there have been cases reported in young girls.

Patients with vulvovaginal LP will often present with complaints of itching, burning, and/or dyspareunia; however, up to 40% may be symptom free.[18]

Erosive lesions are seen in half of patients with genital involvement. Furthermore, up to two-thirds will display atrophy, most commonly in the context of erosions, and about a quarter present with plaques. Papular and reticular lesions are seen less frequently.[18]

On physical examination, erosive vulvovaginal LP presents with well-demarcated pink to red erosions with a white, hyperkeratotic linear border or reticulate plaque and is most commonly seen at the vaginal introitus (90%) followed by the vagina (20%–38%), vulva (37%), and perianal skin (8%)[19,20] (**Fig. 4**).

Similar to LS, longstanding, untreated disease is often complicated by scarring and atrophy due to resorption of normal anatomic landmarks. Agglutination of the clitoris is common as is the development of adhesions and midline fusion of

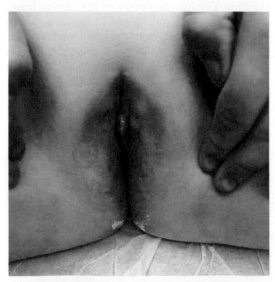

Fig. 3. Hypopigmentation and petechial macules in a young girl presenting with LS.

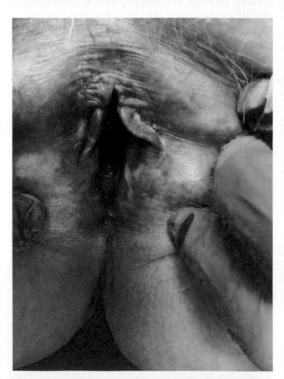

Fig. 4. Erythematous erosions with hyperkeratotic white borders involving the vaginal introitus.

the vestibule resulting in a narrowed vaginal introitus (**Fig. 5**).

Genital erosive LP may be difficult to distinguish from LS, mucous membrane pemphigoid, pemphigus vulgaris, blistering drug eruptions, and plasma cell vulvitis (PCV).

Histologically, LP classically demonstrates a dense bandlike lymphocytic infiltrate with interface changes often obscuring the dermoepidermal junction. The International Society for the Study of Vulvovaginal Disease published criteria for the diagnosis of vulvar LP based on both clinical and histologic findings (**Table 1**).[21]

Psoriasis

According to a multicenter observational study of 354 adult psoriasis patients, 38% noted current genital involvement, whereas 63% reported having experienced genital involvement at some point in their disease course.[22–27]

Women with psoriasis affecting the vulva often present primarily with a complaint of pruritus. They may also report associated pain, burning, and dyspareunia. Whether predominantly concerned about pruritus or appearance, genital psoriasis causes great mental angst and appears to be the most distressing site of involvement among patients with psoriasis.[22] Patients may or may not have a known history of psoriasis on extensor skin or in other intertriginous sites. Inverse psoriasis is a well-described clinical variant and is typified by involvement of intertriginous sites, including the axillae, inframammary skin, inguinal creases, and anogenital skin.

Given the inherent differences in vulvar skin compared with extensor skin, vulvar psoriasis often lacks the typical silvery scale seen in classic psoriatic plaques. Psoriasis of the vulva is often characterized by well-demarcated, shiny, or glazed-appearing brightly erythematous patches and plaques. Plaques of vulvar psoriasis preferentially involve hair-bearing sites, with the most common site affected being the labia majora (**Fig. 6**).[22] Further examination of the anogenital region may reveal similar involvement of the intergluteal cleft. In addition, more classic psoriasiform plaques with micaceous scale can be observed on the mons pubis.

Other papulosquamous dermatoses such as seborrheic dermatitis can clinically mimic genital psoriasis. Seborrheic dermatitis affecting the vulva may share several overlapping features with vulvar psoriasis, including the primary complaint of itch. In these cases, the term "sebopsoriasis" may be most appropriate.

Tinea cruris is often considered because of the scaling associated with psoriasis. Superficial dermatophytosis can be distinguished by a scaly, advancing border with or without pustule formation and extension onto the buttocks/medial thigh. The presence of tinea pedis or tinea unguium as well as examination of scale with potassium hydroxide (KOH) would make the distinction clear.

Erythrasma often presents with pruritic, erythematous, scaly patches and plaques involving the skin folds and may be confused with inverse psoriasis. Delineation is easily made by coral red fluorescence with Wood's lamp and a negative KOH preparation.

Plasma Cell Vulvitis

PCV, Zoon vulvitis, vulvitis circumscripta plasmacellularis, and idiopathic lymphoplasmacellular mucositis-dermatitis are interchangeable terms referring to a benign, chronic, inflammatory dermatosis of the vulva. PCV appears to be a distinct entity both clinically and histopathologically; however, the cause remains unknown.[28] Clinically, lesions are solitary, deeply erythematous, shiny plaques mostly involving the vestibule, labia minora, and rarely, the clitoris. Patients primarily complain of pruritus, burning, and soreness.[29,30] On histology, the epidermis is atrophic and spongiotic with a bandlike dermal infiltrate

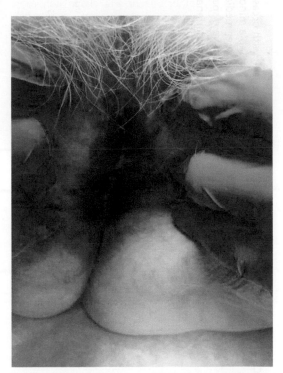

Fig. 5. Midline fusion in a patient with longstanding, untreated erosive LP.

Table 1
Inflammatory causes of female genital itch

Diagnosis	Clinical Features	Location	Cause	Histopathology/Diagnostic Findings
AD	Poorly demarcated erythematous edematous plaques with vesicles Erythematous patches or plaques Lichenified plaques	Mons pubis, labia majora perineal skin with possible extension to groin areas and upper medial thighs	Interaction between genetic, immune, and environmental factors	Early Spongiosis, intraepidermal edema with microvesiculation or macrovesiculation and inflammatory infiltrates composed of lymphocytes, eosinophils, and mast cells As the lesion progresses, spongiosis persists but vesiculation disappear Late Acanthosis
LSC	Ill-defined, erythematous to hyperpigmented, lichenified plaques	Labia majora (MC) with occasional extension to the labia minora, mons pubis, or upper medial thighs. Vagina is always spared	Several inciting factors that ultimately result in the itch-scratch cycle	Psoriasiform hyperplasia, compact orthokeratosis, hypergranulosis, and dermal fibrosis
LS	Well-demarcated white plaques in a "figure-of-8" pattern; petechiae and erosions variable	Vulva, perineum, and perianal skin Spares other mucosal sites Extragenital lesions rare	Unknown, autoimmune, genetic, infectious, traumatic	Early Superficial dermal edema with vacuolar degeneration at the DEJ and a lichenoid infiltrate Late Pale, homogenized papillary dermis, dilated vessels and hemorrhage, hyperkeratosis variable
LP	Well-demarcated pink to red erosions with a white, hyperkeratotic linear border or reticulate plaque	Vaginal introitus > vagina, vulva, and perianal skin May have oral or cutaneous involvement	Unknown, T cell–mediated, autoinflammatory	Interface dermatitis with dense bandlike lymphocytic infiltrate often obscuring the DEJ, erosive lesions may be nonspecific

Psoriasis	Erythematous, sharply marginated plaques with a glazed appearance	Most commonly symmetric involvement of the labia majora. Also the mons, inguinal creases, and perianal/presacral skin. Other intertriginous sites may be involved	Multifactorial, environmental genetic and immune factors	Regular acanthosis, parakeratosis containing neutrophils and dilated vessels in the papillary dermis; spongiosis is a classic feature of vulvar lesions
Seborrheic dermatitis	Erythematous patches and plaques with overlying greasy scale	Areas rich in sebaceous glands. Classic extragenital involvement	Genetic, possible immune response to *Malasezzia furfur*	Psoriasiform, spongiotic dermatitis with superficial perivascular and perifollicular lymphocytic infiltrate, neutrophilic scale at shoulder of follicular ostium
PCV	Solitary, deeply erythematous, shiny plaques	Vestibule, labia minora, and rarely the clitoris	Unknown, traumatic, infectious, and autoimmune causes proposed	Atrophic and spongiotic epidermis with a bandlike dermal infiltrate composed primarily of plasma cells (>50). Loss of the granular layer and stratum corneum as well as proliferation of blood vessels with red blood cell extravasation are frequently observed
Mucous membrane pemphigoid	Tense blisters and erosions that heal with scarring; desquamative vaginal discharge	Genital and anal mucosae, will likely have ocular and/or oral mucosal involvement	Autoimmune, circulating autoantibodies against basement membrane proteins	H&E (lesional) Subepidermal vesiculation with variable inflammation and few eosinophils. DIF (perilesional) Linear deposition of IgG and C3 along the DEJ
Pemphigus vulgaris	Flaccid bullae or painful erosions with irregular, ill-defined border	Vaginal mucosa; essentially all patients will have oral involvement, some with cutaneous lesions	Autoimmune, circulating autoantibodies against desmoglein 1 or 3 (MC)	H&E (lesional) Suprabasilar split giving intact basal keratinocytes a "tombstone row" appearance. Tracking down hair follicles, superficial lymphocytic infiltrate, few eosinophils. DIF (perilesional) Intercelluluar deposition of IgG and C3 between keratinocytes in lower epidermis in a "netlike" pattern

Abbreviations: DEJ, dermoepidermal junction; H&E, hematoxylin and eosin; IgG, immunoglobulin; MC, most common.

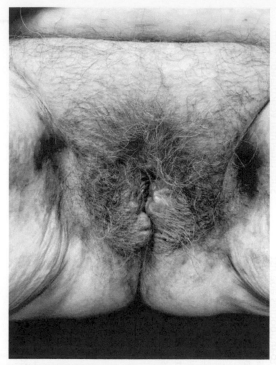

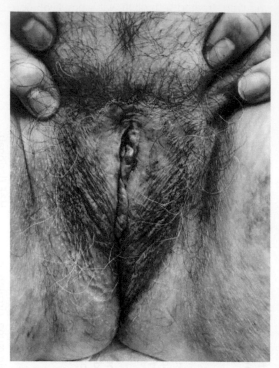

Fig. 6. Erythematous plaques involving the labia majora. Note involvement of the inguinal creases bilaterally as well as the mons pubis.

Fig. 7. Ill-defined erythema and edema of the external genitalia.

composed primarily of plasma cells, often comprising greater than 50% of the inflammatory infiltrate (see **Table 1**).

ENVIRONMENTAL
Irritant Contact Dermatitis

Irritant contact dermatitis (ICD) in the genital area is common in children and adults; the main symptoms are a burning sensation and pruritus. It may develop rapidly, within minutes to hours. Common irritant products include wipes, diapers, pads, and the use of washcloths, harsh soaps, and talcum powder.[31,32] Clinically, ICD is characterized by a well-demarcated erythematous vesicular plaque or a scaly patch corresponding to the area of contact (**Fig. 7**).[3] Special attention should be paid to patients with urinary or fecal incontinence, which often complicates these cases.

Allergic Contact Dermatitis

ACD, in contrast to ICD, takes longer to develop, usually 24 to 48 hours. The list of potential allergens is long and has been previously reviewed.[33,34] Not surprisingly, neomycin sulfate is the most common antibiotic allergen, a common product used by women in the genital area.[35–37]

In the evaluation of a patient with possible ACD, a complete clinical history, which includes a list of all over-the-counter and prescription products used by the patient, is paramount. A high level of suspicion and access to appropriate patch testing are crucial (**Table 2**).

NEOPLASTIC

Albeit rare, genital pruritus may herald the presence of a vulvar neoplasm and should be considered in the differential, especially when a presumed inflammatory process does not respond to first-line treatments.

Vulvar Intraepithelial Neoplasia and Vulvar Squamous Cell Carcinoma

Bowen disease, Bowenoid papulosis, and carcinoma in situ were all once interchangeable terms that are now more correctly referred to together as vulvar intraepithelial neoplasia (VIN). The incidence of VIN is on the increase, and the most common presentation is that of well-demarcated flat-topped papules or plaques that may be erythematous or hyperpigmented. Lesions may be solitary or multifocal and can cause itching and display varying degrees of scale, crust, and erosion.

Table 2
Environmental causes of female genital itch

Diagnosis	Clinical Features	Cause	Diagnosis
ICD	Well-demarcated erythematous vesicular plaque or a scaly patch corresponding to the area of contact. Difficult to distinguish based on clinical features	Any irritant, most commonly: wipes, wash cloths, panty liners, sanitary napkins, pads	Biopsy is most useful on acute lesions: spongiosis, mixed inflammatory dermal infiltrate composed of lymphocytes, histiocytes, and eosinophils. Vesiculation is present in severe reactions
ACD		Most common allergens: neomycin, Balsam of Peru, fragrance mix, nickel sulfate, terconazole, clotrimazole, benzoic acid, benzocaine, conjugate estrogen, sodium lauryl sulfate	Patch test is the gold standard for the diagnosis of ACD

Other malignant neoplasms that may cause pruritus in the genital area are verrucous carcinoma and extramammary Paget of the vulva, both rare neoplastic processes affecting primarily postmenopausal women. Two-thirds of patients endorse moderate to severe pruritus.[38–52] Given the rarity of these conditions and nonspecific clinical appearance, the diagnosis is often delayed, and patients are instead treated for an eczematous process, psoriasis, or superficial fungal infection.

Benign neoplasms such as syringomas may also result in vulvar pruritus in the absence of other findings (**Table 3**).

NEUROPATHIC

Neuropathic pruritus appears to be a consequence of nerve fiber damage affecting cutaneous nerves or larger-caliber neurons of the peripheral and central nervous system. More commonly encountered causes of neuropathic pruritus in the genital area include postherpetic neuralgia, diabetic neuropathy, lumbosacral arthritis, and spinal injuries or surgeries.

Although obtaining a history of shingles in the involved area as well as previous spinal injuries or surgeries is rather straightforward, the effects of diabetic neuropathy and lumbosacral arthritis may not be as readily apparent. Imaging studies may be useful in identifying lumbosacral nerve or nerve root compression. If radiculopathy is diagnosed, there have been reports of improvement in symptoms with paravertebral injection of triamcinolone mixed with lidocaine.[53]

INFECTIONS AND INFESTATIONS

Acute onset pruritus and the presence of itch in bed partners often suggest an infectious cause or infestation (**Table 4**).

Table 3
Neoplastic causes of female genital itch

Diagnosis	Clinical Features	Cause
VIN/squamous cell carcinoma	Solitary or multifocal, well-demarcated flat-topped, erythematous, or hyperpigmented papules or plaques	HPV-associated (-6, -18, -33, -35, and -52) LS and LP associated: possible role for p53/CDKN2a mutations
Verrucous carcinoma	Exophytic mass and complaint of associated pruritus or pain	Possible role for HPV
Extramammary Paget	Well-demarcated, erythematous plaque with overlying scale crust, erosion, or ulceration	Unknown
Syringoma	Skin-colored, asymptomatic, or pruritic papules involving the labia majora	Unknown, benign eccrine neoplasm

Abbreviation: HPV, human papillomavirus.

HORMONAL

Estrogen receptors have been identified on keratinocytes; therefore, temporal hormonal changes contribute greatly to age-related differences in the characteristics of vulvar epithelium with resultant effects on vaginal pH and microflora composition.[54] These changes are reflected in the most common causes of genital itch across age groups with atopic and irritant dermatitis, psoriasis, and LS being the most common in prepubertal girls, whereas vulvovaginal candidiasis (VVC), ACD/ICD, LSC, psoriasis, and LS represent the most common diagnoses in women of reproductive age. Last, atrophic vulvovaginitis, LS, ICD, and squamous cell carcinoma account for most cases of genital itch in postmenopausal women.[55]

Vulvovaginal atrophic vaginitis will affect most postmenopausal women to some extent with almost half of the women developing at least one debilitating symptom, commonly pruritus.[56] The vulvovaginal epithelium appears pale and shiny with loss of rugae and occasionally petechiae. Given that several of the inflammatory, environmental, and neoplastic causes of genital itch occur primarily in postmenopausal women, it is important to assume some contribution of atrophic vaginitis to ongoing pruritus, and this should be addressed. Topical estrogen therapy is the mainstay of treatment of atrophic vaginitis, and 1 to 2 weeks of application can reverse atrophy to premenopausal levels.[57]

MANAGEMENT
General Vulvar Care

A thorough discussion of general vulvar care is mandatory during an initial evaluation, and periodic reminders are often necessary throughout the follow-up and maintenance periods. First and foremost, any and all potential irritants and/or allergens should be identified and discontinued. Washing of anogenital skin should be done with water and hands only. If desired, the use of a gentle, fragrance-free, dye-free soap is acceptable. Avoidance of harsh exfoliating loofahs or washcloths should be emphasized. The use of any vaginal cleansing products, including soaps, foams, sprays, wipes, douches, as well as any antibacterial creams or ointments, should be discontinued. If an emollient is desired, plain white petrolatum ointment or similar commercial preparations may be considered and can be applied multiple times daily for dryness, itch, or irritation as well as after topical corticosteroid (TCS) application.

Modifying vulvar hygiene practices may be more difficult in patients who suffer from incontinence. These patients strongly desire some form of premoistened wipe for cleanliness and comfort in situations away from the home. If necessary, every effort should be made to find an allergen-free brand, and use should be limited to emergencies only.

Similarly, menstruating women and those with incontinence issues may also insist on some form of panty liner, sanitary napkin, or tampon. If unavoidable, consider reusable cloth pads or an allergen-free disposable brand and again minimize use as much as possible.

Last, patients should be advised to avoid tight-fitting clothing and reduce behaviors or stimuli that result in excessive friction or sweating.

Medications

Regardless of the cause of female genital itch or the stage at which it presents, treatment of both primary and secondary causes of vulvar pruritus is managed similarly, at least initially, and it is therefore appropriate to initiate antipruritic therapy even before establishing a definitive diagnosis so as not to prolong suffering. Because most of the conditions discussed occur in postmenopausal women, it is important to consider the addition of a topical or intravaginal estrogen to mitigate discomfort and scar formation if a concomitant atrophic vaginitis is appreciated on speculum examination.

Topicals
Topical medications are first-line therapy for most inflammatory vulvar dermatoses. As with all prescribed treatments, patient education is the key. A detailed discussion of the amount, frequency, and where to apply the medication is paramount to compliance and outcomes. A handheld mirror or clinical photographs can be used to demonstrate where medication should be applied. In general, a small or pea-sized amount of ointment per application is generally sufficient.

Corticosteroids Super-potent and high-potency (class I or II) TCSs are first line for most causes of vulvar pruritus. Ointments are the preferred vehicle, and common choices include clobetasol propionate (0.05%), halobetasol propionate, betamethasone dipropionate (0.05%) in an augmented vehicle and fluocinonide (0.05%). With severe disease or during acute flares, application twice daily is recommended. For moderate to mild disease at presentation, once daily application is appropriate.

Treatment outcomes for the inflammatory dermatoses are fairly consistent, and regardless of

Table 4
Infections and infestations causing female genital itch

	Diagnosis	Causative Agent	Clinical Features	Diagnostic Features	Treatment
Infections	VVC	*Candida albicans* (>90%) Other *Candida* species, specifically *Candida glabrata* (<10%)	Erythema, edema, and a white discharge	Wet preparation with visualization of fungal elements, culture, or polymerase chain reaction (PCR). Normal vaginal pH	Intravaginal or systemic antifungal azoles
	Perianal streptococcal infection	Group A β-hemolytic streptococcus	Pruritic, erythematous patches and plaques involving the perianal area but may extend to the vulva and perineum	Bacterial cultures	Penicillin, amoxicillin, cephalexin (if PCN allergic)
	Trichomonas	*Trichomonas vaginalis*	Erythema and edema of the mucous membranes, in particular the vestibule with grossly purulent vaginal discharge	Wet mount with pathognomonic mobile flagellate organisms or PCR	Oral azoles
	Bacterial vaginitis	GBS, alpha-hemolytic streptococcus, *Staphylococcal aureus*, and *Escherichia coli*	Vestibular erythema and edema and purulent vaginal secretions	Microscopic examination showing increased neutrophils, parabasal cells, and absent lactobacilli, culture, complete response to antibiotic therapy	Oral antibiotic
	Erythrasma	*Corynebacterium minutissimum*	Well-demarcated pink, scaly plaques on the proximal medial thighs, other intertriginous sites may be involved	Coral red fluorescence with Wood's lamp, negative KOH	Oral or topical erythromycin, topical clindamycin
	Dermatophytosis	*Tricophyton rubrum* (MC), *Tricophyton mentagrophytes*, or *Epidermophyton floccosum*	Well-demarcated, scaling, annular red plaques with a raised advancing edge; primarily involve the inguinal creases, keratinized vulvar skin and may extend onto the proximal medial thighs	Fungal elements on KOH, culture, or response to therapy	Topical imidazoles or allylamines. If involvement of the hair follicles, oral griseofulvin or oral terbinafine is required for 2–4 wk

(continued on next page)

Table 4
(continued)

	Diagnosis	Clinical Features	Causative Agent	Diagnostic Features	Treatment
Infestations	Pediculosis pubis	Perifollicular erythema, excoriations, crab lice clinging to the base of hairs	*Pthirus pubis*	Visualization of the lice or nits adherent to hair shafts	Topical insecticides, most commonly permethrin, treat partners
	Scabies	Small erythematous papules with variable degree of excoriation	*Sarcoptes scabiei var hominis*	Visualization of the mite or scybala on mineral oil preparation of skin scrapings	Topical permethrin cream or oral ivermectin; treatment of linens and clothes with high heat
	Enterobiasis	Primarily perianal erythema and pruritus but can cause vulvovaginitis	*Enterobius vermicularis*	Visualization of eggs using adhesive cellophane tape pressed against perianal skin	Mebendazole Albendazole Pyrantel pamoate

Data from Edwards L. Vaginitis. In: Black M, Ambros-Rudolph C, Lidbby E, et al, editors. Obstetric and gynecologic dermatology. 3rd edition. China: Elsevier Limited; 2008. p. 301–16.

cause, should include subjective relief of associated symptoms and induction and maintenance of normal skin color and texture. Although patients may be tempted to become lax with application once pruritus or pain has been relieved, it is important to encourage continued application until both endpoints have been achieved. This is particularly important in LS and erosive LP to reduce the risk of scarring and oncogenesis.[11]

Once disease control is achieved, tapering to daily, every other day, or 3 times weekly application is sufficient. Tapering may also include deescalating the potency of the topical used. Transitioning to a class III or IV steroid such as triamcinolone acetonide (0.1% ointment) to be used 3 times weekly is a suitable maintenance regimen. Patients can always resume more frequent application or return to more potent topical preparations for acute flares.

TCSs are generally well tolerated and safe with little to no risk of significant systemic absorption. Use of topical or intravaginal corticosteroids alone or in combination with estrogen preparations may increase risk for VVC. An anticandidal regimen is often required until disease control is achieved and topical medications can be tapered.

Calcineurin inhibitors Topical calcineurin inhibitors (TCI) are nonsteroidal anti-inflammatory preparations that have recently gained popularity because of a lack of the attendant side effects commonly associated with TCS use, such as atrophy and striae. The 2 products currently available are tacrolimus (0.03% and 0.1% ointment) and pimecrolimus (1% cream).

Although the side-effect profile may be more appealing, TCIs have limited efficacy in conditions such as LSC because they are comparable to a low- or mid-potency corticosteroid. They may be an option for patients who have failed TCS or have a contraindication to their use. They are also not an ideal choice for erosive conditions because patients frequently report a stinging or burning sensation upon application. Furthermore, these products are often cost prohibitive for patients.

Mention must be made of the "black-box" warning for malignancy risk included on all TCIs as mandated by the US Food and Drug Administration (FDA). This warning causes apprehension with long-term use in conditions such as LS and LP because they already carry an inherent risk for malignant transformation.[58]

In an effort to bypass the above limitations of the TCIs, these authors have found benefit from dissolving a tacrolimus capsule in 0.5 L of water, soaking a gauze pad in the solution, and applying this to the affected area. This can be repeated multiple times daily, and the solution can be used for up to a week if stored in the refrigerator. Tacrolimus capsules are affordable, and there is no burning or stinging with application of the prepared solution. This is a helpful adjunct to treatment in erosive vulvar diseases but rarely results in complete remission when used as monotherapy.

Anesthetics Temporary and transient relief may be obtained by the use of topical anesthetic preparations. Specifically, pramoxine (1% cream) and lidocaine (2% jelly), which both have a low sensitizing potential, are efficacious and safe when used in small amounts to a localized area.[59] These agents should not be used as monotherapy nor should they be used long term.

Intralesional

When vulvar pruritus proves to be resistant to topical therapies or if only a partial response is achieved, intralesional injection of triamcinolone acetonide may be considered for the management of inflammatory vulvar dermatoses. Up to 6 months of relief has been accomplished with local subcutaneous injection of 1.5 to 2 mL of 10 mg/mL triamcinolone acetonide with minimal discomfort and no untoward adverse effects.[60–62]

Systemic therapies

Antihistamines Antihistamines are a helpful adjunct to relieve pruritus caused by several of the causes discussed and are particularly helpful in addressing nighttime itch. Nighttime itch not only disrupts sleep but also perpetuates the itch-scratch cycle and may reverse any progress made with other therapeutic interventions. Although their antipruritic effects through histamine blockade actually appear to contribute very little to their efficacy, it is the sedative effects of antihistamines that ultimately decrease the likelihood of nighttime scratching. Commonly used sedating antihistamines include hydroxyzine (10–25 mg) and cyproheptadine (4–8 mg).[59] Dosing should occur 1 to 2 hours before bed and judiciously increased until nighttime itching stops or intolerance, usually oversedation or anticholinergic effects, develops.

Often, addressing the nighttime itch will have mitigating effects on daytime itch, and daytime dosing is not required. In situations wherein breakthrough itching occurs during the night or persists into the day, nighttime doses can be increased as tolerated.

Corticosteroids Systemic corticosteroids are extremely effective in achieving rapid disease control and are used frequently in inflammatory vulvar dermatoses for immediate relief of pruritus and as a bridging therapy to other systemic treatments. Prednisone and other oral preparations should never be considered a long-term therapy because of the unacceptable adverse effects associated with chronic use.

Neuropathic/psychiatric medications Although the neurophysiology of itch is beyond the scope of this article, it is well established that there is a complex and intimate relationship between the nervous system, psyche, and the perception of pruritus. Psychological factors, stress, and social support can greatly influence a patient's experience of pruritus. Symptoms of depression and anxiety are commonly reported in patients suffering from chronic pruritus, and whether they are contributory or consequential, this neuropathic component often requires attention.

Anticonvulsants
Gabapentin and pregabalin are structural analogues of the neurotransmitter γ-aminobutyric acid used primarily to treat neuropathic pain. The evidence supporting its use in vulvar pruritus is largely anecdotal.

Antidepressants
Doxepin is a tricyclic antidepressant (TCA) with extremely high affinity for both H_1 and H_2 histamine receptors, making it an excellent option for patients with nighttime pruritus refractory to hydroxyzine. Amitriptyline, like doxepin, is a TCA that may be used to manage pruritus. Amitriptyline may be preferred over doxepin when symptoms of pain and burning are present in addition to pruritus. The dosing and safety profile are similar to that of doxepin. Topical formulations containing amitriptyline compounded with ketamine have also been used to achieve substantial relief of localized pain and pruritus.[63,64]

The selective serotonin reuptake inhibitors, specifically paroxetine, have shown a modest benefit in the treatment of pruritus from various causes and may have a role in vulvar itch.[65,66]

Mirtazapine is a noradrenergic and specific serotonergic antidepressant that has been effective in relieving nighttime itch.[67]

Immune modulators
When the inflammatory causes of genital pruritus prove refractory to topical treatment and antihistamines, systemic immunotherapies may be considered. In fact, anywhere from 25% to 40% of patients with erosive LP may not respond to topical therapy, and systemic treatments are required.[20,21] Controlling the underlying inflammation often alleviates the attendant pruritus to some extent and certainly decreases the risks of scarring, deformity,

and malignant transformation. Several therapies have been used to treat erosive LP, with the most common being methotrexate, mycophenolate mofetil, and hydroxychloroquine. Although there are no currently published, randomized controlled trials comparing systemic treatments head to head, investigators are actively addressing this deficiency in the literature.[68] All of these medications require regular monitoring, and with no data comparing efficacy, physician comfort and cost of treatment tend to dictate the initial agent chosen. Similarly, the use of methotrexate, with or without a prednisone taper, has been reported to stabilize symptoms and prevent disease progression in refractory vulvar LS.[69]

In patients with psoriasis affecting the genital area, systemic immunotherapies are often warranted. Although there are no currently published reports documenting its efficacy, clinical trials investigating the interleukin-17A inhibitor ixekizumab are underway and preliminary data reported have been encouraging. Ixekizumab has shown superior efficacy compared with placebo in achievement of clear or almost clear status in 73% of treated patients as well as clinically meaningful improvement in genital itch for 60% of treated patients. Improving clinical involvement and symptoms of genital itch in these patients appears to greatly improve quality of life and sexual health[70] (**Table 5**).

Photodynamic therapy
Photodynamic therapy (PTD) is a noninvasive treatment modality that is FDA approved for the treatment of precancerous and selected cancerous lesions. Although off label, there are some data to suggest a modest benefit with PDT for vulvar LP. In a randomized controlled trial, hexyl 5-aminolevulinate hydrochloride–PDT was compared with TCS use alone and no significant difference in mean reduction of pain or pruritus in patients with erosive LP of the vulva was found. However, patients in the PDT treatment group reported using less TCS at follow-up.[71] Another study reported good response rates with the use of aminolevulinic acid (ALA)-PDT for the treatment of papulosquamous lesions of genital LP.[72–74]

More recently, the use of ALA-PDT has been investigated in patients with vulvar LS with significant improvement. Treatment-related pain, sometimes requiring sedation, and prolonged photosensitivity are the most commonly reported adverse effects.

Behavioral modification
Behavioral modification may complement pharmacologic therapy in select patients with genital itch.

Table 5
Treatment of female genital itch

Route	Class	Drug	Dosing	Indication	Adverse Effects
Topical	Corticosteroids	Clobetasol propionate (0.05% ointment) Halobetasol propionate ointment Betamethasone dipropionate (0.05% in an augmented vehicle) Fluocinonide (0.05% ointment) Triamcinolone (0.1% ointment)	Severe disease/acute flares: twice daily application Mild to moderate disease: once daily application Maintenance: 3 times weekly application	First-line therapy for AD, LSC, LS, LP, psoriasis, seborrheic dermatitis (medium to low potency), contact dermatitis	Striae, cutaneous atrophy, and steroid dermatitis, more commonly seen when inappropriately applied to adjacent, nonaffected keratinized skin and skin folds
	Calcineurin inhibitors	Tacrolimus (0.1% or 0.03% ointment) Pimecrolimus (1% cream)	Twice daily application	Option for patients who have failed TCS or have a contraindication to their use	Stinging or burning with application, black-box warning for malignancy risk
	Anesthetics	Pramoxine (1% or 2.5% cream) Lidocaine (2% jelly)	Small amounts multiple times daily as needed (ie, before intercourse or voiding)	Temporary relief, not to be used long term or as monotherapy	Irritation at site of application, systemic absorption and toxicity if used over large surface area
Intralesional	Corticosteroids	Triamcinolone acetonide	1.5–2.0 mL of 10 mg/mL solution to affected areas as needed	Partial response or refractory to TCS, severe lichenification	Localized atrophy

(continued on next page)

Table 5
(continued)

Route	Class	Drug	Dosing	Indication	Adverse Effects
Systemic	Antihistamines	Hydroxyzine	10–50 mg nightly or divided four times daily	Nighttime itch	Sedation, dry mouth
		Cyproheptadine	4–8 mg nightly		
	Corticosteroids	Prednisone	Variable taper regimens	For rapid control of acute flares and/or as a bridging therapy to other systemic treatment	Weight gain, insomnia, anxiety, glucose intolerance, edema, hypokalemia, hypertension, Cushingoid features
		Triamcinolone acetonide	Intramuscularly 80 mg		With long-term use: osteoporosis, glaucoma, cataracts, diabetes, immunosuppression
	Anticonvulsants	Gabapentin	100–3600 mg once nightly or divided 3 times daily	Adjunct when neuropathic component is suspected	Drowsiness, constipation, peripheral edema, weight gain
		Pregabalin	25–200 mg twice daily		
	Antidepressants	Doxepin	10–100 mg once nightly or divided 3 times daily	Nighttime pruritus refractory to hydroxyzine	Drowsiness, urinary retention
		Amitriptyline	25–150 mg once nightly or divided up to 3 times daily	When pruritus is accompanied by pain, burning, stinging	Anticholinergic side effects
		Paroxetine	10–40 mg once daily	Helpful if psychogenic component of pruritus is suspected	Insomnia, sexual dysfunction
		Mirtazapine	7.5–15 mg once daily	Nocturnal pruritus	Drowsiness, dry mouth, increased appetite, weight gain
	Immune modulators	Methotrexate	5–25 mg once weekly	Erosive LP or LS refractory to topicals	Pancytopenia, hepatotoxicity
		Mycophenolate mofetil	500–2000 mg daily divided twice daily		Dose-dependent gastrointestinal distress and cytopenias
		Hydroxychloroquine	200 mg twice daily		Reversible ocular effects, irreversible retinopathy, cutaneous hyperpigmentation

Data from Yosipovitch G, Bernhard JD. Clinical practice. Chronic pruritus. N Engl J Med 2013;368:1625–34.

SUMMARY

Female genital itch is a common problem and a source of significant suffering for many patients. As health care professionals, we must work to expand our knowledge and develop a level of comfort with the diagnosis and management of vulvar pruritus. These patients often require a multidisciplinary care team, including family and primary practice physicians, dermatologists, gynecologists, urologists, and on occasion, mental health providers. Early diagnosis and treatment, centered on the suppression of inflammation, can improve quality of life and minimize risk of complications and permanent dysfunction.

REFERENCES

1. Sullivan A, Staughair G, Marwood R, et al. A multidisciplinary vulva clinic: the role of genito-urinary medicine. J Eur Acad Dermatol 1999;13(1):36–40.
2. Meeuwis K, van de Kerkhof P, Massuger L, et al. Patient's experience of psoriasis in the genital area. Dermatology 2012;224(3):271–6.
3. Pichardo-Geisinger R. Atopic and contact dermatitis of the vulva. Obstet Gynecol Clin North Am 2017; 44(3):371–8.
4. Lynch PJ. Vulvar pruritus and lichen simplex chronicus. In: Black M, Ambros-Rudolph CM, Edwards L, et al, editors. Obstetric and gynecologic dermatology. 3rd edition. China: Elsevier Limited; 2008. p. 157–66.
5. Lynch P. Lichen simplex chronicus (atopic/neurodermatitis) of the anogenital region. Dermatol Ther 2004;17(1):8–19.
6. Powell J, Wojnarowska F, Winsey S, et al. Lichen sclerosus premanarche: autoimmunity and immuno-genetics. Br J Dermatol 2000;142(3):481–4.
7. Chan I, Oyama N, Neill S, et al. Characterization of IgG autoantibodies to extracellular matrix protein 1 in lichen sclerosus. Clin Exp Dermatol 2004;29(5):499–504.
8. Kreuter A, Kryvosheyeva Y, Terras S, et al. Association of autoimmune diseases with lichen sclerosus in 532 male and female patients. Acta Derm Venereol 2013;93(2):238–41.
9. Goldstein A, Marinoff S, Christopher K, et al. Prevalence of vulvar lichen sclerosus in a general gynecology practice. J Reprod Med 2005;50(7):477–80.
10. Cheung S, Gach J, Lewis F. A retrospective study of the referral patterns to a vulval clinic: highlighting educational needs in this subspecialty. J Obstet Gynaecol 2006;26(5):435–7.
11. Lee A, Bradford J, Fischer G. Long-term management of adult vulvar lichen sclerosus: a prospective cohort study of 507 women. JAMA Dermatol 2015; 151(10):1061–7.
12. Funaro D. Lichen sclerosus: a review and practical approach. Dermatol Ther 2004;17(1):28–37.
13. Longinotti M, Scheiffer Y, Kaufman R. Lichen sclerosus involving the vagina. Obstet Gynecol 2005; 106(5 Pt 2):1217–9.
14. Edwards L. Lichen sclerosus with vaginal involvement: report of 2 cases and review of the literature. JAMA Dermatol 2013;149(10):1199–202.
15. Regauer S, Liegl B, Reich O. Early vulvar lichen sclerosus: a histopathological challenge. Histopathology 2007;47(4):340–7.
16. Powell J, Wojnarowska F. Lichen sclerosus. Lancet 1999;353(9166):1777–83.
17. Eisen D. The clinical features, malignant potential, and systemic associations of oral lichen planus: a study of 723 patients. J Am Acad Dermatol 2002; 46(2):207–14.
18. Belfiore P, DiFede O, Cabibi D, et al. Prevalence of vulval lichen planus in a cohort of women with oral lichen planus: an interdisciplinary study. Br J Dermatol 2006;155(5):994–8.
19. Bradford J, Fischer G. Management of vulvovaginal lichen planus: a new approach. J Low Genit Tract Dis 2013;17(1):28–32.
20. Simpson R, Littlewood S, Cooper S, et al. Real-life experience of managing vulval erosive lichen planus: a case-based review and U.K. multicenter case note audit. Br J Dermatol 2012; 167(1):85–91.
21. Simpson R, Thomas K, Leighton P, et al. Diagnostic criteria for erosive lichen planus affecting the vulva: an international electronic-Delphi consensus exercise. Br J Dermatol 2013; 169(2):337–43.
22. Ryan C, Sadlier M, De Vol E, et al. Genital psoriasis is associated with significant impairment in quality of life and sexual functioning. J Am Acad Dermatol 2015;72(6):978–83.
23. Fan X, Yang S, Sun L, et al. Comparison of clinical features of HLA-Cw*0602-positive and -negative psoriasis patients in a Han Chinese population. Acta Derm Venereol 2007;87(4):335–40.
24. Guinot C, Latreille J, Perrussel M, et al. Psoriasis: characterization of six different clinical phenotypes. Exp Dermatol 2009;18(8):712–9.
25. Herron M, Hinckley M, Hoffman M, et al. Impact of obesity and smoking on psoriasis presentation and management. Arch Dermatol 2005;141(12):1527–34.
26. Stadler R, Schaumberg-Lever G, Orfanos C. Histology. In: Mier P, van d Kerkhof P, editors. Textbook of psoriasis. 1st edition. Edinburgh (United Kingdom): Churchill Livingstone; 1986. p. 40–54.
27. Garnier G. Benign plasma cell erythroplasia. Br J Dermatol 1957;69(3):77–81.

28. Hoang M, Reuter J, Papalas J, et al. Vulvar inflammatory dermatoses: an update and review. Am J Dermatopathol 2014;36(9):689–704.

29. Toeima E, Sule M, Warren R, et al. Diagnosis and treatment of Zoon's vulvitis. J Obstet Gynaecol 2011;31(6):473–5.

30. Brix W, Nassau S, Patterson J. Idiopathic lymphoplasmacellular mucositis-dermatitis. J Cutan Pathol 2010;37(4):426–31.

31. Erekson E, Martin D, Brousseau E, et al. Over-the-counter treatments and perineal hygiene in postmenopausal women. Menopause 2014;21(3):281–5.

32. Kamarashev J, Vassileva S. Dermatologic diseases of the vulva. Clin Dermatol 1997;15(1):53–65.

33. Marren P, Wojnarowska F, Powell S. Allergic contact dermatitis and vulvar dermatoses. Br J Dermatol 1992;126(1):52–6.

34. Corazza M, Miscioscia R, Lauriola M, et al. Allergic contact dermatitis due to Cineraria hybrid in an amateur gardener housewife. Contact Dermatitis 2008;59(2):128–9.

35. O'Gorman S, Torgerson R. Allergic contact dermatitis of the vulva. Dermatitis 2013;24(2):64–72.

36. Pincus S. Vulvar dermatoses and pruritus vulvae. Dermatol Clin 1992;10(2):297–308.

37. Ueda Y, Enomot T, Miyatake T, et al. Analysis of clonality and HPV infection in benign, hyperplastic, premalignant, and malignant lesions of the vulvar mucosa. Am J Clin Pathol 2004;122(2):266–74.

38. Lynch PJ. Vulvar neoplasms and cysts. In: Black M, Ambros-Rudolph C, Edwards L, et al, editors. Obstetric and gynecologic dermatology. 3rd edition. China: Elsevier Limited; 2008. p. 267–99.

39. Soufir N, Queille S, Liboutet M, et al. Inactivation of the CDKN2A and the p53 tumor suppressor genes in external genital carcinomas and their precursors. Br J Dermatol 2007;156(3):448–53.

40. van Seters M, van Beurden M, de Craen A. Is the assumed natural history of vulvar intraepithelial neoplasia based on enough evidence? A systematic review of 3322 published patients. Gynecol Oncol 2005;97(2):645–51.

41. Jones R, Rowan D, Stewart A. Vulvar intraepithelial neoplasia: aspects of the natural history and outcome in 405 women. Obstet Gynecol 2005; 106(6):1319–26.

42. Zawislak A, Price J, Dobbs S, et al. The management of vulval intraepithelial neoplasia in Northern Ireland. Int J Gynecol Cancer 2006;16(2):780–5.

43. Hillemanns P, Wang X, Staehle S, et al. Evaluation of different treatment modalities for vulvar intraepithelial neoplasia (VIN): CO(2) laser vaporization, photodynamic therapy, excision and vulvectomy. Gynecol Oncol 2006;100(2):271–5.

44. Hart W, Norris H, Helwig E. Relation of lichen sclerosus et atrophicus of the vulva to development of carcinoma. Obtet Gynecol 1975;45(4):369–77.

45. Wallace H. Lichen sclerosus et atrophicus. Trans St Johns Hosp Dermatol Soc 1971;57(1):9–30.

46. Carlson J, Ambros R, Malfetano J, et al. Vulvar lichen sclerosus and squamous cell carcinoma: a cohort, case control, and investigational study with historical perspective, implications for chronic inflammation and sclerosis in the development of neoplasia. Hum Pathol 1998;29(9):932–48.

47. Franck J, Young AJ. Squamous cell carcinoma in situ arising within lichen planus of the vulva. Dermatol Surg 1995;21(10):890–4.

48. Lewis F, Harrington C. Squamous cell carcinoma arising in vulval lichen planus. Br J Dermatol 1994; 131(5):703–5.

49. Schwartz R. Verrucous carcinoma of the skin and mucosa. J Am Acad Dermatol 1995;32(1):1–21.

50. Fan L, Zhu J, Tao X, et al. Intraepithelial extramammary Paget's disease of the vulva: the clinicopathological characteristics, management, and outcome in a study of 18 female patients. Dermatol Surg 2016;42(10):1142–6.

51. Huang Y, Chuang Y, Kuo T, et al. Vulvar syringoma: a clinicopathologic and immunohistologic study of 18 patients and the results of treatment. J Am Acad Dermatol 2003;48(5):735–9.

52. Stumpf A, Ständer S. Neuropathic itch: diagnosis and management. Dermatol Ther 2013;26(2):104–9.

53. Cohen A, Vander T, Medvendovsky E, et al. Neuropathic scrotal pruritus: anogenital pruritus is a symptom of lumbosacral radiculopathy. J Am Acad Dermatol 2005;52(1):61–6.

54. Raine-Fenning N, Brincat M, Muscat-Baron Y. Skin aging and menopause?: implications for treatment. Am J Clin Dermatol 2003;4(6):371–8.

55. Rimoin L, Kwatra S, Yosipovitch G. Female-specific pruritus from childhood to postmenopause: clinical features, hormonal factors, and considerations. Dermatol Ther 2013;26(2):157–67.

56. Stika C. Atrophic vaginitis. Dermatol Ther 2010; 23(5):514–22.

57. Wines N, Willsteed E. Menopause and the skin. Australas J Dermatol 2001;42(3):149–60.

58. Bunker C. Male genital lichen sclerosus and tacrolimus. Br J Dermatol 2007;157(5):1079–80.

59. Weichert G. An approach to the treatment of anogenital pruritus. Dermatol Ther 2004;17(1):129–33.

60. Kelly R, Foster D, Woodruff J. Subcutaneous injection of triamcinolone acetonide in the treatment of chronic vulvar pruritus. Am J Obstet Gynecol 1993; 169(3):568–70.

61. Matsuda K, Sharma D, Schonfeld A, et al. Gabapentin and pregabalin for the treatment of chronic pruritus. J Am Acad Dermatol 2016; 75(3):619–25.e6.

62. Greaves M. Antihistamines. In: Wolverton S, editor. Comprehensive dermatologic drug therapy. 3rd edition. Elsevier; 2013. p. 343–52.

63. Poterucha T, Sinead L, Paola S, et al. Topical amitriptyline combined with topical ketamine for the management of recalcitrant localized pruritus: a retrospective pilot study. J Am Acad Dermatol 2013;69(2):320–1.

64. Poterucha T, Murphy S, Rho R, et al. Topical amitriptyline-ketamine for treatment of rectal, genital, and perineal pain and discomfort. Pain Physician 2012;15(6):485–8.

65. Ständer S, Böckenholt B, Schürmeyer-Horst F, et al. Treatment of chronic pruritus with the selective serotonin reuptake inhibitors paroxetine and fluvoxamine: results of an open-labelled, two-arm proof-of-concept study. Acta Derm Venereol 2009;89(1):45–51.

66. Zylicz Z, Krajnik M, Sorge A, et al. Paroxetine in the treatment of severe non-dermatological pruritus: a randomized, controlled trial. J Pain Symptom Manag 2003;26(6):1105–12.

67. Hundley J, Yosipovitch G. Mirtazapine for reducing nocturnal itch in patients with chronic pruritus: a pilot study. J Am Acad Dermatol 2004;50(6):889–91.

68. Mauskar M. Erosive lichen planus. Obstet Gynecol Clin North Am 2017;44(3):407–20.

69. Nayeemuddin F, Yates V. Lichen sclerosus et atrophicus responding to methotrexate. Clin Exp Dermatol 2008;33(5):651–2.

70. Jancin B. Ixekizumab has a profound impact on genital psoriasis. Dermatol News 2017. Available at: http://www.mdedge.com/edermatologynews/article/149233/psoriasis/ixekizumab-has-profound-impact-genital-psoriasis. Accessed November 27, 2017.

71. Helgesen A, Warloe T, Pripp A, et al. Vulvovaginal photodynamic therapy vs. topical corticosteroids in genital erosive lichen planus: a randomized-controlled trial. Br J Dermatol 2015;173(5):1156–62.

72. Fan Z, Zhang L, Wang H, et al. Treatment of cutaneous lichen planus with ALA-mediated topical photodynamic therapy. J Innov Opt Heal Sci 2015;8(1):1–7.

73. Maździarz A, Osuch B, Kowalska M, et al. Photodynamic therapy in the treatment of vulvar lichen sclerosus. Photodiagnosis Photodyn Ther 2017;19:135–9.

74. Shi L, Miao F, Zhang L, et al. Comparison of 5-aminolevulinic acid photodynamic therapy and clobetasol propionate in treatment of vulvar lichen sclerosus. Acta Derm Venereol 2016;96(5):684–8.

Pruritus in Cutaneous T-Cell Lymphoma and Its Management

Linda Serrano, MD[a],
Maria Estela Martinez-Escala, MD, PhD[b],
Xiaolong A. Zhou, MD[c], Joan Guitart, MD[d],*

KEYWORDS

- Cutaneous T-cell lymphoma • Interleukins • Pruritus • Substance P • Antidepressants
- Histone deacetylase inhibitors • Aprepitant • Visual analog scale

KEY POINTS

- In cutaneous T-cell lymphoma (CTCL), pruritus is experienced in approximately 62% to 88% of patients and is more common in late-stage mycosis fungoides, Sézary syndrome, and folliculotropic mycosis fungoides.
- The pathogenesis of CTCL-related pruritus is not completely understood; however, it seems that malignant T-cell clones, along with their accompanying dermal infiltrate, play an important role in CTCL-related pruritus.
- Different mediators of pruritus have been described in CTCL patients, including interleukin-31, nerve growth factor, and substance P.
- Worsening pruritus is associated with disease progression, relapse, or superinfection of CTCL patients. Repeated clinical pruritus assessments are warranted to assess disease status.
- Management of pruritus in CTCL patients should include effective disease therapy, neurotropic medication, proper skin care, and psychological support.

INTRODUCTION

Pruritus of lymphoma is commonly associated with both Hodgkin lymphoma (HL) and cutaneous T-cell lymphoma (CTCL) and may precede any other symptoms.[1] The prevalence of chronic itch in HL has been reported in up to 30% of patients and its specific pathogenesis is not well known. Currently, management includes supportive care along with disease therapy.[2] In CTCL, pruritus is experienced in approximately 62% to 88% of patients and is more common in late-stage mycosis fungoides (MF), Sézary syndrome (SS), and folliculotropic MF (FMF), a variant of MF distinguished by infiltration of pilosebaceous units.[3–8] In recent years, new mechanisms of pruritus in CTCL have been discovered and new therapies have been developed.[6,9,10] Because of the impact this

---

Disclosure: J. Guitart is the principal investigator, and L. Serrano, M.E. Martinez-Escala and X.A. Zhou are sub-investigators of a multicenter clinical trial on topical naloxone sponsored by Elorac (NCT02811783), mentioned in this article.
a Department of Dermatology, Northwestern University, Feinberg School of Medicine, 645 North Michigan Avenue, Suite 1050, Chicago, IL 60611, USA; b Department of Dermatology, Northwestern University, Feinberg School of Medicine, 676 North Saint Clair Street, Suite 1765, Chicago, IL 60611, USA; c Department of Dermatology, Northwestern University, Feinberg School of Medicine, 676 North Saint Clair Street, Suite 1600, Chicago, IL 60611, USA; d Department of Dermatology, Northwestern University, Feinberg School of Medicine, 676 North Saint Clair Street, Suite 1765, Chicago, IL 60611, USA
* Corresponding author.
E-mail address: j-guitart@northwestern.edu

Dermatol Clin 36 (2018) 245–258
https://doi.org/10.1016/j.det.2018.02.011
0733-8635/18/

symptom has on patient quality of life (QOL), this article focuses on the pathogenesis, management, and treatment of CTCL-associated pruritus.

PATHOPHYSIOLOGY IN CUTANEOUS T-CELL LYMPHOMA PRURITUS

The pathophysiology of CTCL-related pruritus has recently made remarkable advances, yet is not completely understood. Pruritus is a complex symptom that includes pruriceptive, neuropathic, neurogenic, and psychogenic causes that originate from different pathways.[11] Pruriceptive pruritus originates from stimulation of sensory nerve terminals with the cell body located in the dorsal root ganglia; thereafter the stimulus is sent to the brain through the spinothalamic cord. The identification of the mediators that participate in the stimulation of sensory nerve terminals has become an active research area for potential therapeutics. That standard treatments for pruritus are frequently ineffective for CTCL patients suggests a distinct mechanism for pruritogenesis arising from the unique cytokine profile generated by the malignant T-cell clones and tumor microenvironment.

The overall T-cell infiltrate in early MF shows a T helper (Th)1 cytokine profile (interleukin [IL]-2, IL-12, and interferon-γ), whereas in advanced MF and SS the predominant cytokine profile is Th2 (IL-4, IL-5, IL-10, and IL-13).[12] The latter cytokine profile is also observed in atopic dermatitis, and promotes immune responses mediated by eosinophils, mast cells, and immunoglobulin (Ig)E isotype.[13] Malignant T cells are also accompanied by a large number of nonmalignant immune cells, which include CD8+ tumor-infiltrating T cells, T cells with regulatory profile, dendritic cells, macrophages, and mast cells. Macrophages and mast cells have shown an important protumorigenic role.[12,14]

Among the different mediators involved in CTCL-related pruritus, interleukins play an important role. IL-2 is produced by activated T cells and promotes proliferation and differentiation of T-cell clones. Intradermal injection of IL-2 causes itchiness and erythema in healthy volunteers.[15] In addition, cyclosporine A is known to block IL-2 production, as well as the release of histamine from mast cells. This may explain the successful use of cyclosporine A in a patient with refractory SS and severe pruritus, which disappeared 2 days after treatment initiation.[16] However, because cyclosporine A causes immunosuppression, it should be avoided in CTCL patients owing to the high risk of disease progression.[17]

As mentioned previously, a predominant Th2 profile is observed in advanced disease and SS

causes increased levels of IL-4, which is also observed in atopic dermatitis. The pathogenic role of IL-4 in CTCL-related pruritus or in CTCL by itself is unknown. Drugs targeting IL-4 have been developed specifically for atopic dermatitis patients; however, data in CTCL patients are not available yet.[18] IgE production is enhanced by IL-4 and increased IgE levels have been reported in CTCL patients. IgE binds to Fc receptors of mast cells, basophils, eosinophils, monocytes, and macrophages, releasing mediators such as histamine and serotonin, among others. The involvement of these mediators in pruritogenesis is well known.

Another interleukin found within a rich Th2-environment is IL-31, which is released by the Th2 cells but also by dendritic cells, mast cells, and keratinocytes. Receptors for IL-31, such as oncotic M receptor beta and receptor alpha, have been described in keratinocytes, as well as in the dorsal root ganglia.[19] Binding to its receptors induces Janus kinase and then activates signal transducers and activators of transcription, mitogen-activated protein kinase and phosphatidylinositol 3-kinase pathways.[20] Increased serum levels of IL-31 have been described in pruritic dermatitis, including atopic dermatitis, prurigo nodularis, and allergic contact dermatitis, as well as in *Staphylococcus aureus* infection.[19,21–26]

IL-31 can be expressed by circulating malignant T-cell clones.[27] Controversial results have been observed regarding serum levels of IL-31 in patients with CTCL and pruritus. Although increased serum levels of IL-31 are higher in patients with advanced disease and severe pruritus, this correlation is not clearly observed in early-stage disease with or without pruritus.[19,20] The latter might be explained by the predominant Th1 cytokine profile and that there are undetectable T-cell clones observed in blood of early-stage MF. Finally, current therapies known to induce pruritus relief, such as mogamulizumab (anti-CCR4 conjugated humanized monoclonal antibody) and histone deacetylase (HDAC) inhibitors, demonstrated decreased circulating lymphocyte IL-31 expression.[28]

Skin biopsies of CTCL samples show an increased expression of IL-31 in the epidermis and in the interstitial lymphocytic infiltrate. Moreover, increased expression of its receptors has been observed, mostly in the epidermis, including in early lesions. The increased expression was associated with significantly higher clinical pruritus scores, yet no differences were observed with regard to disease stage.[19]

Chemoattractant cytokines (with C-C motif) or chemokines are involved in CTCL-related pruritus, including CCL1 (C-C motif ligand 1) and CCL26.

CCL1 has a unique receptor, CCR8, which is expressed in Th2 cells. It is a potent attractant for Th2 cells and serum levels have been significantly higher in CTCL patients with severe clinical pruritus scores. The latter chemokine, CCL26, and its receptor, CCR3, are expressed in Th2 cells. High serum levels of CCL26 have also been detected in CTCL patients with high pruritus scores. In addition, high messenger RNA levels of CCL26 are observed in skin biopsies of advanced CTCL when compared with skin biopsies of early-stage disease.[29,30]

The nerve growth factor (NGF) is a member of the neurotrophins and it is mainly produced by keratinocytes. It stimulates the proliferation of nerve fibers and modulates the synthesis of neuropeptides. Increased serum levels of NGF have been described in patients with atopic dermatitis.[30] One group analyzed the immunohistochemical expression of NGF and the increase of dermal nerve fibers through the expression of protein gene product 9.5 in skin lesions of patch, plaque, tumor MF, and SS. They found a significant increase of NGF expression, as well as in the number of dermal nerve fibers in lesional skin biopsies of SS when compared with patch, plaque, and tumor MF. Serum NGF levels were significantly higher in SS and stage IV MF than in early-stage MF. Furthermore, pruritus severity was associated with high serum levels of NGF. Therefore, this group suggested that NGF expression may be essential for the development and survival of nerve fibers, and that it is associated with increased pruritus. Because NGF has been suggested to stimulate T-cell and mast cell proliferation, a protumorigenic role of NGF in SS has been proposed.[30]

NGF also modulates the synthesis of a neuropeptide, substance P. Substance P is released by cutaneous nociceptive nerve terminals (C and Aδ nerve fibers) and affects vascular remodeling and alters immune responses involved in neurogenic inflammation. It has been found to localize to mast cells.[31] Neurokinin-1 is a receptor of substance P expressed in keratinocytes and the dorsal horn neurons. Initially, substance P was thought to induce itch by releasing histamine from mast cells; however, a histamine-independent pathway has been demonstrated by inducing itch (scratching behavior) in mast cell–deficient mice.[32]

Possible involvement of substance P in CTCL-related pruritus has been suggested by the improvement of the pruritus in patients treated with aprepitant, an antagonist of the neurokinin-1 receptor. This led to the investigation of the expression of substance P and its receptor in the skin and blood. Although neurokinin-1 receptor was expressed in the circulating T cells of CTCL patients, expression of its receptor was not observed in the T cells of skin MF lesions. The investigators suggested the existence of diverse isoforms of the neurokinin-1 receptor, which may not be recognizable by the currently available monoclonal antibodies and may justify the different expression observed in tissue and blood. Regarding substance P, high serum levels were found in CTCL patients and those correlated with disease stage.[33,34] Increased serum levels of SP did not correlate with increased numbers of terminal nerves in the dermis. Due to the retrospective method of the study, a correlation with pruritus severity could not be performed.

Finally, another mediator related to pruritus in MF and SS is the vascular endothelial growth factor (VEGF)-A. It is a proangiogenic factor with receptors located in endothelial cells. It is secreted by MF or SS tumor cells and its expression has been correlated with CCL27 (chemoattractant of skin-homing T cells, CTCL marker).[29] Another VEGF, VEGF-C, which is also involved in the development of MF or SS, modulates lymphangiogenesis. Higher serum levels of VEGF-A (but not VEGF-C) have been detected in erythrodermic MF or SS patients when compared with early stages of MF or healthy controls, these levels also correlated with pruritus score severity. In addition, serum levels of VEGF-A correlated with NGF levels and IgE levels.[35] VEGF increases expression of adhesion molecules on endothelial cells, such as vascular cell adhesion molecule 1 or intercellular adhesion molecule 1, which are involved in the pathogenesis of erythroderma.[36,37] Therefore, increased serum levels of VEGF-A may result in increased dermal vascularity, which helps explain the erythroderma seen in advanced CTCL rather than its pruritus symptoms.

ASSESSMENT TOOLS FOR CUTANEOUS T-CELL LYMPHOMA PRURITUS

Severe pruritus has been observed in 68% to 74% of patients with FMF and in 93% of patients with SS.[3,5,6] In addition, 63% of patients with MF and SS have S aureus skin colonization, which promotes inflammation via S aureus-toxin and Th2 cytokines, such as IL-31. It also correlates with worsening erythroderma and pruritus, which improves after antibiotic therapy.[38] Clinical assessments of pruritus are necessary to determine the clinical course. If a patient develops worsening pruritus, progression, recurrence, or superinfection should be suspected. Pruritus in CTCL patients may affect physical, social, and emotional functioning, including depression, sleep disturbances, frustration, and anger.[9,39]

Itch assessments have been validated and used both clinically and in clinical trials in CTCL. The visual analog scale (VAS), numerical rating scale (NRS), and the verbal rating scale (VRS) are all validated subjective assessments of itch.[40] The VAS is a 10-cm ruler-like scale with 0 meaning no itch and 10 being the worst itch imaginable. The patient draws a perpendicular line at the point at which they feel their itch corresponds and it is then measured by the provider. The NRS is similar to the VAS with a 0 to 10 scale of 11 boxes. The VRS is a list of adjectives asking the patient to describe the symptoms experienced (**Fig. 1**).[40]

These 3 scales were originally developed and validated for pain but were adapted for use in pruritus.[41] VAS scores below 4 are mild, between 4 and 6.9 are moderate, and 7 is considered severe, with scores equal to or greater than 9 indicating very severe itch.[42–44] The VRS asks the patient what number their itch corresponds with: 0 is none, 1 is mild, 2 is moderate, and 3 is severe.[40] An 11-point verbal NRS (VNRS-11), with 0 being no itch, 5 being moderate itch, and 10 being the worst imaginable itch, correlates to the 4-question VRS; it is also used clinically.[44]

The VAS is the most commonly used assessment in clinical trials for CTCL and is a reliable and a rapid assessment; however, NRS correlates strongly with VAS and is easier for patients to understand. VAS scores of 92 patients with CTCL surveyed ranged from 0 to 10, with a mean score of 3.35. Early-stage patients had a mean of 2.9 and advanced-stage patients had a mean of 3.9.

Eighty percent of participants reported some pruritus the day they took the survey and 17% reported more severe pruritus, greater than 7.[8] Some limitations of the VAS scale include a possible discrepancy between races, usage for intensity only, and difficulty for patients with motor or cognitive impairments.[43]

The VAS, NRS, and VRS all have a strong correlation; however, there are slightly higher NRS scores when directly compared.[40,43] A sustained decrease of at least 3 points on the VAS or NRS indicates clinical improvement and has been used as meaningful endpoint in clinical trials.[45–47] VAS has correlated with multiple dermatology-validated QOL surveys, including the SkinDex29 and the Dermatology Life Quality Index (DLQI), which are specific to skin-related diseases, indicating a worse QOL with worse pruritus.[8,46]

These itch scales are not comprehensive and do not measure the impact of pruritus on QOL. Generic scales, cancer-specific, and skin-specific QOL assessments exist but do not specifically address pruritus. A nocturnal itch VAS has been developed to assess the effect on sleep: 0 is no sleep loss and 10 is cannot sleep at all.[48] This can be a quick method to assess an aspect of QOL that is missed with the itch assessment alone.

The ItchyQoL questionnaire, a 22-item survey that takes about 3 minutes to complete, is a validated tool for clinicians and in research.[49,50] It determines the impact on functioning, emotions, and symptoms, and is measured by both the frequency and the bother of itch.[49] The DLQI and VAS correlate with the ItchyQoL, although the DLQI was

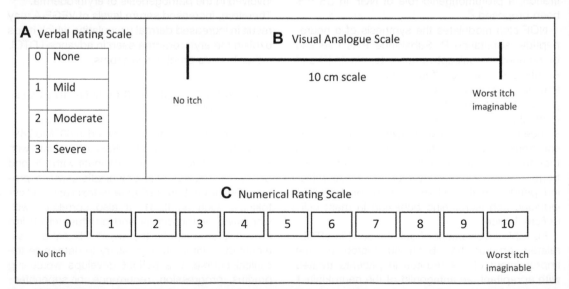

Fig. 1. Examples of different scales used for the assessment of pruritus in CTCL: A, VRS; B, VAS; and C, NRS. (*Courtesy of* Ngoc Quan Phan, MD, Münster, Germany.)

developed for noticeable skin lesions and not pruritus.[51]

QOL is an important endpoint considered secondary only to survival in clinical trials.[9] Itch severity, frequency, duration, and anatomic location correlate directly with QOL.[52] Beynon and colleagues[53] conducted interviews with CTCL patients to explore how their QOL is affected by the disease. They interviewed 19 patients, 16 of whom described pruritus and 13 described severe pruritus. Their itch was exacerbated by a lack of heat regulation, which also caused them to sleep in different beds than their partners. They also endorsed trouble sleeping directly related to their pruritus. The frequency, intensity, and QOL of pruritus can be measured by reliable assessment tools, which are important in the clinical setting. The authors recommend using the VNRS-11 to assess pruritus at every clinic visit to monitor symptom relief or progression. This is easy for patients to understand and a quick assessment that can be monitored over time. There is a correlation of pruritus and QOL in CTCL; however, the extent has not yet been comprehensively assessed.

THERAPEUTICS FOR CUTANEOUS T-CELL LYMPHOMA PRURITUS

Several topical and systemic agents are recommended by the National Comprehensive Cancer Network (NCCN) to treat CTCL-associated pruritus (**Box 1**). Topical therapies include moisturizers and emollients, topical corticosteroids, topical camphor or menthol, and topical pramoxine formulations. Systemic agents are divided into first line (antihistamine, doxepin, gabapentin, pregabalin), second line (aprepitant, mirtazapine, selective serotonin reuptake inhibitors), and third line (naltrexone).[54] The evidence for the use of these pruritus-specific agents are mostly based on other pruritic dermatologic disorders but anecdotally have shown benefit in CTCL. Data from large-scale trials are lacking. Specifically for CTCL, mirtazapine and gabapentin has been used with success by Demierre and colleagues[55] but no study on its clinical efficacy has been performed. Naltrexone was found to be beneficial in 50% of 10 malignancy-associated pruritus subjects (including 7 with CTCL) in a German study looking at the efficacy of naltrexone on pruritus of various causes.[56] There is currently a multicenter, double-blind, randomized, crossover clinical trial investigating the use of topical naloxone for pruritus in MF and SS (NCT02811783). Aprepitant has been proposed to be a possible treatment of pruritus in CTCL. It showed significant improvement in 4 of 4 cases in 1 series and varied response on

---

Box 1
Therapeutic ladder recommended by National Comprehensive Cancer Network guidelines

Topical agents

Topical steroids plus or minus occlusion

Moisturizers and emollients

Anti-itch creams or lotions: camphor or menthol, pramoxine

Optimize skin-directed and systemic therapy

Systemic agents

First line

- Antihistamines
- Doxepin
- Gabapentin

Second line

- Aprepitant
- Mirtazapine
- Selective serotonin reuptake inhibitors

Third line

- Naltrexone

Data from National Comprehensive Cancer Network (NCCN). T-cell lymphomas (Version 1.2018). NCCN 2018.

---

review of the literature, which was attributed to discrepancies in dose, timing of regimens, and outcome measures.[57]

Although pruritus control is an important component of CTCL management, the primary goal is still controlling the primary process (CTCL), which by itself may be the most effective way of decreasing the itching sensation. However, the authors have observed dissociation between the clinical improvement and resolution of pruritus, which can linger even after skin improvement. Besides the pruritus-specific therapies mentioned in the NCCN guidelines, other CTCL skin-directed therapies may be effective.[54] In phototherapy (eg, psoralen and ultraviolet A [PUVA], ultraviolet [UV] B), PUVA is 1 of the best studied and oldest treatments for CTCL pruritus and is effective in early-stage CTCL.[58] Nitrogen mustard derivatives (eg, mechlorethamine and carmustine) have also shown some pruritus benefit but carry the risk of contact dermatitis that at least temporarily worsens pruritus.[13,59,60]

Systemic therapies for CTCL are rapidly evolving with new treatments that decrease the burden of disease and often help decrease the pruritus. **Table 1** describes some of the systemic

Table 1
Summary of pruritus data from clinical trials of therapies for cutaneous T-cell lymphoma

Drug	Author, Year	Study Design	Dose	Number of Subjects	Disease Type and Stage	Assessment Method	Pruritus Response	Concomitant Antipruritic Treatment	Comments
Naltrexone	Brune et al,[56] 2004	Single-arm, open-label, single-center	50–100 mg	133 (7 CTCL)	CTCL (unknown stage)	VAS	Pruritus response: 5 of 10 subjects with malignancies (50%)	Unknown	—
Aprepitant	Song et al,[57] 2017	Case series	Variable	4	CTCL (unknown stage)	NRS	All subjects with response	Unknown	—
	Booken et al,[46] 2011	Open-label pilot	125 mg day 1 80 mg days 2 and 3	5	Erythrodermic MF or SS IIA-IVB (3 SS, 2 MF)	VAS	Mean reduction 4.5 ($P = .125$)	—	—
Belinostat	Foss et al,[64] 2015	Single-arm, open-label, multicenter, phase II	1000–1400 mg/m²/d	29	MF or SS IB-IVB	Scale 0–10 (scale not specified)	Response: 46.7 Severe pruritus response: 50%	Unknown	—

	Dose	Reference	Study design	N	Diagnosis	Pruritus scale	ORR/Response		Notes
Panobinostat	20 mg/d	Duvic et al,[63] 2013	Single-arm, open-label, multicenter, phase II	139	MF or SS IB–IVA	Scale 0–10 (scale not specified)	ORR: 24.7%	Unknown	Divided into subjects with previous exposure to bexarotene (n = 79) or bexarotene-naive (n = 60)
Quinostat	8–12 mg TIW	Child et al,[65] 2016	Single-arm, multi-center open-label, phase II	26	MF or SS IB–IVA	Pruritus method not described	ORR: 40% 67% responders 32% nonresponders	Unknown	—
Romidepsin	14 mg/m²/wk	Whittaker et al,[47] 2010	Single-arm, open-label, multicenter, phase II	96	MF or SS IB–IVA	VAS	60/65 (92%) reported reduction in VAS (mean change of −38 mm) Response: 43% of moderate to severe pruritus subjects, 53% of severe pruritus subjects	Not permitted	—

(continued on next page)

Table 1
(continued)

Drug	Dose	Author, Year	Study Design	Number of Subjects	Disease Type and Stage	Assessment Method	Pruritus Response	Concomitant Antipruritic Treatment	Comments
Vorinostat	400 mg/d or 300 mg bid 3–5 d/wk or 300 mg bid for 2 wk, 1 wk off, then 200 mg tid	Duvic et al,[62] 2007	Single-arm, open-label, single center, phase II	33	MF or SS IA to IVB	Scale 0–10 (scale not specified)	Response: 45% Complete relief 10%	Antihistamines and topical steroids permitted if stable dose at C2	—
	400 mg/d	Olsen et al,[81] 2007	Single-arm, open-label multicenter, phase IIB	74	MF or SS IB–IVB	VAS	ORR: 32.3% Severe pruritus response: 43.3%	Anti-histamines permitted; topical steroids and systemic steroids (for SS) used for 3 mo were allowed to continue	
	200–400 mg	Dummer et al,[76] 2012	Single arm, open-label, multicenter, phase I	23	MF/SS IB to IVB	VAS	ORR at each dose vorinostat or bexarotene (mg) 200/150: 33% 300/150: 20% 200/225: 0% 200/300: 33% 400/150: 60% 400/225: 33%	Unknown	Combination with bexarotene 150–300 mg

Bexarotene	6.5 or 300 mg/m²/d	Duvic et al,[77] 2001	Randomized open-label, multicenter, phase II–III	58	IA to IIA	Scale not specified	Pruritus consistently improved	Permitted	—
	300 mg/m²/d	Duvic et al,[77] 2001	Single-arm, open-label, multicenter, phase II–III	94	MF or SS IIB–IVB	Scale of 0–8 for ≤5 representative index lesions	Pruritus consistently improved	Permitted	
	Variable	Sepmeyer et al,[67] 2007	Single-arm, open-label, single center, phase pilot	4	MF or SS IB–IVA	VAS	Response: 75%	Unknown	Bexarotene given with rosiglitazone
	300 mg/m²/d	Straus et al,[68] 2014	Single-arm, open-label multicenter, phase II	37	MF or SS IB–IVA	VAS	Response: 60% post bexarotene	Topical steroids permitted	Liposomal doxorubicin followed by bexarotene
Alemtuzumab	3–30 mg as tolerated	Lundin et al,[69] 2003	Single-arm, open-label, multicenter, phase II	22	MF or SS IIA–IVB	VAS	Mean of 8 to mean of 2, including in 50% of subjects without a response to treatment	Subjects received antihistamine 30 min before infusion. Use of systemic steroids during week 1 optional	—
	3–30 mg as tolerated	Kennedy et al,[80] 2003	Single-arm, open-label, single-center, phase II	8	MF or SS IIB–IVB	Self-assessment on scale of 0–8	Response: 50% regardless of tumor response	Promethazine and hydrocortisone permitted for infusion	—

(continued on next page)

Table 1 (continued)

Drug	Dose	Author, Year	Study Design	Number of Subjects	Disease Type and Stage	Assessment Method	Pruritus Response	Concomitant Antipruritic Treatment	Comments
Extracorporeal photopheresis	—	Bouwhuis et al,[70] 2002	Retrospective, single-center	55	MF or SS III–IVB	Scale not specified	Good response: 60% PR: 7%	Unknown	—
Denileukin diftitox	9 or 18 µg/kg/d	Duvic et al,[78] 2002	Phase III, multicenter, open-label	64	Stage IB-III disease MF or SS following ≥4 prior treatments or stage IVA recurrent or persistent after at least 1 prior therapy	VAS	Relief: 53.1% >50% relief: 42.2% Complete relief: 10.1%	Hydroxyzine, topical emollients, bath additives were permitted	—
Valproic acid	30 mg/kg tid	Espinoza-Zamora et al,[79] 2017	Single-center, open-label, phase II	14	MF or SS ≥IB Lymphomatoid papulosis	VAS	CR: 93% PR: 7%	Given with hydralazine 83 mg or 182 mg	—

Abbreviations: C2, cycle 2; CR, complete remission; ORR, overall rate response; PR, partial response; TIW, 3 times a week.
Data from Refs.[47,76–81]

therapies for which pruritus has been measured and the level of evidence for each.

HDAC inhibitors are a class of medications that have shown to have significant pruritus benefit in patients with advanced CTCL. Although the exact mechanism of action is unknown, they are known to alter epigenetic pathways important for cancer growth and progression. Romidepsin is approved for CTCL patients who have received at least 1 prior systemic therapy. In a phase II study of 96 subjects with stage IB to IVA CTCL, almost all subjects with moderate to severe pruritus (60 out of 65, 92%) reported sustained reduction in VAS scores (mean change of −38 mm). Clinically meaningful reduction in pruritus is seen in 28 out of 65 subjects (43%) with moderate to severe pruritus at baseline, including 19 out of 36 subjects (53%) with severe pruritus at baseline.[61] Vorinostat showed a mean pruritus score improvement of 3 points and 45% of patients with baseline pruritus had symptomatic relief.[62] Newer HDAC inhibitors also show a pruritus benefit, including, panobinostat (25%), quisinostat (40%), and belinostat (47%).[63–65]

Bexarotene is a synthetic nuclear retinoid X receptor-selective retinoid approved by the US Food and Drug Administration for the treatment of refractory CTCL in all stages and is available in oral and topical formulations. In a pivotal phase II to III clinical trial of oral bexarotene in refractory early-stage CTCL, index lesion pruritus consistently decreased from mild-moderate at baseline to absent-mild by week 16. Pruritus even continued to improve in later weeks independent of antihistamine or antipruritic use.[66] Some studies that have attempted to combine bexarotene with other agents (eg, liposomal doxorubicin and rosiglitazone) have also found significant improvements in pruritus.[67,68]

Alemtuzumab is a humanized monoclonal antibody against CD52, which is abundantly expressed on normal and malignant T lymphocytes. Pruritus was reduced from a median of 8 (at baseline) to 2 (at the end of treatment period) in 1 study.[69]

Extracorporeal photopheresis (ECP) is a form of apheresis whereby blood is treated first with a photosensitizer and then exposed to UVA rays to induce apoptosis of malignant T lymphocytes. This procedure has also been shown to be beneficial for pruritus. In retrospective study, 60% of the subjects with good response to ECP had a pruritus improvement of greater than 50%.[70]

Zanolimumab is an investigational fully human anti-CD4 monoclonal antibody specific to the CD4 receptor on T lymphocytes. The antibody prevents interaction between the CD4 receptor and the major histocompatibility complex class II molecule, thus blocking T cell activation. Among 13 CTCL subjects responding to zanolimumab treatment, 11 subjects (85%) reported improvement in severity of pruritus; 52% of nonresponders (n = 25) also had some improvement in pruritus.[71]

Mogamulizumab, an anti-CCR4 monoclonal antibody, is a promising therapeutic option to control IL-31 expression in CTCL. Most IL-31–producing malignant T cells express CCR4. Cedeno-Laurent and colleagues,[28] found a single mogamulizumab infusion decreased pruritus significantly. Clinical trials have not yet assessed pruritus in CTCL.[72,73] Dupilumab, an anti–IL-4 and anti–IL-13 human monoclonal antibody, and nemolizumab, an anti-IL-31 receptor A antibody, have also shown promise in reducing pruritus in atopic dermatitis, although studies in CTCL are necessary to determine if they have role in treatment.[74,75] In addition, CTCL clinical trials with other drugs and outcomes in pruritus relief are listed in **Table 1**.

SUMMARY

Pruritus is the most commonly experienced symptom in CTCL and critically affects the QOL of patients. Understanding the pruritogenesis in CTCL has led to development of new therapeutic agents with promising outcomes in the management of this recalcitrant symptom. Repeated clinical assessments are warranted because they may support the evaluation of treatment response, the presence of new flares, or the recurrence of disease. Severe pruritus scores may require further investigation of emotional distress, including sleep disturbances and depression, for a better patient approach. Besides the need to treat the disease more effectively with modern therapeutic options, dermatologists will play a key role in the treatment of pruritus in CTCL patients by guiding the patient in the importance of preserving the integrity of the skin barrier with proper skin care instructions and emollient creams. These measures will reduce the inflammation, bacterial colonization, and infection known to contribute to worsening pruritus and disease progression.

REFERENCES

1. Yosipovitch G. Chronic pruritus: a paraneoplastic sign. Dermatol Ther 2010;23(6):590–6.
2. Wang H, Yosipovitch G. New insights into the pathophysiology and treatment of chronic itch in patients with end-stage renal disease, chronic liver disease, and lymphoma. Int J Dermatol 2010; 49(1):1–11.

3. Gerami P, Rosen S, Kuzel T, et al. Folliculotropic mycosis fungoides: an aggressive variant of cutaneous T-cell lymphoma. Arch Dermatol 2008; 144(6):738–46.

4. Hodak E, Amitay-Laish I, Atzmony L, et al. New insights into folliculotropic mycosis fungoides (FMF): a single-center experience. J Am Acad Dermatol 2016;75(2):347–55.

5. Lehman JS, Cook-Norris RH, Weed BR, et al. Folliculotropic mycosis fungoides: single-center study and systematic review. Arch Dermatol 2010;146(6):607–13.

6. Vij A, Duvic M. Prevalence and severity of pruritus in cutaneous T cell lymphoma. Int J Dermatol 2012; 51(8):930–4.

7. Willemze R, Jaffe ES, Burg G, et al. WHO-EORTC classification for cutaneous lymphomas. Blood 2005;105(10):3768–85.

8. Wright A, Wijeratne A, Hung T, et al. Prevalence and severity of pruritus and quality of life in patients with cutaneous T-cell lymphoma. J Pain Symptom Manage 2013;45(1):114–9.

9. Demierre MF, Gan S, Jones J, et al. Significant impact of cutaneous T-cell lymphoma on patients' quality of life: results of a 2005 National Cutaneous Lymphoma Foundation Survey. Cancer 2006; 107(10):2504–11.

10. Sampogna F, Frontani M, Baliva G, et al. Quality of life and psychological distress in patients with cutaneous lymphoma. Br J Dermatol 2009;160(4):815–22.

11. Potenzieri C, Undem BJ. Basic mechanisms of itch. Clin Exp Allergy 2012;42(1):8–19.

12. Rubio Gonzalez B, Zain J, Rosen ST, et al. Tumor microenvironment in mycosis fungoides and Sezary syndrome. Curr Opin Oncol 2016;28(1):88–96.

13. Ahern K, Gilmore ES, Poligone B. Pruritus in cutaneous T-cell lymphoma: a review. J Am Acad Dermatol 2012;67(4):760–8.

14. Rabenhorst A, Schlaak M, Heukamp LC, et al. Mast cells play a protumorigenic role in primary cutaneous lymphoma. Blood 2012;120(10):2042–54.

15. Wahlgren CF, Tengvall Linder M, Hagermark O, et al. Itch and inflammation induced by intradermally injected interleukin-2 in atopic dermatitis patients and healthy subjects. Arch Dermatol Res 1995; 287(6):572–80.

16. Ryan C, Amor KT, Menter A. The use of cyclosporine in dermatology: part II. J Am Acad Dermatol 2010; 63(6):949–72 [quiz: 73–4].

17. Quereux G, Renaut JJ, Peuvrel L, et al. Sudden onset of an aggressive cutaneous lymphoma in a young patient with psoriasis: role of immunosuppressants. Acta Derm Venereol 2010;90(6):616–20.

18. Tsianakas A, Stander S. Dupilumab: a milestone in the treatment of atopic dermatitis. Lancet 2016; 387(10013):4–5.

19. Nattkemper LA, Martinez-Escala ME, Gelman AB, et al. Cutaneous T-cell lymphoma and pruritus: the expression of IL-31 and its receptors in the skin. Acta Derm Venereol 2016;96(7):894–8.

20. Mobs M, Gryzik S, Haidar A, et al. Analysis of the IL-31 pathway in Mycosis fungoides and Sezary syndrome. Arch Dermatol Res 2015;307(6):479–85.

21. Kato A, Fujii E, Watanabe T, et al. Distribution of IL-31 and its receptor expressing cells in skin of atopic dermatitis. J Dermatol Sci 2014;74(3): 229–35.

22. Maier E, Werner D, Duschl A, et al. Human Th2 but not Th9 cells release IL-31 in a STAT6/NF-kappaB-dependent way. J Immunol 2014;193(2):645–54.

23. Neis MM, Peters B, Dreuw A, et al. Enhanced expression levels of IL-31 correlate with IL-4 and IL-13 in atopic and allergic contact dermatitis. J Allergy Clin Immunol 2006;118(4):930–7.

24. Nobbe S, Dziunycz P, Muhleisen B, et al. IL-31 expression by inflammatory cells is preferentially elevated in atopic dermatitis. Acta Derm Venereol 2012;92(1):24–8.

25. Sonkoly E, Muller A, Lauerma AI, et al. IL-31: a new link between T cells and pruritus in atopic skin inflammation. J Allergy Clin Immunol 2006;117(2): 411–7.

26. Niebuhr M, Mamerow D, Heratizadeh A, et al. Staphylococcal alpha-toxin induces a higher T cell proliferation and interleukin-31 in atopic dermatitis. Int Arch Allergy Immunol 2011;156(4):412–5.

27. Singer EM, Shin DB, Nattkemper LA, et al. IL-31 is produced by the malignant T-cell population in cutaneous T-Cell lymphoma and correlates with CTCL pruritus. J Invest Dermatol 2013;133(12):2783–5.

28. Cedeno-Laurent F, Singer EM, Wysocka M, et al. Improved pruritus correlates with lower levels of IL-31 in CTCL patients under different therapeutic modalities. Clin Immunol 2015;158(1):1–7.

29. Miyagaki T, Sugaya M, Fujita H, et al. Eotaxins and CCR3 interaction regulates the Th2 environment of cutaneous T-cell lymphoma. J Invest Dermatol 2010;130(9):2304–11.

30. Suga H, Sugaya M, Miyagaki T, et al. Association of nerve growth factor, chemokine (C-C motif) ligands and immunoglobulin E with pruritus in cutaneous T-cell lymphoma. Acta Derm Venereol 2013;93(2): 144–9.

31. Toyoda M, Makino T, Kagoura M, et al. Immunolocalization of substance P in human skin mast cells. Arch Dermatol Res 2000;292(8):418–21.

32. Andoh T, Nagasawa T, Satoh M, et al. Substance P induction of itch-associated response mediated by cutaneous NK1 tachykinin receptors in mice. J Pharmacol Exp Ther 1998;286(3):1140–5.

33. Misery L, Bourchanny D, Kanitakis J, et al. Modulation of substance P and somatostatin receptors in cutaneous lymphocytic inflammatory and tumoral infiltrates. J Eur Acad Dermatol Venereol 2001;15(3): 238–41.

34. Tuzova M, Conniff T, Curiel-Lewandrowski C, et al. Absence of full-length neurokinin-1 receptor protein expression by cutaneous T cells: implications for substance P-mediated signaling in mycosis fungoides. Acta Derm Venereol 2015; 95(7):852–4.

35. Sakamoto M, Miyagaki T, Kamijo H, et al. Serum vascular endothelial growth factor A levels reflect itch severity in mycosis fungoides and Sezary syndrome. J Dermatol 2018;45(1):95–9.

36. Kim I, Moon SO, Kim SH, et al. Vascular endothelial growth factor expression of intercellular adhesion molecule 1 (ICAM-1), vascular cell adhesion molecule 1 (VCAM-1), and E-selectin through nuclear factor-kappa B activation in endothelial cells. J Biol Chem 2001;276(10):7614–20.

37. Miyamoto D, Sotto MN, Otani CS, et al. Increased serum levels of vascular endothelial growth factor in pemphigus foliaceus patients with erythroderma. J Eur Acad Dermatol Venereol 2017;31(2):333–6.

38. Talpur R, Bassett R, Duvic M. Prevalence and treatment of Staphylococcus aureus colonization in patients with mycosis fungoides and Sezary syndrome. Br J Dermatol 2008;159(1):105–12.

39. Beynon T, Radcliffe E, Child F, et al. What are the supportive and palliative care needs of patients with cutaneous T-cell lymphoma and their caregivers? A systematic review of the evidence. Br J Dermatol 2014;170(3):599–608.

40. Phan NQ, Blome C, Fritz F, et al. Assessment of pruritus intensity: prospective study on validity and reliability of the visual analogue scale, numerical rating scale and verbal rating scale in 471 patients with chronic pruritus. Acta Derm Venereol 2012;92(5): 502–7.

41. Williamson A, Hoggart B. Pain: a review of three commonly used pain rating scales. J Clin Nurs 2005;14(7):798–804.

42. Kido-Nakahara M, Katoh N, Saeki H, et al. Comparative cut-off value setting of pruritus intensity in visual analogue scale and verbal rating scale. Acta Derm Venereol 2015;95(3):345–6.

43. Reich A, Heisig M, Phan NQ, et al. Visual analogue scale: evaluation of the instrument for the assessment of pruritus. Acta Derm Venereol 2012;92(5): 497–501.

44. Jenkins HH, Spencer ED, Weissgerber AJ, et al. Correlating an 11-point verbal numeric rating scale to a 4-point verbal rating scale in the measurement of pruritus. J Perianesth Nurs 2009;24(3):152–5.

45. Reich A, Riepe C, Anastasiadou Z, et al. Itch assessment with visual analogue scale and numerical rating scale: determination of minimal clinically important difference in chronic itch. Acta Derm Venereol 2016;96(7):978–80.

46. Booken N, Heck M, Nicolay JP, et al. Oral aprepitant in the therapy of refractory pruritus in erythrodermic cutaneous T-cell lymphoma. Br J Dermatol 2011; 164(3):665–7.

47. Whittaker SJ, Demierre MF, Kim EJ, et al. Final results from a multicenter, international, pivotal study of romidepsin in refractory cutaneous T-cell lymphoma. J Clin Oncol 2010;28(29):4485–91.

48. Furue M, Ebata T, Ikoma A, et al. Verbalizing extremes of the visual analogue scale for pruritus: a consensus statement. Acta Derm Venereol 2013; 93(2):214–5.

49. Desai NS, Poindexter GB, Monthrope YM, et al. A pilot quality-of-life instrument for pruritus. J Am Acad Dermatol 2008;59(2):234–44.

50. Krause K, Kessler B, Weller K, et al. German version of ItchyQoL: validation and initial clinical findings. Acta Derm Venereol 2013;93(5):562–8.

51. Stumpf A, Pfleiderer B, Fritz F, et al. Assessment of quality of life in chronic pruritus: relationship between ItchyQoL and dermatological life quality index in 1,150 patients. Acta Derm Venereol 2018;98(1): 142–3.

52. Carr CW, Veledar E, Chen SC. Factors mediating the impact of chronic pruritus on quality of life. JAMA Dermatol 2014;150(6):613–20.

53. Beynon T, Selman L, Radcliffe E, et al. 'We had to change to single beds because I itch in the night': a qualitative study of the experiences, attitudes and approaches to coping of patients with cutaneous T-cell lymphoma. Br J Dermatol 2015;173(1): 83–92.

54. Network NCC. T-cell lymphomas (Version 1.2018). 2018.

55. Demierre MF, Taverna J. Mirtazapine and gabapentin for reducing pruritus in cutaneous T-cell lymphoma. J Am Acad Dermatol 2006;55(3):543–4.

56. Brune A, Metze D, Luger TA, et al. Antipruritic therapy with the oral opioid receptor antagonist naltrexone. Open, non-placebo controlled administration in 133 patients. Hautarzt 2004;55(12): 1130–6 [in German].

57. Song JS, Tawa M, Chau NG, et al. Aprepitant for refractory cutaneous T-cell lymphoma-associated pruritus: 4 cases and a review of the literature. BMC Cancer 2017;17(1):200.

58. Querfeld C, Rosen ST, Kuzel TM, et al. Long-term follow-up of patients with early-stage cutaneous T-cell lymphoma who achieved complete remission with psoralen plus UV-A monotherapy. Arch Dermatol 2005;141(3):305–11.

59. Lessin SR, Duvic M, Guitart J, et al. Topical chemotherapy in cutaneous T-cell lymphoma: positive results of a randomized, controlled, multicenter trial testing the efficacy and safety of a novel mechlorethamine, 0.02%, gel in mycosis fungoides. JAMA Dermatol 2013;149(1):25–32.

60. Heald P, Mehlmauer M, Martin AG, et al. Topical bexarotene therapy for patients with refractory or

persistent early-stage cutaneous T-cell lymphoma: results of the phase III clinical trial. J Am Acad Dermatol 2003;49(5):801–15.

61. Kim YH, Demierre MF, Kim EJ, et al. Clinically meaningful reduction in pruritus in patients with cutaneous T-cell lymphoma treated with romidepsin. Leuk Lymphoma 2013;54(2):284–9.

62. Duvic M, Talpur R, Ni X, et al. Phase 2 trial of oral vorinostat (suberoylanilide hydroxamic acid, SAHA) for refractory cutaneous T-cell lymphoma (CTCL). Blood 2007;109(1):31–9.

63. Duvic M, Dummer R, Becker JC, et al. Panobinostat activity in both bexarotene-exposed and -naive patients with refractory cutaneous T-cell lymphoma: results of a phase II trial. Eur J Cancer 2013;49(2): 386–94.

64. Foss F, Advani R, Duvic M, et al. A Phase II trial of Belinostat (PXD101) in patients with relapsed or refractory peripheral or cutaneous T-cell lymphoma. Br J Haematol 2015;168(6):811–9.

65. Child F, Ortiz-Romero PL, Alvarez R, et al. Phase II multicentre trial of oral quisinostat, a histone deacetylase inhibitor, in patients with previously treated stage IB-IVA mycosis fungoides/Sezary syndrome. Br J Dermatol 2016;175(1):80–8.

66. Duvic M, Martin AG, Kim Y, et al. Phase 2 and 3 clinical trial of oral bexarotene (Targretin capsules) for the treatment of refractory or persistent early-stage cutaneous T-cell lymphoma. Arch Dermatol 2001; 137(5):581–93.

67. Sepmeyer JA, Greer JP, Koyama T, et al. Open-label pilot study of combination therapy with rosiglitazone and bexarotene in the treatment of cutaneous T-cell lymphoma. J Am Acad Dermatol 2007;56(4):584–7.

68. Straus DJ, Duvic M, Horwitz SM, et al. Final results of phase II trial of doxorubicin HCl liposome injection followed by bexarotene in advanced cutaneous T-cell lymphoma. Ann Oncol 2014;25(1):206–10.

69. Lundin J, Hagberg H, Repp R, et al. Phase 2 study of alemtuzumab (anti-CD52 monoclonal antibody) in patients with advanced mycosis fungoides/Sezary syndrome. Blood 2003;101(11):4267–72.

70. Bouwhuis SA, el-Azhary RA, Gibson LE, et al. Effect of insulin-dependent diabetes mellitus on response to extracorporeal photopheresis in patients with Sezary syndrome. J Am Acad Dermatol 2002; 47(1):63–7.

71. Kim YH, Duvic M, Obitz E, et al. Clinical efficacy of zanolimumab (HuMax-CD4): two phase 2 studies in refractory cutaneous T-cell lymphoma. Blood 2007;109(11):4655–62.

72. Duvic M, Pinter-Brown LC, Foss FM, et al. Phase 1/2 study of mogamulizumab, a defucosylated anti-CCR4 antibody, in previously treated patients with cutaneous T-cell lymphoma. Blood 2015;125(12): 1883–9.

73. Ogura M, Ishida T, Hatake K, et al. Multicenter phase II study of mogamulizumab (KW-0761), a defucosylated anti-cc chemokine receptor 4 antibody, in patients with relapsed peripheral T-cell lymphoma and cutaneous T-cell lymphoma. J Clin Oncol 2014; 32(11):1157–63.

74. Beck LA, Thaci D, Hamilton JD, et al. Dupilumab treatment in adults with moderate-to-severe atopic dermatitis. N Engl J Med 2014;371(2):130–9.

75. Ruzicka T, Mihara R. Anti-interleukin-31 receptor A antibody for atopic dermatitis. N Engl J Med 2017; 376(21):2093.

76. Dummer R, Beyer M, Hymes K, et al. Vorinostat combined with bexarotene for treatment of cutaneous T-cell lymphoma: in vitro and phase I clinical evidence supporting augmentation of retinoic acid receptor/retinoid X receptor activation by histone deacetylase inhibition. Leuk Lymphoma 2012; 53(8):1501–8.

77. Duvic M, Hymes K, Heald P, et al. Bexarotene is effective and safe for treatment of refractory advanced-stage cutaneous T-cell lymphoma: multinational phase II-III trial results. J Clin Oncol 2001; 19(9):2456–71.

78. Duvic M, Kuzel TM, Olsen EA, et al. Quality-of-life improvements in cutaneous T-cell lymphoma patients treated with denileukin diftitox (ONTAK). Clin Lymphoma 2002;2(4):222–8.

79. Espinoza-Zamora JR, Labardini-Mendez J, Sosa-Espinoza A, et al. Efficacy of hydralazine and valproate in cutaneous T-cell lymphoma, a phase II study. Expert Opin Investig Drugs 2017;26(4): 481–7.

80. Kennedy GA, Seymour JF, Wolf M, et al. Treatment of patients with advanced mycosis fungoides and Sezary syndrome with alemtuzumab. Eur J Haematol 2003;71(4):250–6.

81. Olsen EA, Kim YH, Kuzel TM, et al. Phase IIb multicenter trial of vorinostat in patients with persistent, progressive, or treatment refractory cutaneous T-cell lymphoma. J Clin Oncol 2007;25(21):3109–15.

Pruritus in Pregnancy and Its Management

Mark A. Bechtel, MD

KEYWORDS

- Pruritus • Pemphigoid gestationis • Polymorphic eruption of pregnancy
- Intrahepatic cholestasis of pregnancy • Atopic eruption of pregnancy

KEY POINTS

- Pemphigoid gestationis often involves the periumbilical region.
- Polymorphic eruption of pregnancy starts in the striae gravidarum.
- Intrahepatic cholestasis of pregnancy has no primary skin lesions, but may produce intense itching of the palms.
- Atopic eruption of pregnancy has the earliest onset during pregnancy, usually the first or second trimester.
- Pemphigoid gestationis has been associated with maternal autoimmune thyroid disease, and intrahepatic cholestasis of pregnancy with maternal hepatobiliary disease, gall stones, and hepatitis C.

Pruritus is the most common dermatologic complaint during pregnancy. It has been reported in 14% to 20% of pregnancies.[1] Most cases of pruritus are mild but some can be severe, interfering with sleep, producing mood changes, and affecting quality of life. The etiologic factors of pruritus during pregnancy can be directly related to pregnancy-specific dermatoses, allergic hypersensitivity reactions, and systemic diseases. Additional important causes of pruritus include atopic dermatitis, psoriasis, lichen sclerosus, lichen planus, vulvovaginal candidiasis, allergic and irritant contact dermatitis, and scabies.[2]

An underlying systemic cause of pruritus is important to consider if there is no specific cutaneous eruption. Considerations should include hepatic and renal disease, poorly controlled diabetes, and an underlying malignancy, such as lymphoma. Intense itching of the palms during the third trimester without a specific eruption may be an indication of intrahepatic cholestasis of pregnancy (ICP).[3] Pruritus during pregnancy in the setting of jaundice may indicate a more serious condition, such as hepatitis, acute fatty liver of pregnancy, severe ICP, or hyperbilirubinemia states.[1]

Many physiologic changes occur during pregnancy that can be exacerbate itching. There is abdominal stretching, edema of the legs, and xerosis. Important complex immunologic mechanisms at the maternal-fetal interface occur during pregnancy. The T helper (Th)-2-type profile predominates, whereas Th1 is downregulated. Important Th2 cytokines include interleukin (IL)-4, IL-5, IL-6. IL-10, IL-13, and transforming growth factor (TGF)-beta. Regulatory T cells, which suppress antigen-specific immune responses, are elevated during pregnancy. The change in the cytokine profile may exacerbate atopic dermatitis but improve psoriasis.[4] There are also fluctuating estrogen and progesterone levels.

Pregnancy-specific dermatoses are an important cause of pruritus during pregnancy and include ICP, atopic eruption of pregnancy (AEP), pemphigoid gestationis (PG), and polymorphic eruption of pregnancy (PEP). Some of the

Disclose: The author has nothing to disclose.
Division of Dermatology, Ohio State University College of Medicine, 540 Officenter Place, #240, Gahanna, OH 43230, USA
E-mail address: dermdocmab@aol.com

Dermatol Clin 36 (2018) 259–265
https://doi.org/10.1016/j.det.2018.02.012

disorders were reclassified, which can lead to confusion[5] (**Table 1**). Many of the pregnancy-specific dermatoses have distinct presentations of their rash and pruritus, as well as time of onset during pregnancy, which can help in diagnosis (**Fig. 1, Table 2**). **Box 1** presents skin rashes in genitals that can cause itch in pregnancy that are nonpregnancy associated.

PREGNANCY-SPECIFIC DERMATOSES
Polymorphic Eruption of Pregnancy

PEP was previously known as pruritic and urticarial papules and plaques of pregnancy (PUPPP syndrome). PEP is one of the most common dermatoses of pregnancy and occurs in approximately 1 in 200 pregnancies.[3] It typically presents in primigravidas late in the third trimester or immediately postpartum. Risk factors include multiple gestation pregnancies and increased maternal weight gain.[6] The pathophysiology of PEP is unknown but may be related to abdominal distention, immunologic factors, fetal cell microchimerism, and hormonal factors.[3] The onset of the eruption typically occurs late in the third trimester at the peak of stretching of abdominal skin. Many patients have multiple gestational pregnancies or excessive maternal weight gain, which maximizes abdominal stretching. A direct relationship with damage of the collagen fibers due to distension and overstretching of the skin is suspected.[7] This is supported by the onset of PEP within the striae gravidarum. One study showed that pregnant women with PEP had a significant reduction in serum cortisol levels, but normal levels of ß-human chorionic gonadotropin.[8] The rash initially presents in the striae distensae (**Fig. 2**) and then spreads to the trunk and proximal thighs. Typically, the rash spares the umbilicus, in contrast to PG. Clinically, the cutaneous lesions may be urticarial papules, eczematoid patches, targetoid lesions, vesicles, and bullae.[6]

Neonates do not develop skin lesions and the maternal and fetal prognosis is not affected.[9] Diagnosis of PEP is based on clinical presentation and history. The cutaneous histopathology is nonspecific and laboratory tests are unremarkable.

Treatment of PEP is symptomatic. Low-potency to mid-potency topical steroids are first-line treatment, along with bland emollients.[10] Oral antihistamines, such as chlorpheniramine and diphenhydramine, are first-line agents for pruritus. Loratadine remains the first choice and cetirizine the second choice among second-generation antihistamines.[11] Severe intractable pruritus can be treated with short courses of systemic steroids or ultraviolet B phototherapy.[8] Folic acid levels should be monitored during phototherapy and avoidance of high heat is advisable.[11] Prednisone is the preferred systemic steroid because placental enzymes limit passage to the embryo.[11] In some cases of PEP unresponsive to other treatments, early delivery may be a treatment of last resort.[12]

Table 1
Diagnostic features of the pregnancy-specific dermatoses

Condition	Onset	Clinical Features	Diagnosis	Treatment
ICP	Late second or third trimester	Pruritus, especially palms No primary skin lesions	Total bile acids >11 µmol/L	Ursodeoxy cholic acid 15 mg/kg/d or 1 gm
PEP	Third trimester or postpartum	Urticarial papules, plaques, vesicles, target lesions Initially involves striae gravidarum, spares umbilicus	No specific laboratory or skin biopsy findings, negative DIF	Topical or oral corticosteroids, antihistamines
PG	Second or third trimester or postpartum	Urticarial papules and bullae Umbilicus usually involved	Linear C_3 deposition along DEJ on DIF antibodies to BP 180	Topical or oral corticosteroids, antihistamines
AEP	First and second trimesters	Widespread eczematous excoriated papules, plaques, prurigo nodularis	Clinical appearance, elevated IgE	Emollients, topical steroids, light therapy, antihistamines

Abbreviations: BP, bullous pemphigoid; DEJ, dermal epidermal junction; DIF, direct immunofluorescence.

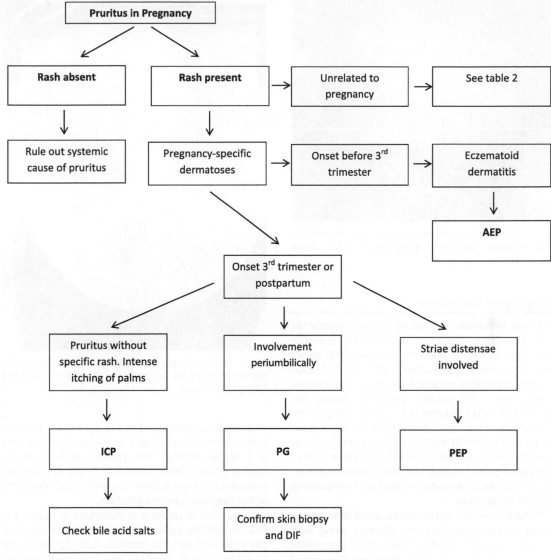

Fig. 1. Diagnostic evaluation of pregnancy pruritus. DIF, direct immunofluorescence.

Table 2
Non pregnancy specific diseases causing pruritus in pregnancy

- Lichen sclerosis
- Infectious vulvovaginitis
- Vulvovaginal candidiasis
- Allergic and irritant contact dermatitis
- Lichen simplex chronicus and neuropathic itch
- Psoriasis
- Drug hypersensitivity reactions
- Hepatic or renal dysfunction
- Underlying malignancy

Box 1
Nonpregnancy-specific skin diseases in women that cause pruritus in pregnancy

- Lichen sclerosis
- Infectious vulvovaginitis
- Vulvovaginal candidiasis
- Allergic and irritant contact dermatitis
- Lichen simplex chronicus and neuropathic itch
- Genital psoriasis
- Drug hypersensitivity reactions

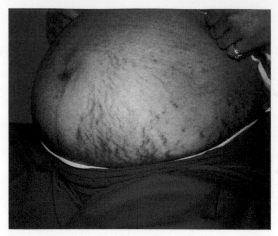

Fig. 2. An early manifestation of PEP is pruritic erythematous urticarial papules of the striae distensae.

Pemphigoid Gestationis

PG was previously known as herpes gestationis and is a rare autoimmune blistering disorder occurring in 1 in 50,000 pregnancies.[3] The disorder has been associated with trophoblastic tumors, including hydatidiform mole and choriocarcinoma.[13] PG usually presents during the second or third trimester but postpartum presentation is also common. Many patients experience flares at the time of delivery. Flares during subsequent menses, with oral contraceptive use, or during subsequent pregnancies have been reported. Fetal risks include preterm labor and intrauterine growth retardation.[14]

Patients present with an acute onset of erythematous urticarial papules and plaques along with vesicles and tense bullae. The lesions are similar to bullous pemphigoid (BP). Initial involvement of skin around the umbilicus and abdomen is common (**Fig. 3**). Umbilical involvement, although common in PG, is not seen in PEP.[10] There is sparing of the face and mucous membranes. An increased risk of Graves disease has been reported.[10]

There is an association with abnormal major histocompatibility complex II expression on amniochorionic stromal cells and trophoblasts, which results in exposure of BP 180 antigen to the maternal immune surveillance.[3] Maternal antiplacental immunoglobulin (Ig)G antibodies cross-react with BP 180 in the skin.[14] There is a high sensitivity of BP 180 enzyme-linked immunosorbent assay (ELISA) in detecting anti-BP-180 antibodies in patients with PG.[15]

The histology depends on the presentation and stage of the disease. In the prebullous stage with

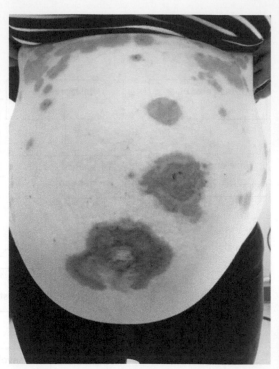

Fig. 3. Periumbilical papules and plaques with initial presentation of PG. (*Courtesy of* Amy Levinson, MSN CRNP, Doylestown, PA.)

erythematous plaques, there is a perivascular infiltrate of lymphocytes and eosinophils in the mid and upper dermis. The bullous stage demonstrates subepidermal blisters.[13] Direct immunofluorescence shows a linear C_3 and/or IgG deposits at the dermoepidermal junction.[15]

Reduction of pruritus is important in managing PG. Emollients containing pramoxine or menthol are safe and provide comfort. Low to moderate strength topical steroids are the treatment of choice but more potent topical steroids for short period of time may be necessary. Mild topical steroids should be used for intertriginous regions.

Systemic steroids to control pruritus and reduce blister formation are often required. Prednisone is the systemic steroid of choice. PG is usually controlled at 20 to 40 mg daily but severe cases require a dosage of 1 to 2 mg/kg[10] per day. Prednisone dosing should not be tapered until new blister formation has been stabilized for 2 weeks. A significant number of patients may flare at the time of delivery, requiring a temporary increase in prednisone. Calcium and vitamin D supplementation is recommended while on systemic steroids. An exacerbation in pregnancy-specific morbidities can occur due to systemic steroid, including gestational diabetes, eclampsia, preeclampsia, and hypertension.[16] Refractory cases of PG can be treated with intravenous IgG, along with systemic steroids. Intravenous IgG is a US Food and Drug Administration pregnancy class C.[16] In severe cases, after delivery and if not breastfeeding, patients can be treated similarly to BP with mycophenolate mofetil, azathioprine, cyclosporine, tetracycline, niacinamide, or (in resistant cases) rituximab.[3,10,16]

Atopic Eruption of Pregnancy

There is a dominant Th2 cytokine production during pregnancy. AEP encompasses prurigo of pregnancy, pruritic folliculitis of pregnancy, and eczema in pregnancy.[5] AEP represents the most common pruritic disorder of pregnancy and most cases present before the third trimester.[3] Although 20% of patients develop an exacerbation of preexisting atopic dermatitis, approximately 80% experience and eczematoid dermatitis for the first time or after a long period of remission.[13]

The most common presentation is an eczematous dermatitis in the classic atopic sites, including the antecubital and popliteal fossae, face, eyelids, and neck. Approximately one-third of patients with AEP present with nonspecific pruritic papules on the neck, trunk, and extremities.[3] Many patients demonstrate severe xerosis, excoriations, and prurigo nodularis.

Histopathology is nonspecific and direct immunofluorescence is negative. Serum IgE levels may be elevated.[13] The eruption may recur with subsequent pregnancies. There is no increased fetal or maternal risk.[3]

Intrahepatic Cholestasis of Pregnancy

ICP is a reversible cholestasis that occurs in genetically predisposed patients late in pregnancy.[13] A striking geographic variation is noted with an incidence as high as 28% in patients of Araucanian Indian ancestry in Chile. The prevalence in Europe is 0.1% to 1.5%.[17] Mutations in the gene adenosine triphosphate cassette canalicular transporter ABCB4 has been studied in ICP and may play an important role in some patients.[18]

Patients with ICP develop a reduction in excretion of bile acids with increased levels of bile acids crossing the placenta. This precipitates severe pruritus in the mother and fetal compromise due to placental anoxia and impaired cardiomyocyte function.[13] If ICP is suspected, it is important to check liver function tests, quantitated bile acid salts, and screen for hepatitis C.

The pregnant patient typically presents with severe pruritus in the late second or third trimester. Severe pruritus of the palms and soles is often the initial finding. There is no specific cutaneous eruption and

excoriations along with prurigo nodularis are often noted.[3] The pruritus usually resolves within 2 to 3 weeks after delivery. ICP may recur with future pregnancies and there is an increased association with hepatitis C and hepatobiliary disease.[19]

Maternal prognosis is favorable in ICP but severe jaundice is associated with an increased risk of bleeding. There is concern for the fetus with increased risk of preterm delivery, meconium-stained amniotic fluid, and stillbirths.[20] The fetal risks correlate with the level of bile acids.

There are significant elevations in IL-17 in severe cases of ICP.[21] Concentrations of progesterone sulfates are associated with itch severity and, in combination with autotaxin, help distinguish ICP from pruritus gravidarum. Progesterone sulfates mediate itch by evoking a Tgr5-dependent scratch response in mice.[22] Increased serum autotaxin activity is a highly specific diagnostic marker of ICP and distinguishes ICP from other pregnancy-related liver diseases.[23]

Lysophosphatidic acid (LPA) is an itch mediator found in cholestatic itch patients. Increased levels of LPA have been noted in patients with ICP. The increased levels of LPA correlate with highly significant increases in serum autotaxin, which correlate with the severity of itch.[24] LPA-induced itch is mediated by LPA5 receptor, phospholipase D, transient receptor potential ankyrin 1 (TRPA1), and vanilloid 1 (TRPV1) signaling. These may represent targets for cholestatic itch therapeutic interventions.[25]

Management of ICP requires an accurate and timely diagnosis. Advanced neonatal-obstetric management is essential. Patients with ICP are at increased risk for recurrence and first-degree relatives of ICP patients are also at increased risk.[3]

The primary goal in management of ICP is to reduce serum bile acid levels. This will reduce pruritus, prolong pregnancy, and reduce fetal risks.[3] Ursodeoxycholic acid (UDCA) is the treatment of choice and reduces maternal pruritus while improving fetal prognosis.[13] The drug is off-label when used in ICP. A dosage of 15 mg/kg/d or 1 g per day is administered as a single dose or divided into 2 to 3 doses before delivery.[10] Pruritus often improves in 2 to 3 weeks, along with decreases in total bile acids and alanine aminotransferase. In an observational study of 98 consecutive subjects treated with UDCA at 14 mg/kg/d, pruritus improved in 76.5% and totally resolved in 25.5% before delivery. Liver enzymes improved. There was no association with clinical response and the presence of ABCB4 gene mutation.[26]

Most stillbirths clustered at the 38th week. Patients with ICP with highly elevated serum bile acids (>40 μmol/L) should be considered for

Box 2
Management of pruritus in pregnancy

- Antihistamines[11]
  - Chlorpheniramine (US Food and Drug Administration [FDA]-B) first-line agent
  - Diphenhydramine (FDA-B) first-line agent
  - Loratadine (FDA-B) first choice of second generation
  - Cetirizine (FDA-B) second choice of second generation
- Systemic steroids[11]
  - Prednisone (preferred choice) limited passage through placenta
  - Increased risk of orofacial clefts
  - Try to limit exposure to dosage greater than 20 mg/d
  - Limit prolonged use to 7.5 mg/d
  - Need vitamin D and calcium supplementation
- Phototherapy[11]
  - Narrowband and broadband ultraviolet B are safe
  - Monitor folic acid levels
  - Avoid high heat

Data from Murase JE, Heller MM, Butler DC. Safety of dermatologic medications in pregnancy and lactation: part I. Pregnancy. J Am Acad Dermatol 2014;70(3):401.e1–14.

delivery at 37 weeks or earlier.[20] This was not associated with increased fetal risks.

SUMMARY

Pruritus in pregnancy is the most common dermatologic complaint during pregnancy and can significantly affect quality of life. Pruritus can be due to pregnancy-specific dermatoses, an exacerbation of preexisting dermatologic disease, or unrelated to pregnancy. It is important to make an accurate early diagnosis of the cause of pruritus and determine any maternal or fetal risks. Management of pruritus in pregnancy should take into consideration fetal risks (**Box 2**). Pruritus without a primary rash should prompt a workup for systemic causes.

REFERENCES

1. Meta N, Chen K, Kroumpouzos G. Skin disease in pregnancy: the approach of the obstetric medicine physician. Clin Dermatol 2016;34:320–6.

2. Rimoin L, Kwata S, Yosipovitch G. Female-specific pruritus from childhood to postmenopause: clinical features, hormonal factors, and treatment consideration. Dermatol Ther 2013;26(2):157–67.

3. Bechtel M, Plotner A. Dermatoses of pregnancy. Clin Obstet Gynecol 2015;58:104–11.

4. Gammill H, Shields LE, Waldorf KMA. Maternal-fetal immunology. In: Gabbe S, Niebyl J, Simpson J, et al, editors. Obstetrics normal and problem pregnancies. 6th edition. Philadelphia: Elsevier/Saunders; 2012. p. 66–82.

5. Ambrose-Rudolph CM, Müllegger RR, Vaughan-Jones SA, et al. The specific dermatoses of pregnancy revisited and reclassified: results of a retrospective two-center study on 505 pregnant patients. J Am Acad Dermatol 2006;54:395–404.

6. Rudolph CM, Al-Fares S, Vaughan-Jones SA, et al. Polymorphic eruption of pregnancy: clinicopathology and potential trigger factors in 181 patients. Br J Dermatol 2006;154:54–60.

7. Lambert J. Pruritus in female patients. Biomed Res Int 2014;2014:1–6.

8. Vaughan-Jones SA, Hern S, Nelson-Piercy C, et al. A prospective study of 200 women with dermatoses of pregnancy correlating clinical findings with hormonal and immunopathological profiles. Br J Dermatol 1999;141:71–81.

9. Ohel I, Levy A, Silerstein T, et al. Pregnancy outcome of patients with urticarial papules and plaques of pregnancy. J Matern Fetal Neonatal Med 2006;19:305–8.

10. Lehrhoff S, Pomeranz MK. Specific dermatoses of pregnancy and their treatment. Dermatol Ther 2015;26:274–84.

11. Murase JE, Heller MM, Butler DC. Safety of dermatologic medications in pregnancy and lactation: part I. Pregnancy. J Am Acad Dermatol 2014; 70(3):401.e1–14.

12. Beltrani VP, Beltrani VS. Pruritic urticarial papules and plaques of pregnancy: a severe case requiring early delivery for relief of symptoms. J Am Acad Dermatol 1992;26:266–7.

13. Ambrose-Rudolf CM. Dermatoses of pregnancy–clues to diagnosis, fetal risk, and therapy. Ann Dermatol 2011;23:265–75.

14. Beard MP, Millington GW. Recent developments in the specific dermatoses of pregnancy. Clin Exp Dermatol 2012;37:1–14.

15. Saif FA, Jouen F, Herbert V, et al. Sensitivity and specificity of BP180 NC16A enzyme-linked immunosorbent assay for the diagnosis of pemphigoid gestationis. J Am Acad Dermatol 2017; 76(3):560–2.

16. Braunstein I, Werth V. Treatment of dermatologic connective tissue disease and autoimmune blistering disorders in pregnancy. Dermatol Ther 2013; 26(4):354–63.

17. Lammert F, Marschall HU, Matern S. Intrahepatic cholestasis of pregnancy, molecular pathogenesis, diagnosis, and management. J Hepatol 2000;33: 1012–21.

18. Dixon PH. The pathophysiology in intrahepatic cholestasis of pregnancy. Clin Res Hepatol Gastroenterol 2016;40(2):141–53.

19. Bergman H, Melamed N, Koren G. Pruritus in pregnancy: treatment of dermatoses unique to pregnancy. Can Fam Physician 2013;59(12): 1290–4.

20. Geenes V, Chappell LC, Seed PT, et al. Association of severe intrahepatic cholestasis of pregnancy with adverse pregnancy outcomes: a prospective population-based case-controlled study. Hepatology 2014;59:1482–91.

21. Kirbas A, Biberoglu E, Ersoy AO, et al. The role of interleukin-17 in intrahepatic cholestasis of pregnancy. J Matern Fetal Neonatal Med 2016; 29(6):977–81.

22. Abu-Hayyeh S, Ovadia C, Lieu T, et al. Prognostic and mechanistic potential of progesterone sulfates in intrahepatic cholestasis of pregnancy and pruritus gravidarum. Hepatology 2016;63:1287–98.

23. Kremer AE, Boiler R, Dixon PH, et al. Autotaxin activity has a high accuracy to diagnose intrahepatic cholestasis of pregnancy. J Hepatol 2015;62(4): 897–904.

24. Elferink R, Bolier R, Beuers U. Lysophosphatidic acid and signaling in sensory neurons. Biochim Biophys Acta 2015;1851:61–5.

25. Kittaka H, Uchida K, Fukuta N, et al. Lysophosphatidic acid-induced itch is mediated by signaling of LPA5 receptor, phospholipase D and TRPA1/TRPV1. J Physiol 2017;595(8):2681–98.

26. Bacq Y, leBesco M, Lecuyer A, et al. Ursodeoxycholic acid therapy in intrahepatic cholestasis of pregnancy: results in real-world conditions and factors predictive of response to treatment. Dig Liver Dis 2017;49(1):63–9.

Pruritus in Autoimmune Connective Tissue Diseases

Gideon P. Smith, MD, MPH, PhD[a], Yahya Argobi, MD[b],*

KEYWORDS

• Pruritus • Itch • Connective tissue • Lupus • Dermatomyositis • Systemic sclerosis • Sjögren

KEY POINTS

• Autoimmune connective tissue diseases (ACTDs) have prominent skin manifestations and commonly present with pruritus.
• Triggers of pruritus in ACTDs are diverse from disease related to medication side effects and malignancy development.
• It's important to work-up pruritus in ACTDs to treat patients appropriately according to the underlying cause independent of disease activity.

INTRODUCTION

The autoimmune connective tissue diseases (ACTDs) are a broad range of diseases (eg, the most common being lupus, dermatomyositis [DM], systemic sclerosis [SSc], and Sjögren syndrome), often with multisystem involvement. Their unifying feature is that a person's own immune system is dysregulated. Although these diseases are commonly primarily managed by rheumatologists, they often have prominent skin manifestations. The primary symptom of skin findings is either pruritus, or burning. Just as the diseases themselves are diverse, however, so are the causes of these symptoms. This article addresses the most common triggers for pruritus in these patients, the appropriate work-up, and the evidence behind different treatment regimens when pruritus occurs, whether dependent on or independent of disease activity.

DERMATOMYOSITIS

Itch and Cutaneous Dermatomyositis

Pruritus is a prominent feature in DM and has a significant impact on patients' quality of life.[1] A pruritus questionnaire of 70 DM subjects showed that subjects had a mean score of 44.6 on the 100-mm visual analog scale (VAS) in response to effect of itching on daily life.[2] A prospective study[3] conducted to compare clinical characteristics of DM, its relationship to malignancy, and treatment between 2 tertiary medical centers in the United States and Singapore reported that itch was the most common initial symptom among both populations, representing 63% and 80% of patients in the United States and Singapore, respectively.

Although photosensitivity in DM is similar to that of SSc lupus erythematosus (SLE),[4] pruritus evaluated by a VAS and a 0 to 10 scale in DM and in cutaneous lupus erythematosus (CLE) populations found that DM produces more pruritus than CLE (P<.0001).[5] This is possibly consistent with the observation that DM patients are more diffusely erythematous than SLE patients even when disease is relatively quiescent. Photoprotection is important and DM patients must be counseled to use broad-spectrum sunscreens that incorporate UV-A and UV-B blocking elements, to reapply

Disclosure Statement: The authors have nothing to disclose.
[a] Department of Dermatology, Connective Tissue Diseases Clinic, MGH, Bartlett Hall 622, Boston, MA 02114, USA; [b] Department of Dermatology, King Khalid University, College of Medicine, PO Box 641, Abha 61421, Saudi Arabia
* Corresponding author.
E-mail address: Yahya.derm@gmail.com

Dermatol Clin 36 (2018) 267–275
https://doi.org/10.1016/j.det.2018.02.013

sunscreen frequently, to remain out of direct sunlight as much as possible (especially between the hours of 10:00 AM and 2:00 PM), and to use physical barriers, such as broad-brimmed hats and long sleeves. The use of topical and SSc immunosuppressants can be helpful, although patients with DM are more likely to have an adverse cutaneous reaction to antimalarial therapy than SLE patients.[6]

Itch and Comorbidity Considerations in Dermatomyositis

The contribution of pharmacotherapy either as itch as a medication side effect or the medications effects on internal organs should be considered in the itchy DM patient (**Fig. 1**). Although DM is significantly associated with malignancy, with up to 30% of patients with DM having an associated malignancy,[7] hemoproliferative forms are extremely rare in DM.

LUPUS
Itch and Cutaneous Systemic Sclerosis Lupus Erythematosus

The term, *lupus*, can refer to disease limited to the skin, such as chronic CLE, also known as discoid lupus erythematosus (DLE); to subacute cutaneous lupus (SCLE), a different skin-only form; or to the SSc multisystem form SLE. Even in SLE, DLE and SCLE may occur. Itch can occur, however, with or without cutaneous involvement.

In a review of 91 SLE patients meeting American College of Rheumatology diagnostic criteria, 81% of SLE patients had clinical photosensitivity. Although some of these were SLE-specific photosensitivity, others had conditions, such as polymorphous light eruptions and solar urticaria.[4] These latter reactions were found more common in SLE than in the general population and it is unclear if the photosensitive triggering of different conditions is a comorbidity or if SLE photosensitivity may itself be more polymorphous in its presentation than previously thought. This same study found, however, that the more severe photosensitive cutaneous findings were associated with more severe disease flares, regardless of the form, possibly supporting the latter contention. Pruritus may be an early warning sign, because questionnaire data suggest that both SLE and DM patients experience skin pruritus on average 9.5 years before diagnosis, a finding not found in the same study in SSc patients.[8] Although some investigators suggest that photosensitivity varies by ethnic origin, with darker skin showing less photosensitivity,[9] others have not found this the case.[4] Recommendations for photoprotection for SLE patients are similar to those for DM patients.

Immunosuppression, topical with corticosteroids, calcineurin inhibitors, or calcipotriene, can assist in decreasing inflammation and thereby the symptom of pruritus, and some patients need SSc suppression with oral corticosteroids or steroid-sparing agents, such as methotrexate, mycopheolate mofetil, azathioprine, and thalidomide, among other options. Minimally

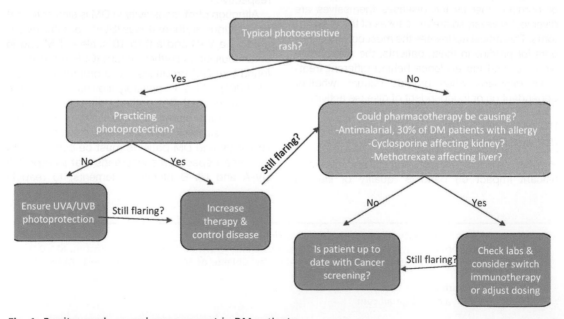

Fig. 1. Pruritus work-up and management in DM patients.

immunosuppressive therapy is also available, such as with antimalarials, dapsone, and retinoids. A full review of these treatment options for cutaneous manifestations of SLE is presented elsewhere.[10,11]

Itch and Medications in Systemic Sclerosis Lupus Erythematosus

If a patient has been well controlled on antimalarials and begins to flare, careful history, including smoking, should be taken because it has been suggested that smoking may flare lupus[12] or make antimalarials less effective,[13] although both of these assertions remain somewhat controversial.

In evaluating patients with well-controlled SSc disease but persistent pruritus, particular attention should be paid to medications (**Fig. 2**). Antimalarials remain a mainstay of SLE treatment, because of their low side-effect profile and because of the suggestion that they can help reduce flares and possibly ameliorate progression to kidney involvement.[14] In a review of 209 patients on antimalarials, however, 76% were found to have cutaneous side effects.[15] The most common is xerosis, followed by hyperpigmentation ($P<.0001$) and pruritus; although pruritus failed to meet statistical significance ($P<.39$) compared with a control group, it has also been reported with strong temporal association with the drug challenge.[16] In addition to nontriggered itch, aquagenic itch

has been specifically cited in association with antimalarials.[17] In some cases, switching from one antimalarial to another can reduce or eliminate side effects.[6]

Pruritus is a major side effect of antimalarial chloroquine use and is an important cause of noncompliance, especially in Africans compared with white populations.[18] It has been shown that chloroquine stimulates itch nerves by activating the G protein–coupled receptor (GPCR) Mrgpr, expressed exclusively in peripheral sensory neurons.[19] *Mrgpr* genes are highly polymorphic, which underlies the ethnic variation in chloroquine induced itch.

Although antimalarials remain the most common medication SLE patients are on, other medications should also be examined in terms of timing and the initiation of pruritus, because not only is pruritus as a side effect common but also other side effects that cause pruritus can occur, such as kidney insufficiency with cyclosporine; liver damage with methotrexate; xerosis, prominent with retinoid use; and neuropathy, in dapsone and thalidomide. All of these should be carefully screened for.

Itch and Systemic Sclerosis Involvement or Comorbidities of Systemic Sclerosis Lupus Erythematosus

Finally, in the review of systems, evaluation of noncutaneous disease involvement causing

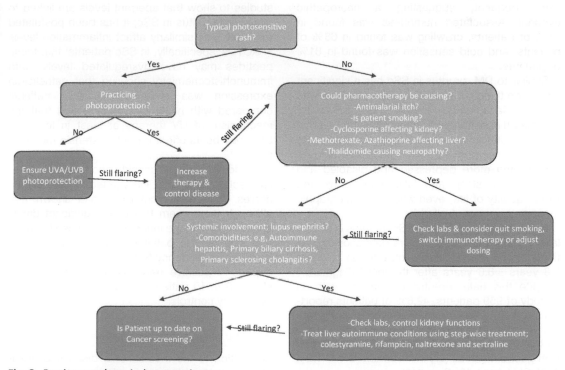

Fig. 2. Pruritus work-up in lupus patients.

pruritus should be evaluated. In SLE, the biggest concern is for SLE nephritis as pruritus can be a prominent component in declining kidney function, occurring in 50% to 90% of patients with end-stage renal disease.[20] Management of this is with close management of kidney function, often cyclophosphamide for active lupus nephritis, and, in cases of end-stage renal disease, optimization of dialysis. Although liver function enzyme abnormalities are common, occurring at some point in their disease course in up to 60% of patients, most commonly this is associated with hepatotoxic drugs or viral infections.[21] Less common in SLE but also possible as an overlap in any of the ACTDs are autoimmune hepatitis, primary sclerosing cholangitis,[22] or primary biliary cirrhosis (PBC).

SYSTEMIC SCLEROSIS
Itch and Cutaneous Systemic Sclerosis

A recent questionnaire[23] of SSc patients who were followed from 2000 to 2015 reported that of 61 patients, 38 (62%) suffered from pruritus. The study found that pruritus was more frequent in the evening and 15 patients (40%) had pruritus at the skin areas affected by SSc. Fatigue, stress, dry skin, and specific clothes increased the intensity of pruritus, whereas rest, sleep, hot water, and hot ambient temperature slightly decreased pruritus. Sensory symptoms on the extremities were frequent, suggesting a neuropathic element. Associated numbness was found in 71% of patients, crawling was found in 68% of patients, and cold sensation was found in 61% of patients.

Similar to DM, pruritus in SSc has a significant impact on the quality of life. A total of 964 patients from the Canadian SSc Research Group Registry completed questionnaires measuring itch severity, pain severity, function, and quality of life.[24] SSc subjects who reported higher itch severity were also feeling more depressed and disabled and having more sleep and fatigue problems and worse quality of life, even when all demographic measures were controlled for.

In contrast to SLE/DM, in SSc, pruritus is often a later finding, with questionnaire data showing patients first recalling this symptom on average 2.8 years ±8.6 years after the initial diagnosis.[8] Despite this data, pruritus is common with, in 1 study of 959 patients, 42.6% of patients reporting pruritus.[25] The pruritus correlated both with the degree of skin involvement (odds ratio [OR] = 1.02; 95% CI, 1.00, 1.04; $P = .017$), and with gastrointestinal (GI) involvement (OR = 1.24; 95% CI, 1.04; 1.48; $P = .018$).

In part, the increased pruritus with skin involvement is likely due to increased damage from sclerotic annihilation of adnexal structures, resulting in lower endogenous cutaneous lubrication production as well as distribution of what is produced throughout a thickened dermis.[26] A prospective, case-controlled study of 68 SSc patients compared with 66 healthy controls showed there is a marked increased rate of hand xerosis in SSc (71%) versus in healthy controls (32%).[27] This can in part be ameliorated by advising good skin care, with shorter, cooler bathing due to the stripping of what little oils are being produced by hot water, use of nondetergent soaps, avoidance of waterless soaps, and copious use of moisturizers. Although prescription moisturizers designed to reduce transepidermal water loss exist, most have been developed in the context of inadequate epidermal function in atopic dermatitis and even in that condition their effectiveness over-the-counter moisturizers is controversial.[28] No products specific to sclerodermatous skin have been scientifically developed, and studies on the utility and comparative effectiveness of those products in existence are still needed in this disease state.

There is evidence, however, that not only may the prevention of transepidermal water loss be important in driving atopic skin but also the change in antimicrobial peptides, such as canthelecidins and beta-defensins.[29] Although there are no studies to show that aberrant levels are linked to increased pruritus in SSc, it has been postulated that they may similarly affect inflammation levels in ACTDs, specifically, in SSc patients; that these peptides may have dysregulated levels, with immunohistochemistry showing that cathelicidin expression was enhanced in SSc patients compared with healthy controls[30]; and that the mechanism of UV therapy at least in localized SSc may be its effect on beta-defensin molecule levels.[31]

In addition to these considerations, the progressive sclerosis is also likely affecting cutaneous nerves. Immunohistochemistry has shown that although there seem to be no significant differences in peptidergic innervation between the forearm skin of SSc patients and healthy controls, there was a tendency to higher density of neuropeptide Y–positive nerve fibers in the forearm skin in 6 to 10 patients compared with only 1 of 10 healthy controls.[32]

Itch and Medications in Systemic Sclerosis

In addition to the medications, discussed previously, calcium channel blockers are commonly prescribed in SSc for Raynaud disease and have been particularly associated in elderly patients with a cause of itch[33,34] (**Fig. 3**).

Itch and Malignancy Considerations in Systemic Sclerosis

SSc has been also associated with an increased risk for various malignancies, including non-Hodgkin lymphoma (NHL) and hematological cancers.[35,36] Anti-RNA polymerase III antibody in particular has been associated with higher risk of malignancy development in SSc.[37–39]

Therapy folr Itch in Systemic Sclerosis

Although antihistamines are often the first, and sometimes only, medication given for itch, a double-blind, randomized controlled trial of ketotifen versus placebo in early diffuse SSc demonstrated that mast cell stabilizing therapy has little effect in pruritus of SSc. This is likely because mast cell dysregulation is not believed a significant component of the itch, and density of mast cells is not increased in pruritic SSc patients over healthy controls.[40]

Although there are no studies to date on the use of UV for itch in SSc sclerodermatous skin, there are studies of UV for the sclerosis of sclerodermatous skin and UV for the symptom of itch. Although the results of the studies of UV for sclerosis of sclerodermatous skin are highly variable, with some cases in the literature reporting near-complete remission of sclerodermatous skin, the majority show limited if any improvement in skin.[41,42] Most of these studies have been done with UV-A, due to its deeper penetration. There is also some evidence for the reduction of itch in localized SSc

(morphea) a clinically distinct yet histopathologically identical condition where sclerotic skin occurs in localized plaques. In studies of morphea skin, status significantly improved on average in all studies, resulting in significant reduction in clinical score.[43] Although low-dose (LD) and medium-dose (MD) UV-A1 produced similar clinical results they were significantly more effective than narrow band UV-B (NBUV-B) when judged on clinical skin score. Only NBUV-B, however, showed improvement in histologic grading (decreased thickness, decreased elastic fibers, and decreased infiltrate). VAS score for tightness and itching significantly decreased in MD UV-A1, but in LD UV-A1 and NBUV-B only tightness improved. Results of UV-A seem independent of skin type.[44] In itch, both UV-A and NBUV-B have been studied, both generally of benefit over a wide range of underlying triggers, whether skin inflammation, such as atopic dermatitis[45]; SSc itch, such as with cholestasis[46]; or renal disease.[47,48]

One therapy for potential multifaceted benefit is serotonin reuptake inhibitors. Not only have they been used effectively in controlling itch in a variety of conditions, including prurigo, atopic dermatitis, cholestasis, psychogenic pruritus, paraneoplastic pruritus, and polycythemia vera,[48] but also they have been shown as effective as nifedipine in the control of Raynaud,[49] which can be a prominent and difficult aspect of SSc and important to ulcer formation and sclerodactyly progression.

In a case series of 3 patients with RNA polymerase III–positive SSc, all 3 failed antihistamines and selective serotonin reuptake inhibitor (sertraline) therapy but responded well to LD naltrexone. Each patient was initiated on 2 mg by mouth at

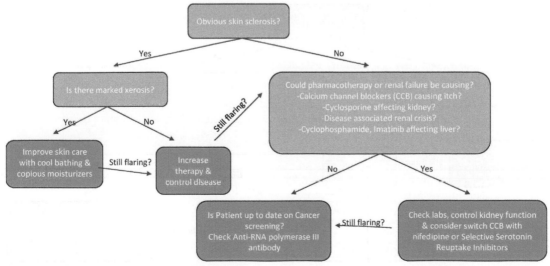

Fig. 3. Work-up of chronic pruritus in SSc.

bedtime for the first month. The dose was increased by 1 mg by mouth at bedtime each week (0.5 mg the final week) up to a maximum dose of 4.5 mg.

SJÖGREN SYNDROME
Itch and Cutaneous Sjögren syndrome

The most well-known features of Sjögren syndrome are dry eyes and dry mouth. In the eyes this dryness can produce a sensation of grittiness, a foreign body, or itch. Beyond artificial tears, a trial of 60 Sjögren syndrome patients showed a statistically significant improvement in subjective and objective measures using cevimeline, 20 mg 3 times daily, a muscarinic acetylcholine receptor agonist, when compared with placebo.[50] In addition, although a less well-known feature, xerosis of the skin seems increased in this condition.[51] A recent questionnaire for the assessment of pruritus of 19 patients with primary Sjögren syndrome showed 90% suffering from xerosis and 53% suffering from chronic itch with VAS 7.7 ± 1.7. The onset of the itch ranged from 11 years prior to diagnosis of primary Sjögren syndrome to 3 years after the diagnosis.[52]

Itch and Systemic Sclerosis and Comorbidities in Sjögren Syndrome

Sjögren syndrome is also the disease most commonly associated autoimmune disease of the GI system, including autoimmune hepatitis[53] and PBC. In 1 study of 322 Chinese PBC patients, 46.6% had 1 or more CTDs, the most common being Sjögren syndrome, which accounted for 36.2% of cases.[54] These diseases also can occur, however, in the context of IgG4 infiltration of these organs in IgG4 disease.[55] Pruritus has been reported in up to 70% of patients with cholestatic liver disease, most commonly in patients with PBC. It is believed to result from accumulation of bile salts in the plasma and tissues and dysregulation of endogenous opioids. Recently, a correlation was found between itching and lysophosphatidic acid, a potent neuronal activator. Unlike in cholestasis of pregnancy, ursodeoxycholic acid does not improve itch in PBC.[56] The American Association for the Study of Liver Diseases and the European Association for the Study of the Liver recommended a stepwise treatment using cholestyramine, rifampicin, naltrexone, and sertraline.[57]

Finally, Sjögren syndrome is also the autoimmune disease most commonly associated with vasculitis and neuropathy[58] and has been shown to have a high prevalence of small fiber polyneuropathy.[59] Although the primary findings in these conditions are burning, allodynia, and pain, itch can also be a component. In such cases, initial treatment is directed at suppressing nerve damage through immunosuppressants or, especially in the case of small fiber polyneuropathy, intravenous immunoglobulin (IVIG).[60,61] Once ongoing damage has been repressed, residual symptoms due to neural damage are best managed with neuromodulatory medications, such as pregabalin and gabapentin, or topical neuromodulators, such as tricyclic antidepressants and ketamine (Fig. 4).

Although urticaria can be a component of multiple SSc autoimmune diseases, its recognition is usually not a diagnostic quandary, and its

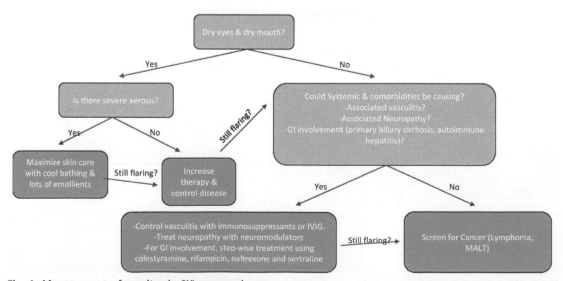

Fig. 4. Management of pruritus in Sjögren syndrome.

management, whether via high-dose antihistamines, immunosuppression, or targeted biologic therapy, is discussed elsewhere.[62]

Itch and Malignancy in Sjögren syndrome

Sjögren syndrome has been associated with hematological malignancy risk. A meta-analysis[63] of 14 studies, including more than 14,523 patients with primary Sjögren syndrome, reported significant increased risk of overall malignancy, NHL, and thyroid cancer. A Spanish study[64] of 1300 consecutive patients with primary Sjögren syndrome showed an 11-fold higher risk of developing hematological cancers than the general population. One-third of the cancers developed during the study were B-cell lymphomas; mucosa-associated lymphoid tissue (MALT) lymphomas accounted for 60% of B-cell lymphomas. Another retrospective study[65] of 25-year outcome of 152 patients with primary Sjögren syndrome reported that malignancy affected 28.3% and NHL affected 10.5%. Hemoproliferative cancers can contribute significantly to pruritus, so a change in this without a change in disease activity should give consideration to re-review of malignancy screening.

MIXED CONNECTIVE TISSUE DISEASE

Mixed connective tissue disease (MCTD) is a SSc autoimmune disease characterized by overlapping features between 2 or more connective tissue diseases and the presence of anti-ribonucleoprotein antibodies. The skin involvement of MCTD usually includes sclerodermatous changes and lupus-like manifestations. MCTD patients can have photosensitivity, pruritus, DLE, SCLE, and vasculitis.[66] Photoprotection and treating the primary skin lesions are recommended.

SUMMARY

ACTDs often present with pruritus that range from tolerable itch to severe intractable itch. Usually the itch is triggered by the disease activity. It can be triggered by other causes, however, including system organ involvement, medications side effects, and malignancy development. Therefore, careful history taking and work-up are crucial. Treatment of the itch in connective tissue diseases is disappointing and there is no single effective therapy. It is important to understand the itch pathogenesis in each case to reach the appropriate therapy.

REFERENCES

1. Hundley JL, Carroll CL, Lang W, et al. Cutaneous symptoms of dermatomyositis significantly impact patients' quality of life. J Am Acad Dermatol 2006; 54(2):217–20.
2. Shirani Z, Kucenic MJ, Carroll CL, et al. Pruritus in adult dermatomyositis. Clin Exp Dermatol 2004; 29(3):273–6.
3. Yosipovitch G, Tan A, LoSicco K, et al. A comparative study of clinical characteristics, work-up, treatment, and association to malignancy in dermatomyositis between two tertiary skin centers in the USA and Singapore. Int J Dermatol 2013; 52(7):813–9.
4. Foering K, Chang AY, Piette EW, et al. Characterization of clinical photosensitivity in cutaneous lupus erythematosus. J Am Acad Dermatol 2013;69(2): 205–13.
5. Goreshi R, Chock M, Foering K, et al. Quality of life in dermatomyositis. J Am Acad Dermatol 2011;65(6): 1107–16.
6. Pelle MT, Callen JP. Adverse cutaneous reactions to hydroxychloroquine are more common in patients with dermatomyositis than in patients with cutaneous lupus erythematosus. Arch Dermatol 2002;138(9): 1231–3 [discussion: 3].
7. Travassos AR, Borges-Costa J, Filipe P, et al. Malignancy associated with dermatomyositis - a retrospective single-center study with 33 patients. Acta Reumatol Port 2013;38(2):92–7.
8. Schroder L, Hertl M, Chatzigeorgakidis E, et al. Chronic pruritus in autoimmune dermatoses : results of a comparative survey. Hautarzt 2012;63(7): 558–66 [in German].
9. Ward MM, Studenski S. Clinical manifestations of systemic lupus erythematosus. Identification of racial and socioeconomic influences. Arch Intern Med 1990;150(4):849–53.
10. Schairer D, Friedman A. Manifestations and treatment of cutaneous lupus erythematosus (Part II of II). J Drugs Dermatol 2011;10(12):1474–6.
11. Schairer D, Friedman A. Manifestations and treatment of cutaneous lupus erythematosus (part I of II). J Drugs Dermatol 2011;10(10):1212–4.
12. Bourre-Tessier J, Peschken CA, Bernatsky S, et al. Association of smoking with cutaneous manifestations in systemic lupus erythematosus. Arthritis Care Res (Hoboken) 2013;65(8):1275–80.
13. Dutz J, Werth VP. Cigarette smoking and response to antimalarials in cutaneous lupus erythematosus patients: evolution of a dogma. J Invest Dermatol 2011;131(10):1968–70.
14. Pons-Estel GJ, Alarcon GS, McGwin G Jr, et al. Protective effect of hydroxychloroquine on renal damage in patients with lupus nephritis: LXV, data from a multiethnic US cohort. Arthritis Rheum 2009; 61(6):830–9.
15. Skare T, Ribeiro CF, Souza FH, et al. Antimalarial cutaneous side effects: a study in 209 users. Cutan Ocul Toxicol 2011;30(1):45–9.

16. Gul U, Cakmak SK, Kilic A, et al. A case of hydroxy-chloroquine induced pruritus. Eur J Dermatol 2006; 16(5):586–7.

17. Jimenez-Alonso J, Tercedor J, Jaimez L, et al. Anti-malarial drug-induced aquagenic-type pruritus in patients with lupus. Arthritis Rheum 1998;41(4): 744–5.

18. Tey HL, Yosipovitch G. Itch in ethnic populations. Acta Derm Venereol 2010;90(3):227–34.

19. Liu Q, Tang Z, Surdenikova L, et al. Sensory neuron-specific GPCR Mrgprs are itch receptors mediating chloroquine-induced pruritus. Cell 2009;139(7): 1353–65.

20. Brewster UC. Dermatological disease in patients with CKD. Am J Kidney Dis 2008;51(2):331–44.

21. Beisel C, Weiler-Normann C, Teufel A, et al. Associ-ation of autoimmune hepatitis and systemic lupus er-ythematodes: a case series and review of the literature. World J Gastroenterol 2014;20(35): 12662–7.

22. Alberti-Flor JJ, Jeffers L, Schiff ER. Primary scle-rosing cholangitis occurring in a patient with sys-temic lupus erythematosus and diabetes mellitus. Am J Gastroenterol 1984;79(11):889–91.

23. Théréné C, Brenaut E, Sonbol H, et al. Itch and sys-temic sclerosis: frequency, clinical characteristics and consequences. Br J Dermatol 2017;176(5): 1392–3.

24. Racine M, Hudson M, Baron M, et al. The impact of pain and itch on functioning and health-related qual-ity of life in systemic sclerosis: an exploratory study. J Pain Symptom Manage 2016;52(1):43–53.

25. Razykov I, Levis B, Hudson M, et al. Prevalence and clinical correlates of pruritus in patients with sys-temic sclerosis: an updated analysis of 959 patients. Rheumatology (Oxford) 2013;52(11):2056–61.

26. Haber JS, Valdes-Rodriguez R, Yosipovitch G. Chronic pruritus and connective tissue disorders: re-view, gaps, and future directions. Am J Clin Derma-tol 2016;17(5):445–9.

27. Serup J, Rasmussen I. Dry hands in scleroderma. Including studies of sweat gland function in healthy individuals. Acta Derm Venereol 1985;65(5):419–23.

28. Nolan K, Marmur E. Moisturizers: reality and the skin benefits. Dermatol Ther 2012;25(3):229–33.

29. Kahlenberg JM, Kaplan MJ. Little peptide, big ef-fects: the role of LL-37 in inflammation and autoim-mune disease. J Immunol 2013;191(10):4895–901.

30. Kim HJ, Cho DH, Lee KJ, et al. LL-37 suppresses sodium nitroprusside-induced apoptosis of systemic sclerosis dermal fibroblasts. Exp Dermatol 2011; 20(10):843–5.

31. Kreuter A, Hyun J, Skrygan M, et al. Ultraviolet A1-induced downregulation of human beta-defensins and interleukin-6 and interleukin-8 correlates with clinical improvement in localized scleroderma. Br J Dermatol 2006;155(3):600–7.

32. Wallengren J, Akesson A, Scheja A, et al. Occur-rence and distribution of peptidergic nerve fibers in skin biopsies from patients with systemic scle-rosis. Acta Derm Venereol 1996;76(2):126–8.

33. Berger TG, Shive M, Harper GM. Pruritus in the older patient: a clinical review. JAMA 2013;310(22): 2443–50.

34. Valdes-Rodriguez R, Stull C, Yosipovitch G. Chronic pruritus in the elderly: pathophysiology, diagnosis and management. Drugs Aging 2015;32(3):201–15.

35. Zhang JQ, Wan YN, Peng WJ, et al. The risk of cancer development in systemic sclerosis: a meta-analysis. Cancer Epidemiol 2013;37(5):523–7.

36. Kaşifoğlu T, Yaşar Bilge Ş, Yıldız F, et al. Risk factors for malignancy in systemic sclerosis patients. Clin Rheumatol 2016;35(6):1529–33.

37. Saigusa R, Asano Y, Nakamura K, et al. Association of anti RNA polymerase III antibody and malignancy in Japanese patients with systemic sclerosis. J Dermatol 2015;42(5):524–7.

38. Airò P, Ceribelli A, Cavazzana I, et al. Malignancies in italian patients with systemic sclerosis positive for Anti-RNA polymerase III antibodies. J Rheumatol 2011;38(7):1329–34.

39. Lazzaroni MG, Cavazzana I, Colombo E, et al. Ma-lignancies in patients with Anti-RNA Polymerase III antibodies and systemic sclerosis: analysis of the EULAR scleroderma trials and research cohort and possible recommendations for screening. J Rheumatol 2017;44(5):639–47.

40. Frech T, Novak K, Revelo MP, et al. Low-dose naltrexone for pruritus in systemic sclerosis. Int J Rheumatol 2011;2011:804296.

41. Rombold S, Lobisch K, Katzer K, et al. Efficacy of UVA1 phototherapy in 230 patients with various skin diseases. Photodermatol Photoimmunol Pho-tomed 2008;24(1):19–23.

42. Pereira N, Santiago F, Oliveira H, et al. Low-dose UVA(1) phototherapy for scleroderma: what benefit can we expect? J Eur Acad Dermatol Venereol 2012;26(5):619–26.

43. Kroft EB, Berkhof NJ, van de Kerkhof PC, et al. Ultra-violet A phototherapy for sclerotic skin diseases: a systematic review. J Am Acad Dermatol 2008; 59(6):1017–30.

44. Jacobe HT, Cayce R, Nguyen J. UVA1 phototherapy is effective in darker skin: a review of 101 patients of Fitzpatrick skin types I-V. Br J Dermatol 2008;159(3): 691–6.

45. Hong J, Buddenkotte J, Berger TG, et al. Manage-ment of itch in atopic dermatitis. Semin Cutan Med Surg 2011;30(2):71–86.

46. Pinheiro NC, Marinho RT, Ramalho F, et al. Refrac-tory pruritus in primary biliary cirrhosis. BMJ Case Rep 2013;2013 [pii:bcr2013200634].

47. Mettang T, Kremer AE. Uremic pruritus. Kidney Int 2014;87(4):685–91.

48. Steinhoff M, Cevikbas F, Ikoma A, et al. Pruritus: management algorithms and experimental therapies. Semin Cutan Med Surg 2011;30(2):127–37.

49. Coleiro B, Marshall SE, Denton CP, et al. Treatment of Raynaud's phenomenon with the selective serotonin reuptake inhibitor fluoxetine. Rheumatology (Oxford) 2001;40(9):1038–43.

50. Ono M, Takamura E, Shinozaki K, et al. Therapeutic effect of cevimeline on dry eye in patients with Sjogren's syndrome: a randomized, double-blind clinical study. Am J Ophthalmol 2004;138(1):6–17.

51. Rashtak S, Pittelkow MR. Skin involvement in systemic autoimmune diseases. Curr Dir Autoimmun 2008;10:344–58.

52. Valdes-Rodriguez R, Rowe B, Lee HG, et al. Chronic pruritus in primary sjögren's syndrome: characteristics and effect on quality of life. Acta Derm Venereol 2017;97(3):385–6.

53. Paredes Millan M, Chirinos Montes NJ, Martinez Apaza A, et al. The most common rheumatic diseases in patients with autoimmune liver disease in the Hospital Arzobispo Loayza from 2008 -2013, Lima, Peru. Rev Gastroenterol Peru 2014;34(4): 305–10 [in Spanish].

54. Wang L, Zhang FC, Chen H, et al. Connective tissue diseases in primary biliary cirrhosis: a population-based cohort study. World J Gastroenterol 2013; 19(31):5131–7.

55. Frider B, Bruno A, Zylberman M, et al. Autoimmune cholangitis associated to IgG4 related sclerosing disease. Acta Gastroenterol Latinoam 2011;41(1): 55–9.

56. Levy C. Management of pruritus in patients with cholestatic liver disease. Gastroenterol Hepatol (N Y) 2011;7(9):615–7.

57. Hegade VS, Kendrick SF, Jones DE. Drug treatment of pruritus in liver diseases. Clin Med (Lond) 2015; 15(4):351–7.

58. Seror R, Theander E, Bootsma H, et al. Outcome measures for primary Sjogren's syndrome: a comprehensive review. J Autoimmun 2014;51:51–6.

59. Fauchais AL, Richard L, Gondran G, et al. Small fibre neuropathy in primary Sjogren syndrome. Rev Med Interne 2011;32(3):142–8 [in French].

60. Wakasugi D, Kato T, Gono T, et al. Extreme efficacy of intravenous immunoglobulin therapy for severe burning pain in a patient with small fiber neuropathy associated with primary Sjogren's syndrome. Mod Rheumatol 2009;19(4):437–40.

61. Oaklander AL, Klein MM. Evidence of small-fiber polyneuropathy in unexplained, juvenile-onset, widespread pain syndromes. Pediatrics 2013; 131(4):e1091–100.

62. Viegas LP, Ferreira MB, Kaplan AP. The maddening itch: an approach to chronic urticaria. J Investig Allergol Clin Immunol 2014;24(1):1–5.

63. Liang Y, Yang Z, Qin B, et al. Primary Sjögren's syndrome and malignancy risk: a systematic review and meta-analysis. Ann Rheum Dis 2014;73(6):1151–6.

64. Brito-Zerón P, Kostov B, Fraile G, et al, SS Study Group GEAS-SEMI. Characterization and risk estimate of cancer in patients with primary Sjögren syndrome. J Hematol Oncol 2017;10(1):90.

65. Abrol E, González-Pulido C, Praena-Fernández JM, et al. A retrospective study of long-term outcomes in 152 patients with primary Sjögren's syndrome: 25-year experience. Clin Med (Lond) 2014;14(2): 157–64.

66. Pope JE. Other manifestations of mixed connective tissue disease. Rheum Dis Clin North Am 2005; 31(3):519–33.

End-Stage Renal Disease Chronic Itch and Its Management

Radomir Reszke, MD, Jacek C. Szepietowski, MD, PhD*

KEYWORDS

- Chronic itch • Chronic kidney disease • Epidemiology • Pathogenesis • Quality of life • Treatment

KEY POINTS

- End-stage renal disease chronic itch is a frequent symptom that bothers patients with advanced stages of chronic kidney disease.
- The pathogenesis of the chronic itch symptom is complex and not yet fully understood and includes many metabolic, immunologic, and neurogenic factors.
- A significant burden of the disease results in decrease of quality of life with sleep impairment, depressive symptoms, and increased mortality of affected individuals.
- No treatment of choice is available; topical therapy (emollients), phototherapy (UV-B), and systemic therapy (antiepileptics, opioid agonists, and antagonists) provide significant relief in varying percentages of patients

INTRODUCTION

Chronic kidney disease (CKD) is a major problem worldwide because it is encountered in approximately 13% of the population (stages 1–5), whereas in 11% it is present in advanced stages 3 to 5.[1] CKD is a problem of growing importance because the elderly population is increasing, along with the number of patients suffering from diabetes or hypertension. CKD is defined as abnormalities of kidney structure or function that are present for more than 3 months.[2] To diagnose CKD, at least one criterion has to be fulfilled: decreased glomerular filtration rate (GFR) (<60 mL/min/1.73 m^2) or markers of kidney damage, such as albuminuria, urine sediment abnormalities, electrolyte and other abnormalities associated with tubular disorders, histologic abnormalities, structural abnormalities detected by imaging, and a history of kidney transplantation.

CKD is divided into 5 stages according to GFR, the fifth being characterized by GFR < 15 mL/min/1.73 m^2, also termed end-stage renal disease (ESRD). CKD is associated with numerous complications, such as anemia, hyperlipidemia, nutrition, osteodystrophy, or cardiovascular risk,[3] to mention just a few. Cutaneous manifestations of CKD are profuse and especially marked in ESRD, including skin color alterations, elastosis, ecchymoses, xerosis, and pruritus, but also specific disorders, such as acquired perforating disorders, disorders with metastatic calcification, or bullous disorders of hemodialysis (HD).[4]

Chronic itch (CI) is a frequent symptom in the general population and systemic diseases, posing a high burden and decrease in quality of life (QoL) of an affected individual.[5] CI is defined as an itch that lasts for more than 6 weeks. According to the International Forum for the Study of Itch (IFSI), the etiologic classification of chronic

Disclosure: The authors have nothing to disclose.
Department of Dermatology, Venereology and Allergology, Wroclaw Medical University, Chalubinskiego Street 1, Wrocław 50-368, Poland
* Corresponding author.
E-mail address: jacek.szepietowski@umed.wroc.pl

Dermatol Clin 36 (2018) 277–292
https://doi.org/10.1016/j.det.2018.02.007

pruritus comprises 6 categories: (I) dermatologic, (II) systemic, (III) neurologic, (IV) psychogenic/psychosomatic, (V) mixed, and (VI) others.[6] One of the most important causes of systemic itch is end-stage renal disease–associated chronic itch (ESRDCI). Since its first description in 1932 coined "uremic itch,"[7] it remains a common problem impairing the QoL of patients and a significant therapeutic challenge for physicians specializing in dermatology and nephrology. Although numerous proposed etiologic factors have been explored, the cause is unclear and may involve several mechanisms.

DISCUSSION
Definition

ESRDCI or another more commonly used term, uremic pruritus, is defined as CI observed in patients with CKD with significant abnormal renal function with advanced stages of renal damage.[8] Establishing the diagnosis is based on exclusion of other possible causes. It is necessary to diagnose CKD beforehand. It must be emphasized that acute kidney injury is not considered an eliciting factor of CI.

Epidemiology

Epidemiologic aspects of ESRDCI vary according to data presented in the literature, especially when newer reports are taken into account. In the early 1970s, 85% of patients on dialysis could have suffered from CI, decreasing to 50% to 60% at the end of 1980s.[9] A large multicenter study by Pisoni and colleagues[10] (Dialysis Outcomes and Practice Patterns Study, DOPPS) of 18,801 hemodialysis patients revealed that 42% of them suffered from CI. Interestingly, pruritus was a predictor of a 17% higher mortality. Weiss and colleagues[11] analyzed the data from 860 HD patients attending German dialysis units. The point prevalence of CI was 25%, and 12-month prevalence reached 27%, whereas lifetime prevalence was estimated to be 35%. Interestingly, patients aged less than 70 years complained of CI more often than those aged 70 and older. One Korean study demonstrated that CI was more prevalent among patients on peritoneal dialysis (PD) (n = 223) than those on HD (n = 425), with the prevalence estimated at 62% and 48%, respectively (P = .001).[12] Regarding patients on PD (n = 30), Tessari and colleagues[13] reported that 52.1% of patients suffered from CI, and these figures were similar to those regarding patients on HD (n = 135). A Polish study revealed that among children suffering from CKD (stages 3–5) (n = 103) CI is present in 20.8% of cases.[14] Moreover, the

percentages were comparable among different treatment methods: 18.4% in conservative treatment group and 23.5% in the group on dialysis (HD or peritoneal). In a study comprising 171 individuals on HD, Heisig and colleagues[15] reported that 52.6% of patients complained of itch in the past, whereas in 46.2% of itch was present within the last 3 days.

Notwithstanding the abundance of ESRDCI reports focusing on patients on HD or PD, there are also epidemiologic reports focusing solely on patients with CKD not yet on dialysis. Solak and colleagues[16] evaluated 402 predialysis patients with CKD stages 2 to 5 and itch was present in 19%, regardless of CKD stage. Another study demonstrated that in stages 4 to 5 of CKD pruritus was reported by 56% of patients.[17] Murtagh and colleagues[18] evaluated 66 patients with CKD stage 5, reporting that itch was experienced by 74% of individuals.

Pathogenesis

Pathogenesis of ESRDCI is not fully understood, and various factors are described as contributing to the development of this symptom (Box 1). Renal failure leads to changes in blood urea nitrogen and creatinine, resulting in a certain "metabolic

---

Box 1
Important factors associated with the development of end-stage renal disease chronic itch

- Metabolic disequilibrium (increased levels of urea, creatinine)
- Xerosis (skin dryness)
- Vitamin A
- Low vitamin D
- Divalent ions (eg, calcium)
- PTH
- Phosphorus
- Mast cells
- Tryptase and chymase
- Histamine
- Serotonin
- Microinflammation (Th1/Th2 lymphocyte dysregulation, abundance of proinflammatory cytokines)
- HCV
- μ-Opioid overexpression and κ-opioid downregulation
- Neuropathy

disequilibrium."[19] Uremic xerosis is a common problem and was historically associated with ESRDCI itch and a predisposing factor for CI. Morton and colleagues[20] assessed 72 patients on dialysis with regard to stratum corneum hydration (measured by corneometer) and itching intensity. These aspects correlated with each other, and consequently, emollient use alleviated itch. Chorążyczewska and colleagues[21] reported that xerosis was more common in the uremic itch group than in controls (80% vs 42%; $P = .002$). Surprisingly, the content of ceramides, cholesterol, free fatty acids, triglycerides, cholesteryl esters, and squalene was comparable in patients with itch and those without it. Yosipovitch and colleagues[22] described worse stratum corneum integrity in patients with ESRD as well as a negative correlation between glycerol content of the stratum corneum and xerosis. However, no correlation between xerosis and itch was determined. Nevertheless, studies have shown that emollient application improves not only uremic xerosis but also ESRDCI,[23–25] and therefore, lipid content and resulting skin barrier integrity contribute to the development of itch. A Japanese study has proven that increased levels of aquaporin-3 are associated with ESRDCI, but not with xerosis.[26]

A Dutch study has evaluated vitamin A levels in patients on HD.[27] Although its levels were increased in all patients (n = 35), no correlation was detected between mean serum vitamin A level and presence of pruritus ($P>.25$). The role of vitamin D, which is frequently decreased in the CKD population, was also investigated.[28,29] Other researchers investigated the role of divalent ions in eliciting CI. Momose and colleagues[30] analyzed calcium ions in skin of patients with moderate to severe itch versus those without itch. The former presented with significantly higher deposition of calcium ions in the extracellular fluid, in the cytoplasm of basal cells, as well as in the extracellular fluid and cytoplasm of spinous cells when compared with patients without this symptom. Similar observations were made by Duque and colleagues,[31] who reported a positive correlation between uremic itch and serum calcium concentration ($P = .04$). In addition, the intensity of itch positively correlated with the increasing months on dialysis ($P = .02$), higher Kt/V parameter ($P = .01$), and skin dryness ($P = .01$). Regarding calcium metabolism, it is important to review the role of parathormone (PTH) in relation to ESRDCI because secondary or tertiary hyperparathyroidism is a frequent complication in ESRD patients. In 1968, Massry and colleagues[32] demonstrated that ESRD patients (n = 7) suffering from chronic, intractable itch have elevated levels of PTH.

Subtotal parathyroidectomy ensued in rapid disappearance of itch. In 2013, Iranian researchers revealed that in HD patients (n = 153) itch was present in 61%, whereas mean itch intensity was higher in patients with hyperparathyroidism.[33] Serum PTH levels also correlated with itch intensity. Iron serum levels also differ between patients with or without pruritus: lower levels are observed in patients with pruritus,[34] whereas statistically significant differences in itchiness severity were observed in patients with lower hemoglobin ($P<.0001$) and higher phosphorus ($P<.0001$) levels.[35] Pisoni and colleagues[10] reported that ESRD patients moderately or extremely bothered by itch were more likely to exhibit increased higher serum levels of phosphorus ($P<.0001$), higher serum levels of calcium ($P = .01$), and lower levels of albumin ($P<.0001$).

The role of mast cells (MC) was extensively studied in the context of ESRDCI in several papers because this cell's release, for example, histamine, is a "classic" itch mediator. In a study by Szepietowski and colleagues,[36] skin samples of ESRD patients on HD were examined. The mean number of tryptase-positive chymase-positive MC was increased in HD patients with itch when compared with controls. The number of MCs per 1 mm^2 was slightly higher in itchy patients than in those free from itch. Therefore, it was proposed that disturbances in chymase and tryptase activity contribute to the pathogenesis of ESRDCI, because chymase degrades substance P. The latter may induce histamine release from dermal MC. Dimković and colleagues[34] reported that MCs in patients with ESRDCI were increased in number, diffusely spread in dermis, and appeared degranulated. The role of MC in eliciting ESDCI was also proved in other reports,[37,38] whereas Mettang and colleagues[39] could not find any relationship between the level of plasma histamine, the number of skin MCs, or the extent of uremic pruritus. In a study by Szepietowski and colleagues,[40] MCs were subjected to broadband and narrowband UV-B radiation, ensuing in apoptosis. The hypothesis that this method might be beneficial in treating ESRDCI was later confirmed in several studies, including a randomized controlled trial.[41] Apart from histamine, the role of other mediators was also investigated. Balaskas and colleagues[42] reported that not only serum histamine levels are increased in patients suffering from ESRDCI (up to 14 times higher than the upper normal limit) but also serotonin is higher than in patients who do not complain of itch (115.6 ± 43.3 ng/mL vs 64 ± 42.3 ng/mL, respectively; $P<.05$). After administration of ondansetron (a 5-HT$_3$ receptor inhibitor), there was marked improvement in pruritus, along with a decrease in serum histamine and serotonin concentration (from 12.9 ± 1.2 to 6.7 ± 5.9 ng/mL, $P<.05$, and from 125.1 ± 47.8 to 59.3 ± 27.5 ng/mL, $P<.05$; respectively).

Newer theories have suggested that ESRDCI is associated with an inflammatory state and immune alteration. CKD is characterized by a microinflammatory state because of postsynthetic modification of proteins, oxidative stress, and dialysis-associated infectious factors.[43] In particular, in ESRDCI, there have been reports of deranged T-helper lymphocyte differentiation. Kimmel and colleagues[44] observed an increased proportion of T-helper 1 (Th1)/T-helper (Th2) lymphocytes (measured by interferon-γ secretion) along with increased serum levels of C-reactive protein, interleukin-6 (IL-6), and tumor necrosis factor-α among HD patients who complained of itch. Fallahzadeh and colleagues[45] have demonstrated that patients with uremic itch present with higher serum levels of IL-2, which is another proinflammatory cytokine. Recently, increased IL-31, a Th2 itchy cytokine, was demonstrated in ESRDCI.[46,47]

Infection with hepatitis C virus (HCV) is a common problem in patients subjected to HD.[48] Chronic HCV infection is associated with CI, due to cholestasis and induction of cytokines (IL-8) and chemokines (CCL2, CXCL1, CXCL5).[49] Unsurprisingly, several studies revealed possible association between HCV infection and developing ESRDCI. The DOPPS study demonstrated that patients with concurrent HCV infection were 1.29 times more likely to experience moderate to severe itch.[10] Chiu and colleagues[50] investigated 321 HD patients among which CI of mild to moderate intensity bothered 44% subjects, whereas 18.7% complained of severe itch. Using a multivariable logistic regression model, HCV infection was significantly associated with severe itch (odds risk = 2.77, P = .014).

Another suggested pathogenic factor for ESRDI is neuropathy that could be both peripherally and centrally mediated. CKD patients frequently suffer from polyneuropathy. Fantini and colleagues[51] described significant reduction in the total number of skin nerve terminals among uremic patients. However, Johansson and colleagues[52] reported that nerve fibers in ESRD patients sprout through the layers of epidermis, in contrast to the healthy controls. Concerning ESRDCI, Jedras and colleagues[53] suggested the association of uremic itch with neuropathy. Another study revealed that the severity of itch is associated with the presence of paraesthesia.[54] In addition, the investigators observed a tendency toward a relationship between the presence of uremic itch and hypohidrosis, altered skin sympathetic response, and restless legs syndrome. Recent brain imaging study of uremic pruritus suggests that central brain neuropathy is associated with ESRDCI.[55] Interestingly, it was also reported that the worsening of ESRDCI intensity might be associated with the concurrent deterioration of uremic neuropathy.[56]

The role of opioid receptors has also been studied in relation to ESRDCI patients. Wieczorek and colleagues[57] demonstrated a statistically significant negative correlation between κ-opioid receptors expression and intensity of ESRDCI. μ-Opioid receptors are considered as promoting the sensation of itch, whereas κ-opioid receptors act conversely. A κ-opioid agonist (nalfurafine) has been successfully used in managing patients with uremic itch.[58] On the other hand, naltrexone (a μ-opioid antagonist) provided mild[59] or no improvement in clinical studies.[60] The depletion of substance P forms peripheral nerve fibers, and prevention of its reaccumulation is a mechanism of treatment of ESRDCI with topical capsaicin, as evaluated in several clinical trials.[61,62] The authors' group has investigated the role of endocannabinoid receptor 1 gene polymorphism, although no associations with ERSDCI were found.[63] Overall, the pruritus in CKD has a "mixed" etiologic classification.

Box 1 lists most important factors associated with ESRDC, although the list is incomplete and expanding.

Clinical Features

ESRDCI is considered one of the most important systemic disorders causing CI. If this situation persists, then the patient might exhibit chronic scratch lesions (group III). Physical examination reveals excoriations, erosions, scars, nodules, hypopigmentation, or hyperpigmentation of variable intensity. In a recent study by Hayani and colleagues,[64] patients on HD concurrently complaining of CI were classified according to the IFSI classification of CI. It must be emphasized that the investigation concerned all patients with concurrent CI and CKD, regardless of causal relationship. Among 177 patients, 43.5% were classified as IFSI II, 37.9% as IFSI III, and 18.6% as IFSI I. In the latter group, most common dermatoses included psoriasis, eczematous disorders, and mycoses. In an Indian study (n = 200), among CKD patients (stages 3–5), dermatologic manifestations were present in 96% of patients, the most common being xerosis (72%), pigmentary changes (50%), pruritus (36%), and infections (29%; mostly onychomycosis, furunculosis, dermatophytosis, pityriasis versicolor, and folliculitis).[65] Rarely, patients presented with perforating disorders (3%) and prurigo nodularis (1%). A study by Masmoudi and colleagues[66] performed on 458 ESRD patients on chronic HD revealed that patients had high rates of xerosis (53%), and eczema in the fistula area (15%).

The mean intensity of CI was assessed in several papers, for example, via using the visual analogue scale (VAS). The authors' group reported that among patients on maintenance HD (n = 171), 52.6% of patients reported CI in the past and 46.2% of patients reported CI within the previous 3 days, whereas the mean VAS score was 4.1 ± 2.0 points. Most patients (52.6%) regarded the symptom as mild, 38.2% regarded the symptom as moderate, whereas severe and most severe cases occurred in 8% and 1%, respectively.[15] Another study (n = 103) reported the mean intensity of approximately 6 points.[67] In a large study by Phan and colleagues[68] (n = 471), 40% described the pruritus intensity as low (which corresponded with mean VAS 1.9), 37% described the pruritus intensity as moderate (mean VAS 5.12), and 8.1% described the pruritus intensity as severe (mean VAS 8.57). In a large cohort of patients (n = 860), Weiss and colleagues[11] observed that the mean CI severity was 4.1 ± 1.7, whereas the severity at the time of the investigation and the worst severity within the last 6 weeks were 4.2 ± 2.6 and 6.5 ± 2.5, respectively.

Regardless of the cause, the location of itch is another relevant clinical aspect. ESRDCI patients report both localized and generalized itch. The authors' group observed that 38% of patients complained of localized location (mostly back, lower extremities, scalp, upper extremities, abdomen; usually of bilateral distribution), 35.4% reported itch in at least 2 locations, whereas generalized itch concerned 26.6% of respondents.[15] In a German study, most frequent location of itch included legs (54.6%), back (52%), and scalp (43.9%).[11] Notably, the mean CI intensity was significantly worse when arms and legs were affected. Another study emphasized the striking symmetry of itchy areas; 83% of patients complained of itch over large, discontinuous regions of skin without dermatomal pattern.[67]

Itch is a dynamic symptom insofar as its characteristic varies over time, for example, because of external factors that influence its course. In one of the authors' studies regarding ESRDCI including 130 patients, it was noted that 46% of patients experienced pruritus within a year of starting HD.[7] In 27%, itch occurred more than 1 year after starting HD, whereas only in 26% was itch present before HD. A significant positive correlation was found between HD period and total score of pruritus (P<.02). Dialysis membranes used in the procedure were also relevant: 58% of patients experienced itch on polysulfone membranes, whereas 35% of patients experienced itch on cuprophane and 31% of patients experienced itch on hemophane. In another study, 29% of patients reported that itch is most prominent during the end or after dialysis.[15] Mathur and colleagues[67] interviewed 103 patients and noticed that the mean worst itching intensity was higher during the 12-hour nighttime period than for the 12-hour daytime period. According to Zucker and colleagues,[69] ESRDCI tends to occur more often and with higher intensity during night. In addition, the intensity of CI may be associated with the intensity of xerosis as well. The authors' group found that patients with very rough skin experienced pruritus more often than those with rough skin and slightly dry skin (56.2% vs 34.5% vs 27%, respectively).[7] Xerosis cutis might be the reason a percentage of patients observe seasonal variations in ESRDCI.[70] In a study on 219 ESRD patients on HD, it was noted that xerosis was the second most common exacerbating factor of CI (reported by 42%), whereas 57% of patients mentioned rest.[69] Other unfavorable factors included heat (35%), sweat (33%), clothing (19%), and stress (19%). Interestingly, among ameliorating factors, patients mentioned activity (57% of respondents), but also sleep (46%), followed by hot showers (44%), cold showers (39%), and cold conditions (28%).

ESRDCI is often characterized by a prolonged course, which was described by several authors. Hayani and colleagues[64] reported that 60.4% of patients with ESRDCI experienced itch for more than 1 year, and some patients suffered from this phenomenon for more than 10 years (9%). In 1982, Gilchrest and colleagues[70] reported that "prolonged bothersome itchiness" was experienced at some point of the study in as much as 78% of patients. In another study, it was stated that ESRDCI might be regarded as unremittent, refractory, and persistent.[67]

Burden of the Disease

CI is a bothersome symptom associated with significant burden manifested with a marked decrease of various health-related quality of life (HRQoL) domains.[71–74] For example, the authors' group evaluated 200 ESRD patients on HD, among which 38% experienced CI.[75] Patients with CI had significantly lower HRQoL score assessed by short form-36 (SF-36) questionnaire compared with patients without CI (93.0 ± 20.4 vs

99.6 ± 19.9 points, $P = .03$). By focusing on different dimensions of the questionnaire, it was noted that general perception of health was worse among patients with CI ($P = .0003$). Beck's Depression Inventory (BDI) was used in order to determine depression prevalence and severity, revealing that the Dermatology Life Quality Index (DLQI) score and intensity of itch assessed with both VAS ($R = 0.56$, $P<.0001$) and the 4-item Itch Questionnaire ($R = 0.48$, $P< .0001$) were positively correlated. Interestingly, no significant difference in BDI scoring and prevalence of clinically relevant depression was noted when comparing the patients with or without CI. A significant positive correlation was found between BDI scores and itch intensity measured by 4-item itch questionnaire. Pisoni and colleagues[10] reported that patients with moderate to extreme itch felt drained more often than patients with no mild or no itching (adjusted odds ratio [AOR] = 2.3 to 5.2, $P<.0001$). Moreover, their sleep quality was poor (AOR $\leq$1.9–4.1, $P = .0002$), physician-diagnosed depression was more common (AOR = 1.3–1.7, $P\leq$.004), whereas QoL mental and composite scores were 3.1 to 8.6 points lower ($P<.0001$). The authors' group observed that 43.5% patients with ESRDCI had slightly impaired QoL according to DLQI, whereas severe and extremely severe impairment concerned 4.8% and 1.5%, respectively.[15] An evaluation of sleep quality was also performed via the Athens Insomnia Scale. Patients suffering from CI experienced problems with sleep induction more often ($P<.001$); the night awakenings occurred more often ($P<.03$), whereas sleep quality ($P<.03$) and functioning capacity ($P = .03$) were impaired. In another study, more than 70,000 ESRD patients on HD were evaluated for CI and, among others, associated QoL characteristics evaluated by Kidney Disease and Quality of Life-36 survey.[35] Sixty percent of patients were bothered by itching to some extent; 14.5% were "very much bothered" or "extremely bothered" by this symptom. With the increasing level of itchiness, a decreasing trend was observed in physical score (39.27–32.12, $P<.0001$), mental score (52.07–43.46, $P<.0001$), the Effect on Daily Life subscore (76.40–51.85, $P<.0001$), Burden of Disease subscale score (57.23–32.71, $P<.0001$), and Symptom and Problem subscale scores (85.73–52.26). In a study by Ibrahim and colleagues[76] of 200 ESRD patients on HD, 100 patients experienced ESRDCI. Various QoL domains were assessed by the World Health Organization Quality of Life Instruments (WHOQOL)-BREF instrument, which is an abbreviated version of the WHOQOL-100 questionnaire. Physical, psychological, and environmental aspects were more

affected in itchy individuals. Concerning the social domain, personal relationship satisfaction was significantly higher ($P = .0007$) in patients not suffering from ESRDCI, although sexual life satisfaction was similar among the groups ($P = .745$). The significant difference in friend support was observed ($P = .0053$) in favor of patients free from itch. Szepietowski and colleagues[77] reported that intensity of ESRDCI decreased the QoL specifically in patients suffering from uremic xerosis.

In a recent study, Heisig and colleagues[78] performed an evaluation of alexithymia (a personality trait characterized by inability to verbalize emotions) among 90 patients on HD (46.7% patients were suffering from CI). To assess alexithymia, researchers used the Bermond-Vorst Alexithymia Questionnaire-40, comprising domains of analyzing, verbalizing, identifying, emotionalizing, and fantasizing. Patients with CI had a significantly lower mean score in the subscale of fantasizing (21.7 ± 8.9 vs 25.9 ± 11.1 points, $P<.05$) and an inverse correlation with itch intensity was determined ($r = -0.33$; $P = .03$).

Treatment

Because of marked complexity of pathogenesis and associated comorbidities, the treatment of ESRDCI remains challenging, despite the abundance of available modalities. Before reviewing therapeutic methods, it should be emphasized that factors associated with the dialysis strongly influence the appearance ESRDCI. For example, increasing the blood flow during HD may reduce the frequency and intensity of itch.[79] Higher Kt/V parameter (a volume of plasma cleared divided by urea distribution volume) is associated with higher intensity of pruritus.[31] Liakopoulos and colleagues[80] observed that patients on PD experienced itch less often after increasing daily dialysate volume. It was also reported that high-permeability HDs were more effective than conventional HD in managing ESRDCI, possibly because of better clearance of PTH and β2-microglobulin.[81] Whether HD or PD elicits itch more often is not determined because the results are inconsistent.[12,29]

Managing ESCRDI begins with applying preventive measures to avoid factors that can exacerbate the itch, such as contact with irritant substances, hot and spicy food, hot and alcoholic beverages, and negative stress, and by encouraging to moisturize the skin to reduce skin dryness.[5] It is recommended to use mild, nonalkaline cleansers and to bath in lukewarm water for no more than 20 minutes. Soft clothing and frequent application of emollients are also beneficial.

Methods specifically assessed in patients with ESRDCI are listed in **Box 2**, whereas for a suggested therapeutic algorithm, refer to **Fig. 1**.

Topical therapy

Because of its high efficacy and safety profile, topical therapy is used frequently in various dermatologic disorders. Topical therapy is often discussed in association with emollients. The latter reduces water loss from stratum corneum and may also contain humectants, physiologic lipids, and antipruritic agents.[148] Balaskas and colleagues[24] performed a randomized, double-blind study on patients with uremic xerosis (n = 99) who were treated with oil in water emulsion containing glycerol 15% and paraffin 10%. Itch was also evaluated by 100-mm VAS, starting from 40.64 ± 3.36 mm on baseline, whereas on day 28 and 56, a marked reduction was noted (13.39 ± 2.19 mm and 10.66 ± 2.14 mm, respectively). On day 56, a significant improvement was also observed in relation to QoL measured by DLQI and SF-12 questionnaires. The authors' study evaluated the use of *endocannabinoids* in managing ESRDCI. These substances may exert their antipruritic effect because of reduction of histamine induced itch, vasodilatation, and downregulation of MCs.[23] In one study, the authors treated 31 ESRDCI patients on HD with a cream containing structural physiologic lipids and endogenous cannabinoids. The combination was applied twice daily for 3 weeks, and 21 patients were included for final analysis. The baseline itch intensity measured by VAS was 6.24 ± 2.19, which decreased to 1.29 ± 1.41 on the 21st day of therapy. On follow-up visit (14 days after discontinuing the therapy), the values increased to 2.43 ± 2.82 (P = .02), but was still significantly lower than at the beginning (P<.001). More than 90% of patients deemed the therapy at least "satisfactory." The authors' group also reported the usefulness of balneological therapy with *polidocanol* in bath oil among ESRDCI patients on HD. Every 2 days, 31 patients were given 150-L baths with the addition of 30 mL of preparation; the duration of bath was 10 to 15 minutes. After 4 weeks of therapy, 87% of patients reported complete disappearance of itch, marked improvement in 10%, and moderate improvement in 3%. Randomized, double-blind, placebo-controlled studies with topical therapy in ESRDCI were performed with *cromolyn* 4% cream, *γ-linolenic acid* 2.2% cream, *sericin* cream, and *pramoxine* 1% lotion, with a statistically significant effect on treated subjects.[82,84,89,149] The data concerning *tacrolimus* ointment are inconsistent; 2 studies demonstrated its efficacy,[85,86] whereas in a randomized, double-

---

Box 2
Therapeutic modalities evaluated in end-stage renal disease chronic itch

Topical therapy

- Glycerol and paraffin[24]
- Urea 10% and dexpanthenole[25]
- γ-Linolenic acid[82]
- Capsaicin[61,62,83]
- Endocannabinoids[23]
- Pramoxine[84]
- Tacrolimus[85–87]
- Calcipotriol[88]
- Sericin[89]
- Polidocanole[90]
- Chia seed oil[91]

Phototherapy

- Broadband UV-B (BB-UV-B)[92–98]
- Narrowband UV-B (NB-UV-B)[41,99–103]

Systemic treatment

- Gabapentin[102,104–110]
- Pregabalin[111–115]
- Nalfurafine[58,116,117]
- Nalbuphine[118,119]
- Naltrexone[59,60,120]
- Ondasetrone[42,114,121,122]
- Sertraline[123–125]
- Cromolyn[126,127]
- Doxepine[128,129]
- Ketotifene[107,130]
- Montelukast[131]
- Mirtazapine[132]
- Pentoxyphylline[133]
- Thalidomide[134]
- Active charcoal[135,136]
- Nicotinamide[137]
- Ergocalciferole[138]
- Nicergoline[139]
- Lidocaine[140]
- Heparin[141]
- Cholestyramine[142]

Miscellaneous

- Chia seed oil[91]
- Turmeric[143]
- Aromatherapy[144]
- Acupuncture[145]
- Parathyroidectomy[32,146,147]

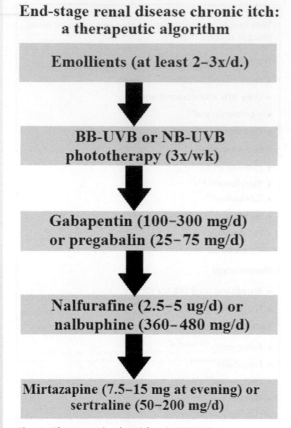

End-stage renal disease chronic itch: a therapeutic algorithm

Emollients (at least 2–3x/d.)

↓

BB-UVB or NB-UVB phototherapy (3x/wk)

↓

Gabapentin (100–300 mg/d) or pregabalin (25–75 mg/d)

↓

Nalfurafine (2.5–5 ug/d) or nalbuphine (360–480 mg/d)

↓

Mirtazapine (7.5–15 mg at evening) or sertraline (50–200 mg/d)

Fig. 1. Therapeutic algorithm in ESRDCI.

blind, vehicle-controlled study by Duque and colleagues,[87] tacrolimus did not provide any improvement in itch intensity.

Despite relative effectiveness and safety of topical therapy in ESRDCI, this method is often very difficult for patients to apply when they have generalized itch and requires assistance of family members and/or caregivers.

Phototherapy
UV radiation exerts its biological effects in dermatologic disorders through several mechanisms. These mechanisms include apoptosis of inflammatory cells, inhibition of Langerhans cells, alteration of cytokine production, antimicrobial activity, improving skin barrier, and positive effect on vitamin D balance.[150] The role of *BB-UV-B* (290- to 320-nm wavelength) radiation in managing uremic pruritus was reported since the 1970s by several investigators, although the number of study participants was low.[92–98] In a study by Blachley and colleagues,[97] 6 patients with severe ESRDCI received BB-UV-B thrice weekly for a total of 6 irradiation treatments. The control group (n = 11) was subjected to UV-A. The baseline

pruritus score of 9.5 ± 1.0 decreased to 2.5 ± 1.1 (assessed by Numerical Rating Scale [NRS]) following the treatment ($P<.001$). In addition, BB-UV-B provided significant reduction in the skin content of phosphorus (0.105 ± 0.009 to 0.047 ± 0.011 mmol/g). Later studies evaluated the efficacy of *NB-UV-B* (311-nm wavelength), because this method is less erythmogenic and provides a better safety profile.[41,99–103] In 2002, Szepietowski and colleagues[40] used BB-UV-B and NB-UV-B and observed that MC apoptosis occurs in a dose-dependent manner using both types of UV-B. The investigators suggested that NB-UV-B, thanks to its ability to penetrate deeper into dermis, might be more effective in reaching MCs and alleviating ESRDCI. Ada and colleagues[99] included 20 patients with ESRDCI who were subjected to NB-UV-B irradiation 3 times a week for 6 weeks. The initial doses were chosen according to the phototype (100 mJ/cm² for phototype I, whereas 500 mJ/cm² for phototype) and increased by 100 mJ/cm² at each session, until a maximum daily dose of 1500 mJ/cm². Among 10 patients who completed the study, the itch intensity measured by VAS decreased by 71%. Seven patients were examined on follow-up after 6 months: of these, 3 were in remission and 4 experienced relapse of symptoms. Ko and colleagues[41] conducted a single-blind, randomized, controlled trial for patients with refractory ESRDCI. NB-UV-B was administered 3 times a week for 6 weeks in 11 patients (starting dose, 210 mJ/cm², increased by 10% with each session), whereas control group (n = 10) was subjected to long-wave UV-A (doses of 1–6 J/cm²). The study was completed by 18 patients (10 in the treatment group and 8 in the control group). The itch intensity score at week 6 (measured by VAS decreased by 3.53 units in NB-UV-B group and 3.38 units in the control group; no statistical significance between the groups was determined). In other reports, patients receiving NB-UV-B obtained statistically significant reduction in itch intensity than control groups.[100,101] In one of these studies,[100] a significant reduction of serum phosphorus and calcium-phosphorus product levels was observed. In a later study by El-Kamel and colleagues,[102] 2 groups of patients with ESRDCI were analyzed, each consisting of 24 patients. One group received NB-UV-B 3 times a week for 6 weeks, with dose characteristic similar to a previous study.[99] Another group received, in addition to NB-UV-B, oral gabapentin 300 mg thrice weekly for 6 weeks (for detailed gabapentin review in ESRDCI, refer to later discussion). Twenty-two patients in the control group and 21 patients in the study group completed the treatment. The baseline 5-D itch score decreased from 18 to 6 points (median) in the control group (P<.0001) and from 19 to 6 points (P = .0001) in the treatment group, although there was no statistically significant difference between the groups.

Systemic therapy

Among numerous systemic treatment modalities of ESRDCI, the significant role of antiepileptic drugs has to be emphasized. *Gabapentin* is a γ-aminobutyric acid structural analogue used to treat epilepsy and neuropathic pain. Gunal and colleagues[104] assessed the efficacy of gabapentin in 25 patients with ESRDCI on HD in a randomized, double-blind, placebo-controlled crossover study. The mean baseline VAS score of itch was 8.4 ± 0.94 points. Gabapentin was administered in a dose of 300 mg thrice weekly for 4 weeks ensuing in a marked itch intensity reduction to 1.2 ± 1.8 points (P = .0001). Mild to moderate adverse events (AE) were somnolence, dizziness, and fatigue, usually subsiding within first 7 days of treatment. In another double-blind, placebo-controlled trial, 34 ESRDCI patients on HD were evaluated.[105] Treatment group received 400 mg of gabapentin twice a week. The mean pruritus score at baseline was 7.2 ± 2.3 points according to VAS. After 4 weeks of treatment, pruritus score was lower in both gabapentin and placebo groups: 6.7 ± 2.6 and 1.5 ± 1.8 points, respectively (P<.001). Most common adverse effects were mild to moderate and included somnolence, dizziness, and nausea, usually subsiding within the first 5 to 10 days of treatment. Marquez and colleagues[106] compared the effectiveness of gabapentin (300 mg 3 times per week) with *desloratadine* (a second-generation antihistamine) 5 mg 3 times per week. Nineteen patients completed the crossover study. Both modalities reduced itch intensity (VAS reduction from 5.95 to 4.6 points with gabapentin; and 5.89–3.4 points with desloratadine), although only the effect associated with desloratadine was statistically significant (P = .004). *Ketotifen*, which is a first-generation antihistamine, was compared with gabapentin in a study by Amirkhanlou and colleagues.[107] Twenty-six patients received ketotifen (1 mg/d for 2 weeks) and 26 received gabapanetin (100 mg/d for 2 weeks). Complete responses in terms of itch were observed in 50% and 53.8% patients, respectively. A previously mentioned study demonstrated that gabapentin does not increase effectiveness of NB-UV-B in ESRDCI patients.[102]

Pregabalin *Pregabalin* is another antiepileptic drug with a similar mechanism of action to gabapentin. It binds to the α2δ subunit of the voltage-dependent calcium channel, thereby blocking calcium influx into nerve terminals.[111] In addition, it decreases the release of neurotransmitter (glutamate, noradrenaline, substance P, and calcitonin gene–related protein). Aperis and colleagues[112] reported that among 12 patients treated with pregabalin (25 mg/d orally before sleep) the mean VAS intensity of itch decreased from 7.44 ± 2.01 to 1.7 ± 1.31 points (P<.0003). Similar results were reported by Shavit and colleagues[111] (n = 12). Khan and colleagues[113] reported that among 51 patients on HD treated with pregabalin (75 mg after dialysis) due to ESRDCI, most common AE included dizziness (47%), somnolence (43.1%), constipation (29.4%), blurred vision (19.6%), and weight gain (11.8%). Yue and colleagues[114] assessed ESRDCI in 62 patients treated with pregabalin (75 mg 2 times per week in PD patients or after dialysis in HD patients), 60 with *ondasetron* in a dose of 8 mg (a potent and selective 5-HT$_3$ receptor) and 57 with placebo. After 12 weeks of follow-up, the mean VAS scale scores dropped from 8.0 ± 2.3 to 1.4 ± 0.2 points (pregabalin), whereas ondasetron (7.9 ± 1.8–5.4 ± 0.6 points) and placebo (7.7 ± 1.5–5.7 ± 0.4 points) provided no significant relief.

Two studies have compared the effectiveness of gabapentin and pregabalin in ESRDCI (**Table 1**).

μ-opioid antagonists and κ-opioid agonists

In a study by Peer and colleagues,[120] 8 patients with ESRDCI received *naltrexone* 50 mg/d (a μ-opioid antagonist) followed by placebo, and 7 patients received placebo followed by naltrexone. A significant itch reduction was noted in comparison to placebo. However, Pauli-Magnus and colleagues[60] reported lack of antipruritic efficacy of naltrexone in comparison to placebo in ERSDCI patients. In addition, AE were also more prevalent (up to 40% of patients on naltrexone experienced loss of appetite and nausea). A French study included 52 patients among which naltrexone (50 mg/d) and *loratadine* (10 mg/d) were administered to 26 patients each.[59] The baseline itch intensity was 4.85 points according to VAS. On the seventh day of treatment, a nonclinical meaningful improvement was observed in both groups: 15 patients on naltrexone experienced 30 adverse effects of nausea and sleep abnormalities.

Activation of different opioid receptors in peripheral nerve endings and brain may result in different outcome concerning itch. μ-Opioid receptor's activation results in increased itching, whereas κ-opioid activation alleviates itch.[58] In a study by Wikström and colleagues,[58] randomized, double-blind, placebo-controlled evaluation of *nalfurafine*,

Table 1
Studies comparing gabapentin and pregabalin in end-stage renal disease chronic itch

Authors, Year	Study Population and Interventions	Outcomes
Rayner et al,[108] 2012	71 patients on gabapentin (starting at 100 mg/d in PD or 100 mg after HD)	66% of patients on gabapentin experienced significant reduction of itch 37% of patients experienced AE, mostly oversedation and dizziness
	15 patients (13 not tolerating gabapentin and 2 experiencing no relief in itch) received pregabalin 25 mg/d (PD) or 25 mg after HD	87% of patients on pregabalin experienced significant reduction of itch Drug discontinuation in 13% due to oversedation
Solak et al,[109] 2012	Each group of 25 patients received gabapentin 300 mg 3 ×/wk or pregabalin 75 mg/d. Before drug switching, a 2-wk washout period was planned. 40 patients completed the study	Gabapentin reduced itch intensity by −4.41 ± 1.78 points (VAS), whereas pregabalin reduced itch intensity by −4.43 ± 2.1 points. No difference between 2 treatment modalities (P = .844). Most common AE: dizziness and sedation. Gabapentin and pregabalin were equally effective in managing neuropathic itch in ESRD patients

a κ-opioid agonist, was administered to ESRDCI patients. In total, 86 patients received nalfurafine (5 μg/d), whereas 58 received placebo. At the second week of treatment, 36% of patients obtained at least a 50% decrease from baseline in terms of "worst itching," as compared with 14% in the placebo group (P = .02). The number of days with nondisturbing itching as well as the number of nights with sound sleep concerned more patients on nalfurafine (P = .04 and P = .0003, respectively). The most common AE associated with nalfurafine included vertigo, vomiting, headache, and insomnia, although the incidence was similar to the placebo group. In a larger cohort of patients, Kumagai and colleagues[116] have also proven the effectiveness and safety of nalfurafine, both 5 μg/d and 2.5 μg/d (n = 114 and n = 112, respectively) in comparison to placebo (n = 111) at the seventh day of treatment (P = .0002 and P = .0001, respectively). The most common AE was insomnia, reported by 14% and 7% patients on nalfurafine, respectively. Another study confirmed that prolonged treatment with nalfurafine (5 μg/d for up to 52 weeks) is well tolerated, and the most frequent AE was insomnia (19.4%), constipation (7.1%), and hyperprolactinemia (3.3%).[117] Nalfurafine has been approved in Japan since 2009 for ESRDCI.

Nalbuphine Nalbuphine is a novel investigational drug undergoing clinical studies and acting as a mixed μ-opioid antagonist and κ-opioid agonist.

Because of its mechanism of action, this substance affects the imbalance between endogenous opiate imbalance associated with the development of ESRDCI–β-endorphin (μ-opioid agonist) and dynorphin A (κ-opioid agonist). Hawi and colleagues[118] evaluated nalbuphine in 14 patients with ESRDCI on HD, compared with 8 healthy controls. Doses were gradually increased, beginning with 30 mg twice daily and ending at 180 twice daily mg over 13 days or 240 mg twice daily over 15 days. The drug effectively reduced itch in 86% of treated patients, with mean itch intensity of 4 points (VAS) at baseline and 1.2 points (180 mg) or 0.4 points (240 mg) at the end of the study. Concomitantly, nalbuphine was well tolerated. A larger phase 2 double-blind study[119] with nalbuphine at a dose of 120 mg twice daily (n = 61) was superior in relieving itch to nalbuphine 60 mg twice daily (n = 63) and placebo (n = 55). In terms of itch intensity (VAS), nalbuphine 120 mg twice daily reduced itch by 49% (6.9–3.5) compared with placebo (P = .017). Itch-related QoL (measured by Skindex-10) and Sleep Disruption (measured by Itch Medical Outcomes Study [MOS]) were also improved by 240 mg/d of nalbuphine. Another promising drug from this therapeutic group includes butorphanol, as well as peripherally acting agents, such as asimadoline or CR845.[151]

An important drug from the selective serotonin reuptake inhibitor group is sertraline. Shakiba and colleagues[123] instigated sertraline in a dose of 50 mg once daily (n = 19). At baseline, 47% of patients deemed itch as moderate, 52% of patients deemed itch as severe, whereas after 4 months of treatment, 58% patients described their itch intensity as weak, 31.5% as moderate, and 11% as severe. These findings were later confirmed by other researchers.[124,125]

Older reports advocated the effectiveness of intravenous *lidocaine*,[140] *heparin*,[141] and *cholestyramine*.[142] *Active charcoal* was evaluated in 2 studies. In 10 out of 11 patients, active charcoal (6 g/d daily for 8 weeks) provided relief in itch ($P = .01$) and was associated with a reduction of scratch-induced skin lesions ($P = .03$).[135] Another report evaluated 23 patients, among which 10 reported complete disappearance of itch and partial effect in another 10 patients.[136] The investigators concluded that this method is safe and low cost, albeit the mechanism of action is unknown. A recent small study has supported the use of *omega-3 polyunsaturated fatty acids* supplementation, because the mean itch score was reduced up to 65% in the treatment group versus 17% in the placebo ($P = .001$).[152]

Miscellaneous

In severe cases of ESRDCI itch with associated secondary hyperparathyroidism, it was observed that *parathyroidectomy* provides relief of symptoms as well as normalization of laboratory parameters.[32,146,147] This method is considered supplementary in severe cases of ESRDCI associated with elevated levels of PTH. Several studies have also supported the use of alternative medicine *acupuncture*,[145,153] *aromatherapy*,[144] and *turmeric*,[143] although these modalities require further studies.

SUMMARY

ESRCDI is an important common symptom especially in advanced stages of CKD disease. Patients often suffer from significant decrease in QoL. The pathogenesis is not fully understood. It is hoped with the recent advances in understanding of mechanisms of neurobiology and immunology of itch and new drug developments that ESRDCI patients will be provided with more effective targeted and safer treatment options.

REFERENCES

1. Hill NR, Fatoba ST, Oke JL, et al. Global prevalence of chronic kidney disease - a systematic review and meta-analysis. PLoS One 2016;11: e0158765.
2. Chapter 1: definition and classification of CKD. Kidney Int Suppl (2011) 2013;3:19–62.
3. Thomas R, Kanso A, Sedor JR. Chronic kidney disease and its complications. Prim Care 2008;35: 329–44, vii.
4. Robinson-Bostom L, DiGiovanna JJ. Cutaneous manifestations of end-stage renal disease. J Am Acad Dermatol 2000;43:975–86 [quiz: 987–90].
5. Weisshaar E, Szepietowski JC, Darsow U, et al. European guideline on chronic pruritus. Acta Derm Venereol 2012;92:563–81.
6. Ständer S, Weisshaar E, Mettang T, et al. Clinical classification of itch: a position paper of the International Forum for the Study of Itch. Acta Derm Venereol 2007;87:291–4.
7. Szepietowski JC, Sikora M, Kusztal M, et al. Uremic pruritus: a clinical study of maintenance hemodialysis patients. J Dermatol 2002;29:621–7.
8. Szepietowski JC, Schwartz RA. Uremic pruritus. Int J Dermatol 1998;37:247–53.
9. Mettang T. Pruritus in renal disease. In: Carstens E, Akiyama T, editors. Itch: mechanisms and treatment. Boca Raton (FL): CRC Press/Taylor & Francis; 2014. p. 47–59.
10. Pisoni RL, Wikström B, Elder SJ, et al. Pruritus in haemodialysis patients: international results from the Dialysis Outcomes and Practice Patterns Study (DOPPS). Nephrol Dial Transpl 2006;21:3495–505.
11. Weiss M, Mettang T, Tschulena U, et al. Prevalence of chronic itch and associated factors in haemodialysis patients: a representative cross-sectional study. Acta Derm Venereol 2015;95:816–21.
12. Min JW, Kim SH, Kim YO, et al. Comparison of uremic pruritus between patients undergoing hemodialysis and peritoneal dialysis. Kidney Res Clin Pract 2016;35:107–13.
13. Tessari G, Dalle Vedove C, Loschiavo C, et al. The impact of pruritus on the quality of life of patients undergoing dialysis: a single centre cohort study. J Nephrol 2009;22:241–8.
14. Wojtowicz-Prus E, Kiliś-Pstrusińska K, Reich A, et al. Chronic kidney disease-associated pruritus in children. Acta Derm Venereol 2016;96:938–42.
15. Heisig M, Reich A, Szepietowski JC. Is uremic pruritus still an important clinical problem in maintenance hemodialysis patients? J Eur Acad Dermatol Venereol 2016;30:e198–9.
16. Solak B, Acikgoz SB, Sipahi S, et al. Epidemiology and determinants of pruritus in pre-dialysis chronic kidney disease patients. Int Urol Nephrol 2016;48: 585–91.
17. Murphy EL, Murtagh FE, Carey I, et al. Understanding symptoms in patients with advanced chronic kidney disease managed without dialysis: use of a short patient-completed assessment tool. Nephron Clin Pract 2009;111:c74–80.
18. Murtagh FE, Addington-Hall JM, Edmonds PM, et al. Symptoms in advanced renal disease: a cross-sectional survey of symptom prevalence in

stage 5 chronic kidney disease managed without dialysis. J Palliat Med 2007;10:1266–76.

19. Kurban MS, Boueiz A, Kibbi AG. Cutaneous manifestations of chronic kidney disease. Clin Dermatol 2008;26:255–64.

20. Morton CA, Lafferty M, Hau C, et al. Pruritus and skin hydration during dialysis. Nephrol Dial Transpl 1996;11:2031–6.

21. Chorążyczewska W, Reich A, Szepietowski JC. Lipid content and barrier function analysis in uraemic pruritus. Acta Derm Venereol 2016;96:402–3.

22. Yosipovitch G, Duque MI, Patel TS, et al. Skin barrier structure and function and their relationship to pruritus in end-stage renal disease. Nephrol Dial Transpl 2007;22:3268–72.

23. Szepietowski JC, Reich A, Szepietowski T. Emollients with endocannabinoids in the treatment of uremic pruritus: discussion of the therapeutic options. Ther Apher Dial 2005;9:277–9.

24. Balaskas E, Szepietowski JC, Bessis D, et al. Randomized, double-blind study with glycerol and paraffin in uremic xerosis. Clin J Am Soc Nephrol 2011;6:748–52.

25. Castello M, Milani M. Efficacy of topical hydrating and emollient lotion containing 10% urea ISDIN® plus dexpanthenol (Ureadin Rx 10) in the treatment of skin xerosis and pruritus in hemodialyzed patients: an open prospective pilot trial. G Ital Dermatol Venereol 2011;146:321–5.

26. Momose A, Funyu T, Wada R, et al. AQP-3 in the epidermis of haemodialysis patients with CKD-associated pruritus is overexpressed. J Clin Exp Nephrol 2016;1:7.

27. de Kroes S, Smeenk G. Serum vitamin A levels and pruritus in patients on hemodialysis. Dermatologica 1983;166:199–202.

28. Gokustun D, Bal AZ, Sezer S, et al. 25-hydroxy vitamin D deficiency may be the secret actor in the pathogenesis of uremic pruritus in hemodialysis patients. J Clin Nephrol Res 2016;3:1053. Available at: https://www.jscimedcentral.com/Nephrology/nephrology-3-1053.pdf.

29. Wu HY, Peng YS, Chen HY, et al. A comparison of uremic pruritus in patients receiving peritoneal dialysis and hemodialysis. Medicine (Baltimore) 2016;95:e2935.

30. Momose A, Kudo S, Sato M, et al. Calcium ions are abnormally distributed in the skin of haemodialysis patients with uraemic pruritus. Nephrol Dial Transpl 2004;19:2061–6.

31. Duque MI, Thevarajah S, Chan YH, et al. Uremic pruritus is associated with higher kt/V and serum calcium concentration. Clin Nephrol 2006;66:184–91.

32. Massry SG, Popovtzer MM, Coburn JW, et al. Intractable pruritus as a manifestation of secondary hyperparathyroidism in uremia. Disappearance of itching after subtotal parathyroidectomy. N Engl J Med 1968;279:697–700.

33. Makhlough A, Emadi N, Sedighi O, et al. Relationship between serum intact parathyroid hormone and pruritus in hemodialysis patients. Iran J Kidney Dis 2013;7:42–6.

34. Dimković N, Djukanović L, Radmilović A, et al. Uremic pruritus and skin mast cells. Nephron 1992;61:5–9.

35. Ramakrishnan K, Bond TC, Claxton A, et al. Clinical characteristics and outcomes of end-stage renal disease patients with self-reported pruritus symptoms. Int J Nephrol Renovasc Dis 2013;7:1–12.

36. Szepietowski J, Thepen T, van Vloten WA, et al. Pruritus and mast cell proliferation in the skin of haemodialysis patients. Inflamm Res 1995;44(Suppl 1):S84–5.

37. Matsumoto M, Ichimaru K, Horie A. Pruritus and mast cell proliferation of the skin in end stage renal failure. Clin Nephrol 1985;23:285–8.

38. Leong SO, Tan CC, Lye WC, et al. Dermal mast cell density and pruritus in end-stage renal failure. Ann Acad Med Singapore 1994;23:327–9.

39. Mettang T, Fritz P, Weber J, et al. Uremic pruritus in patients on hemodialysis or continuous ambulatory peritoneal dialysis (CAPD). The role of plasma histamine and skin mast cells. Clin Nephrol 1990;34:136–41.

40. Szepietowski JC, Morita A, Tsuji T. Ultraviolet B induces mast cell apoptosis: a hypothetical mechanism of ultraviolet B treatment for uraemic pruritus. Med Hypotheses 2002;58:167–70.

41. Ko MJ, Yang JY, Wu HY, et al. Narrowband ultraviolet B phototherapy for patients with refractory uraemic pruritus: a randomized controlled trial. Br J Dermatol 2011;165:633–9.

42. Balaskas EV, Bamihas GI, Karamouzis M, et al. Histamine and serotonin in uremic pruritus: effect of ondansetron in CAPD-pruritic patients. Nephron 1998;78:395–402.

43. Kaysen GA. The microinflammatory state in uremia: causes and potential consequences. J Am Soc Nephrol 2001;12:1549–57.

44. Kimmel M, Alscher DM, Dunst R. The role of microinflammation in the pathogenesis of uraemic pruritus in haemodialysis patients. Nephrol Dial Transpl 2006;21:749–55.

45. Fallahzadeh MK, Roozbeh J, Geramizadeh B, et al. Interleukin-2 serum levels are elevated in patients with uremic pruritus: a novel finding with practical implications. Nephrol Dial Transpl 2011;26:3338–44.

46. Ko MJ, Peng YS, Chen HY, et al. Interleukin-31 is associated with uremic pruritus in patients receiving hemodialysis. J Am Acad Dermatol 2014;71:1151–9.e1.

47. Pelc M, Kozioł M, Szepietowski JC. Expression of IL-31 in uraemic pruritus. 9th World Congress of Itch, 15-17 October, Wroclaw, Poland. Acta Derm Venereol 2017;97:1040. PP059.

48. Ozer Etik D, Ocal S, Boyacioglu AS. Hepatitis C infection in hemodialysis patients: a review. World J Hepatol 2015;7:885–95.

49. Alhmada Y, Selimovic D, Murad F, et al. Hepatitis C virus-associated pruritus: etiopathogenesis and therapeutic strategies. World J Gastroenterol 2017;23:743–50.

50. Chiu YL, Chen HY, Chuang YF, et al. Association of uraemic pruritus with inflammation and hepatitis infection in haemodialysis patients. Nephrol Dial Transpl 2008;23:3685–9.

51. Fantini F, Baraldi A, Sevignani C, et al. Cutaneous innervation in chronic renal failure patients. An immunohistochemical study. Acta Derm Venereol 1992;72:102–5.

52. Johansson O, Hilliges M, Ståhle-Bäckdahl M. Intra-epidermal neuron-specific enolase (NSE)-immuno-reactive nerve fibres: evidence for sprouting in uremic patients on maintenance hemodialysis. Neurosci Lett 1989;99:281–6.

53. Jedras M, Zakrzewska-Pniewska B, Wardyn K, et al. Uremic neuropathy–II. Is pruritus in dialyzed patients related to neuropathy? Pol Arch Med Wewn 1998;99:462–9 [in Polish].

54. Zakrzewska-Pniewska B, Jedras M. Is pruritus in chronic uremic patients related to peripheral somatic and autonomic neuropathy? Study by R-R interval variation test (RRIV) and by sympathetic skin response (SSR). Neurophysiol Clin 2001;31:181–93.

55. Papoiu AD, Emerson NM, Patel TS, et al. Voxel-based morphometry and arterial spin labeling fMRI reveal neuropathic and neuroplastic features of brain processing of itch in end-stage renal disease. J Neurophysiol 2014;112:1729–38.

56. Chirchiglia D, Della Torre A, Caserta C, et al. Can the aggravation of pruritus be a sign of worsening peripheral neuropathy in uremic disease? A clinical and neurophysiological study. Int J Neurol Brain Disord 2016;3:1–4.

57. Wieczorek A, Kozioł M, Szepietowski JC. Expression of opioid receptors in the skin of patients with uremic pruritus. 8th World Congress on Itch (WCI). September 27-29, 2015, Nara, Japan. Acta Derm Venereol 2015;95:894. OP54.

58. Wikström B, Gellert R, Ladefoged SD, et al. Kappa-opioid system in uremic pruritus: multicenter, randomized, double-blind, placebo-controlled clinical studies. J Am Soc Nephrol 2005;16:3742–7.

59. Legroux-Crespel E, Clèdes J, Misery L. A comparative study on the effects of naltrexone and loratadine on uremic pruritus. Dermatology 2004;208:326–30.

60. Pauli-Magnus C, Mikus G, Alscher DM, et al. Naltrexone does not relieve uremic pruritus: results of a randomized, double-blind, placebo-controlled crossover study. J Am Soc Nephrol 2000;11:514–9.

61. Breneman DL, Cardone JS, Blumsack RF, et al. Topical capsaicin for treatment of hemodialysis-related pruritus. J Am Acad Dermatol 1992;26:91–4.

62. Makhlough A, Ala S, Haj-Heydari Z, et al. Topical capsaicin therapy for uremic pruritus in patients on hemodialysis. Iran J Kidney Dis 2010;4:137–40.

63. Heisig M, Łaczmański Ł, Reich A, et al. Uremic pruritus is not associated with endocannabinoid receptor 1 gene polymorphisms. Biomed Res Int 2016;2016:3567527.

64. Hayani K, Weiss M, Weisshaar E. Clinical findings and provision of care in haemodialysis patients with chronic itch: new results from the German Epidemiological Haemodialysis Itch study. Acta Derm Venereol 2016;96:361–6.

65. Khanna D, Singal A, Kalra OP. Comparison of cutaneous manifestations in chronic kidney disease with or without dialysis. Postgrad Med J 2010;86:641–7.

66. Masmoudi A, Hajjaji Darouiche M, Ben Salah H, et al. Cutaneous abnormalities in patients with end stage renal failure on chronic hemodialysis. A study of 458 patients. J Dermatol Case Rep 2014;8:86–94.

67. Mathur VS, Lindberg J, Germain M, et al. A longitudinal study of uremic pruritus in hemodialysis patients. Clin J Am Soc Nephrol 2010;5:1410–9.

68. Phan NQ, Blome C, Fritz F, et al. Assessment of pruritus intensity: prospective study on validity and reliability of the visual analogue scale, numerical rating scale and verbal rating scale in 471 patients with chronic pruritus. Acta Derm Venereol 2012;92:502–7.

69. Zucker I, Yosipovitch G, David M, et al. Prevalence and characterization of uremic pruritus in patients undergoing hemodialysis: uremic pruritus is still a major problem for patients with end-stage renal disease. J Am Acad Dermatol 2003;49:842–6.

70. Gilchrest BA, Stern RS, Steinman TI, et al. Clinical features of pruritus among patients undergoing maintenance hemodialysis. Arch Dermatol 1982;118:154–6.

71. Reich A, Hrehorów E, Szepietowski JC. Pruritus is an important factor negatively influencing the well-being of psoriatic patients. Acta Derm Venereol 2010;90:257–63.

72. Erturk IE, Arican O, Omurlu IK, et al. Effect of the pruritus on the quality of life: a preliminary study. Ann Dermatol 2012;24:406–12.

73. Zachariae R, Lei U, Haedersdal M, et al. Itch severity and quality of life in patients with pruritus: preliminary validity of a Danish adaptation of the itch severity scale. Acta Derm Venereol 2012;92:508–14.

74. Carr CW, Veledar E, Chen SC. Factors mediating the impact of chronic pruritus on quality of life. JAMA Dermatol 2014;150:613–20.

75. Suseł J, Batycka-Baran A, Reich A, et al. Uraemic pruritus markedly affects the quality of life and

depressive symptoms in haemodialysis patients with end-stage renal disease. Acta Derm Venereol 2014;94:276–81.

76. Ibrahim MK, Elshahid AR, El Baz TZ, et al. Impact of uraemic pruritus on quality of life among end stage renal disease patients on dialysis. J Clin Diagn Res 2016;10:WC01–5.

77. Szepietowski JC, Balaskas E, Taube KM, et al. Quality of life in patients with uraemic xerosis and pruritus. Acta Derm Venereol 2011;91:313–7.

78. Heisig M, Reich A, Szepietowski JC. Alexithymia in uraemic pruritus. Acta Derm Venereol 2016;96: 699–700.

79. Aliasgharpour M, Zabolypour S, Asadinoghabi A, et al. The effect of increasing blood flow rate on severity of uremic pruritus in hemodialysis patients: a single clinical trial. J Natl Med Assoc 2017. https://doi.org/10.1016/j.jnma.2017.04.008.

80. Liakopoulos V, Krishnan M, Stefanidis I, et al. Improvement in uremic symptoms after increasing daily dialysate volume in patients on chronic peritoneal dialysis with declining renal function. Int Urol Nephrol 2004;36:437–43.

81. Chen ZJ, Cao G, Tang WX, et al. A randomized controlled trial of high-permeability haemodialysis against conventional haemodialysis in the treatment of uraemic pruritus. Clin Exp Dermatol 2009; 34:679–83.

82. Chen YC, Chiu WT, Wu MS. Therapeutic effect of topical gamma-linolenic acid on refractory uremic pruritus. Am J Kidney Dis 2006;48:69–76.

83. Tarng DC, Cho YL, Liu HN, et al. Hemodialysis-related pruritus: a double-blind, placebo-controlled, crossover study of capsaicin 0.025% cream. Nephron 1996;72:617–22.

84. Young TA, Patel TS, Camacho F, et al. A pramoxine-based anti-itch lotion is more effective than a control lotion for the treatment of uremic pruritus in adult hemodialysis patients. J Dermatolog Treat 2009;20:76–81.

85. Pauli-Magnus C, Klumpp S, Alscher DM, et al. Short-term efficacy of tacrolimus ointment in severe uremic pruritus. Perit Dial Int 2000;20:802–3.

86. Kuypers DR, Claes K, Evenepoel P, et al. A prospective proof of concept study of the efficacy of tacrolimus ointment on uraemic pruritus (UP) in patients on chronic dialysis therapy. Nephrol Dial Transpl 2004;19(7):1895–901.

87. Duque MI, Yosipovitch G, Fleischer AB Jr, et al. Lack of efficacy of tacrolimus ointment 0.1% for treatment of hemodialysis-related pruritus: a randomized, double-blind, vehicle-controlled study. J Am Acad Dermatol 2005;52(3 Pt 1):519–21.

88. Jung KE, Woo YR, Lee JS, et al. Effect of topical vitamin D on chronic kidney disease-associated pruritus: an open-label pilot study. J Dermatol 2015;42:800–3.

89. Aramwit P, Keongamaroon O, Siritientong T, et al. Sericin cream reduces pruritus in hemodialysis patients: a randomized, double-blind, placebo-controlled experimental study. BMC Nephrol 2012;13:119.

90. Wasik F, Szepietowski J, Szepietowski T, et al. Relief of uraemic pruritus after balneological therapy with a bath oil containing polidocanol (Balneum Hernial Plus). An open clinical study. J Dermatol Treat 1996;7:231–3.

91. Jeong SK, Park HJ, Park BD, et al. Effectiveness of topical chia seed oil on pruritus of end-stage renal disease (ESRD) patients and healthy volunteers. Ann Dermatol 2010;22:143–8.

92. Gilchrest BA, Rowe JW, Brown RS, et al. Relief of uremic pruritus with ultraviolet phototherapy. N Engl J Med 1977;297:136–8. Available at: www.tandfonline.com/doi/abs/10.3109/0954663960908955.

93. Gilchrest BA, Rowe JW, Brown RS, et al. Ultraviolet phototherapy of uremic pruritus. Long-term results and possible mechanism of action. Ann Intern Med 1979;91:17–21.

94. Schultz BC, Roenigk HH Jr. Uremic pruritus treated with ultraviolet light. JAMA 1980;243:1836–7.

95. Simpson NB, Davison AM. Ultraviolet phototherapy for uraemic pruritus. Lancet 1981;1:781.

96. Berne B, Vahlquist A, Fischer T, et al. UV treatment of uraemic pruritus reduces the vitamin A content of the skin. Eur J Clin Invest 1984;14: 203–6.

97. Blachley JD, Blankenship DM, Menter A, et al. Uremic pruritus: skin divalent ion content and response to ultraviolet phototherapy. Am J Kidney Dis 1985;5:237–41.

98. Hsu MM, Yang CC. Uraemic pruritus responsive to broadband ultraviolet (UV) B therapy does not readily respond to narrowband UVB therapy. Br J Dermatol 2003;149:888–9.

99. Ada S, Seçkin D, Budakoğlu I, et al. Treatment of uremic pruritus with narrowband ultraviolet B phototherapy: an open pilot study. J Am Acad Dermatol 2005;53:149–51.

100. Ragab BF, Youssef SS, Abou Seif KH, et al. Evaluation of serum levels of calcium and phosphorus in uremic pruritus patients before and after narrow band ultraviolet B phototherapy. J Egypt Women Dermatol Soc 2013;10:160–5.

101. Wang TJ, Lan LC, Lu CS, et al. Efficacy of narrow-band ultraviolet phototherapy on renal pruritus. J Clin Nurs 2014;23:1593–602.

102. El-Kamel MF, Alghobary M, Eid E. Treatment of hemodialysis-associated pruritus with narrow band ultraviolet B phototherapy (NB-UVB) alone vs. combined NB-UVB and gabapentin. Asian J Dermatol 2014;6:16–24. Available at: https://journals.lww.com/jewds/Abstract/2013/09000/Evaluation_of_serum_levels_of_calcium_and.9.aspx.

103. Sherjeena PB, Binitha MP, Rajan U, et al. A controlled trial of narrowband ultraviolet B phototherapy for the treatment of uremic pruritus. Indian J Dermatol Venereol Leprol 2017;83:247–9.

104. Gunal AI, Ozalp G, Yoldas TK, et al. Gabapentin therapy for pruritus in haemodialysis patients: a randomized, placebo-controlled, double-blind trial. Nephrol Dial Transpl 2004;19:3137–9 . Available at: https://scialert.net/abstract/?doi=ajd.2014.16.24.

105. Naini AE, Harandi AA, Khanbabapour S, et al. Gabapentin: a promising drug for the treatment of uremic pruritus. Saudi J Kidney Dis Transpl 2007; 18:378–81.

106. Marquez D, Ramonda C, Lauxmann JE, et al. Uremic pruritus in hemodialysis patients: treatment with desloratidine versus gabapentin. J Bras Nefrol 2012;34:148–52.

107. Amirkhanlou S, Rashedi A, Taherian J, et al. Comparison of gabapentin and ketotifen in treatment of uremic pruritus in hemodialysis patients. Pak J Med Sci 2016;32:22–6.

108. Rayner H, Baharani J, Smith S, et al. Uraemic pruritus: relief of itching by gabapentin and pregabalin. Nephron Clin Pract 2012;122:75–9.

109. Solak Y, Biyik Z, Atalay H, et al. Pregabalin versus gabapentin in the treatment of neuropathic pruritus in maintenance haemodialysis patients: a prospective, crossover study. Nephrology (Carlton) 2012; 17:710–7.

110. Lau T, Leung S, Lau W. Gabapentin for uremic pruritus in hemodialysis patients: a qualitative systematic review. Can J Kidney Health Dis 2016;3:14.

111. Shavit L, Grenader T, Lifschitz M, et al. Use of pregabalin in the management of chronic uremic pruritus. J Pain Symptom Manage 2013;45:776–81.

112. Aperis G, Paliouras C, Zervos A, et al. The use of pregabalin in the treatment of uraemic pruritus in haemodialysis patients. J Ren Care 2010;36: 180–5.

113. Khan TM, Alhafez AA, Syed Sulaiman SA, et al. Safety of pregabalin among hemodialysis patients suffering from uremic pruritus. Saudi Pharm J 2015;23:614–20.

114. Yue J, Jiao S, Xiao Y, et al. Comparison of pregabalin with ondansetron in treatment of uraemic pruritus in dialysis patients: a prospective, randomized, double-blind study. Int Urol Nephrol 2015;47:161–7.

115. Khan TM, Aziz A, Suleiman AK. Effectiveness of posthemodialysis administration of pregabalin (75 mg) in treatment resistance uremia pruritus. J Pharm Bioallied Sci 2016;8:74–6.

116. Kumagai H, Ebata T, Takamori K, et al. Effect of a novel kappa-receptor agonist, nalfurafine hydrochloride, on severe itch in 337 haemodialysis patients: a phase III, randomized, double-blind,

placebo-controlled study. Nephrol Dial Transpl 2010;25:1251–7.

117. Kumagai H, Ebata T, Takamori K, et al. Efficacy and safety of a novel κ-agonist for managing intractable pruritus in dialysis patients. Am J Nephrol 2012;36: 175–83.

118. Hawi A, Alcorn H Jr, Berg J, et al. Pharmacokinetics of nalbuphine hydrochloride extended release tablets in hemodialysis patients with exploratory effect on pruritus. BMC Nephrol 2015;16:47.

119. Kumar J, Crawford P, Mathur V, et al. Nalbuphine ER tablets in hemodialysis patients with severe uremic pruritus: multicenter, randomized, double-blind, placebo-controlled trial. Am J Kidney Dis 2016;67:A65.

120. Peer G, Kivity S, Agami O, et al. Randomised crossover trial of naltrexone in uraemic pruritus. Lancet 1996;348:1552–4.

121. Ashmore SD, Jones CH, Newstead CG, et al. Ondansetron therapy for uremic pruritus in hemodialysis patients. Am J Kidney Dis 2000;35:827–31.

122. Murphy M, Reaich D, Pai P, et al. A randomized, placebo-controlled, double-blind trial of ondansetron in renal itch. Br J Dermatol 2003;148:314–7.

123. Shakiba M, Sanadgol H, Azmoude HR, et al. Effect of sertraline on uremic pruritus improvement in ESRD patients. Int J Nephrol 2012;2012: 363901.

124. Chan KY, Li CW, Wong H, et al. Use of sertraline for antihistamine-refractory uremic pruritus in renal palliative care patients. J Palliat Med 2013;16: 966–70.

125. Pakfetrat M, Malekmakan L, Hashemi N, et al. Sertraline can reduce the uremic pruritus in hemodialysis patient: a double blind randomized clinical trial from Southern Iran. Hemodial Int 2018;22(1): 103–9.

126. Rosner MH. Cromolyn sodium: a potential therapy for uremic pruritus? Hemodial Int 2006;10:189–92.

127. Vessal G, Sagheb MM, Shilian S, et al. Effect of oral cromolyn sodium on CKD-associated pruritus and serum tryptase level: a double-blind placebo-controlled study. Nephrol Dial Transpl 2010;25: 1541–7.

128. Foroutan N, Etminan A, Nikvarz N, et al. Comparison of pregabalin with doxepin in the management of uremic pruritus: a randomized single blind clinical trial. Hemodial Int 2017;21:63–71.

129. Pour-Reza-Gholi F, Nasrollahi A, Firouzan A, et al. Low-dose doxepin for treatment of pruritus in patients on hemodialysis. Iran J Kidney Dis 2007;1: 34–7.

130. Francos GC, Kauh YC, Gittlen SD, et al. Elevated plasma histamine in chronic uremia. Effects of ketotifen on pruritus. Int J Dermatol 1991;30:884–9.

131. Nasrollahi AR, Miladipour A, Ghanei E, et al. Montelukast for treatment of refractory pruritus in

patients on hemodialysis. Iran J Kidney Dis 2007;1: 73–7.

132. Davis MP, Frandsen JL, Walsh D, et al. Mirtazapine for pruritus. J Pain Symptom Manage 2003;25: 288–91.

133. Mettang T, Krumme B, Bohler J, et al. Pentoxifylline as treatment for uraemic pruritus–an addition to the weak armentarium for a common clinical symptom? Nephrol Dial Transpl 2007;22:2727–8.

134. Silva SR, Viana PC, Lugon NV, et al. Thalidomide for the treatment of uremic pruritus: a crossover randomized double-blind trial. Nephron 1994;67: 270–3.

135. Pederson JA, Matter BJ, Czerwinski AW, et al. Relief of idiopathic generalized pruritus in dialysis patients treated with activated oral charcoal. Ann Intern Med 1980;93:446–8.

136. Giovannetti S, Barsotti G, Cupisti A, et al. Oral activated charcoal in patients with uremic pruritus. Nephron 1995;70:193–6.

137. Omidian M, Khazanee A, Yaghoobi R, et al. Therapeutic effect of oral nicotinamide on refractory uremic pruritus: a randomized, double-blind study. Saudi J Kidney Dis Transpl 2013;24:995–9.

138. Shirazian S, Schanler M, Shastry S, et al. The effect of ergocalciferol on uremic pruritus severity: a randomized controlled trial. J Ren Nutr 2013;23: 308–14.

139. Bousquet J, Rivory JP, Maheut M, et al. Double-blind, placebo-controlled study of nicergoline in the treatment of pruritus in patients receiving maintenance hemodialysis. J Allergy Clin Immunol 1989;83:825–8.

140. Tapia L, Cheigh JS, David DS, et al. Pruritus in dialysis patients treated with parenteral lidocaine. N Engl J Med 1977;296:261–2.

141. Yatzidis H, Digenis P, Tountas C, et al. Heparin treatment of uremic itching. JAMA 1972;222:1183.

142. Silverberg DS, Iaina A, Reisin E, et al. Cholestyramine in uraemic pruritus. Br Med J 1977;1:752–3.

143. Pakfetrat M, Basiri F, Malekmakan L, et al. Effects of turmeric on uremic pruritus in end stage renal disease patients: a double-blind randomized clinical trial. J Nephrol 2014;27:203–7.

144. Cürcani M, Tan M. The effect of aromatherapy on haemodialysis patients' pruritus. J Clin Nurs 2014; 23:3356–65.

145. Che-Yi C, Wen CY, Min-Tsung K, et al. Acupuncture in haemodialysis patients at the Quchi (LI11) acupoint for refractory uraemic pruritus. Nephrol Dial Transpl 2005;20:1912–5.

146. Hampers CL, Katz AI, Wilson RE, et al. Disappearance of "uremic" itching after subtotal parathyroidectomy. N Engl J Med 1968;279:695–7.

147. Chou FF, Ho JC, Huang SC, et al. A study on pruritus after parathyroidectomy for secondary hyperparathyroidism. J Am Coll Surg 2000;190:65–70.

148. Moncrieff G, Cork M, Lawton S, et al. Use of emollients in dry-skin conditions: consensus statement. Clin Exp Dermatol 2013;38:231–8.

149. Feily A, Dormanesh B, Ghorbani AR, et al. Efficacy of topical cromolyn sodium 4% on pruritus in uremic nephrogenic patients: a randomized double-blind study in 60 patients. Int J Clin Pharmacol Ther 2012;50:510–3.

150. Ring J, Alomar A, Bieber T, et al. Guidelines for treatment of atopic eczema (atopic dermatitis) Part II. J Eur Acad Dermatol Venereol 2012;26: 1176–93.

151. Cowan A, Kehner GB, Inan S. Targeting itch with ligands selective for κ opioid receptors. Handb Exp Pharmacol 2015;226:291–314.

152. Ghanei E, Zeinali J, Borghei M, et al. Efficacy of omega-3 fatty acids supplementation in treatment of uremic pruritus in hemodialysis patients: a double-blind randomized controlled trial. Iran Red Crescent Med J 2012;14:515–22.

153. Duo LJ. Electrical needle therapy of uremic pruritus. Nephron 1987;47:179–83.

Management of Chronic Hepatic Itch

Miriam M. Düll, MD, Andreas E. Kremer, MD, PhD, MHBA*

KEYWORDS

- Autotaxin • Bile salt • Cholestasis • Liver • Lysophosphatidic acid • Management • Pruritus

KEY POINTS

- The palms and soles are predilection sites for itching specific to the immune-mediated disorders primary biliary cholangitis and primary sclerosing cholangitis; however, pruritus often generalizes.
- Autotaxin activity correlates with itch intensity in patients with hepatic pruritus.
- Cholestyramine is the only drug licensed to treat hepatic itch.
- Rifampicin at a dosage between 150 and 600 mg/d strongly attenuates hepatic itch.
- Bezafibrate at a dosage of 400 mg/d may represent a valuable alternative treatment option for hepatic itch.

INTRODUCTION

Various hepatobiliary disorders are frequently accompanied by chronic pruritus, particularly if cholestasis is an inherent feature of the underlying disease.[1] In these hepatic disorders, cholestasis can be caused by different mechanisms[2]:

- Hepatocellular cholestasis: impaired hepatocellular secretion
  For example, intrahepatic cholestasis of pregnancy (ICP), benign recurrent intrahepatic cholestasis, progressive familial intrahepatic cholestasis type, toxin-induced or drug-induced cholestasis, acute or chronic viral hepatitis
- Cholangiocellular cholestasis: intrahepatic bile duct damage
  For example, primary biliary cholangitis (PBC), primary sclerosing cholangitis (PSC), and secondary sclerosing cholangitis (SSC), or Alagille syndrome

- Obstructive cholestasis: obstruction of the intrahepatic or extrahepatic bile duct
  For example, gallstone disease, biliary atresia, enlarged lymph nodes, cholangiocellular adenoma or carcinoma, or pancreatic head carcinoma.

Pruritus is frequently observed in all these conditions and significantly reduces the quality of life of these patients and affects their sleep. In some patients, itching became so severe that liver transplantation was considered, even in absence of liver failure.[3] Several pruritogens, including bile salts, endogenous opioids, histamine, serotonin, progesterone metabolites, and lysophosphatidic acid (LPA),[4] have been hypothesized to be involved in the pathogenesis of hepatic itch; however, the definite mechanisms have not yet been revealed. Management involves a stepwise approach that tends to be insufficient in some patients. This review summarizes state-of-the-art treatment, demonstrates alternative regimens

Disclosure Statement: The authors have nothing to disclose.
This work was supported by a grant from the Deutsche Forschungsgemeinschaft (KR4391/1-1) and grants E20 and E27 of the IZKF in Erlangen to A.E. Kremer.
Department of Medicine 1, Friedrich-Alexander-University Erlangen-Nürnberg, Ulmenweg 18, Erlangen 91054, Germany
* Corresponding author.
E-mail address: andreas.kremer@uk-erlangen.de

Dermatol Clin 36 (2018) 293–300
https://doi.org/10.1016/j.det.2018.02.008

in patients who are difficult to treat, and summarizes current clinical trials that may represent future treatment options.

CLINICAL ASPECTS OF HEPATIC PRURITUS
Prevalence

Epidemiologic data on hepatic pruritus are scarce. Pruritus is commonly observed in hepatobiliary disorders with cholestatic features, albeit to different extents depending on the underlying condition. Approximately 70% of patients with PBC, PSC, or SSC report on pruritus at some point during their course of disease.[5,6] The prevalence of pruritus in PBC patients in an extensive online survey of 577 participants was as high as 56% (A.E. Kremer and colleagues, unpublished, 2018). In women with ICP, pruritus is even part of the definition criteria of the condition. Obstruction of intrahepatic or extrahepatic biliary tracts is less commonly associated with hepatic itch, with 45% of affected patients with malignant obstruction, such as carcinoma of the pancreatic head, and 16% of affected patients with benign biliary obstruction, such as choledocholithiasis.[7] Between 5% and 15% of untreated patients with chronic hepatitis C virus infections reported itching.[8] In contrast, hepatic itch is rarely observed in patients with chronic hepatitis B virus infections, alcoholic or nonalcoholic fatty liver disease, or alcoholic or nonalcoholic steatohepatitis (NASH), even in case of cholestasis.[9]

Clinical Picture

In immune-mediated hepatobiliary diseases such as PBC and PSC, hepatic pruritus often initially presents at the limbs, particularly at the palms and soles,[5] before itching spreads over other body parts. A circadian rhythm has been conclusively shown by displaying the scratch activity in patients with PBC using piezoelectric electrode attached to the fingernail.[10] The highest rating of itch intensity is commonly reported in the evening and early at night,[11] although this is an usual pattern in chronic pruritus that is often aggravated by warmth and limited sensory input during the night. Patients with hepatic itch do not present with primary lesions of the skin; however, enduring scratching may result in secondary skin alterations; for example, excoriations and prurigo nodularis. These phenomena might cause difficulties in distinguishing hepatic itch from a primary dermatologic condition. Pruritus can have a burdensome impact on the quality of life of patients with hepatic disorders, among other consequences, by inducing sleep deprivation and resulting in exhaustion, fatigue, and depression.[12] Finally, women suffering from hepatic itch show increased symptoms before menstruation, as well as during late pregnancy or hormone replacement therapy.

Pathogenesis of Hepatic Pruritus

Despite the extensive itch research in animals, the underlying pathogenetic mechanisms of chronic pruritus in humans remain largely elusive. This also holds true for the pathogenesis of chronic hepatic itch, although several potential mediators have been controversially discussed to be involved in cholestatic disorders, such as bile salts, histamine, serotonin, endogenous opioids, and progesterone metabolites. LPA, a small phospholipid, was recently identified as a novel candidate pruritogen in hepatobiliary disorders.[13]

Bile Salts

More than 2000 years ago the Greek physician Aretaeus the Cappadocian already suggested "prickly bilious particles" as cause for pruritus in jaundiced patients. Even today his theory still holds true, at least in part: removing bile from the human body; for example, by nasobiliary or transcutaneous drainage, is often very effective in attenuating severe and long-lasting hepatic itch.[14] Bile salts and certain subspecies, which are present in bile in high concentrations, have long been suggested as potential pruritogens. This bile salt hypothesis has recently experienced clinical support by the observation that the novel semisynthetic bile salt obeticholic acid induced or worsened pruritus in PBC and NASH subjects in clinical trials. GSK2330672, a novel inhibitor of the ileal bile acid transporter (IBAT), prevents the reuptake of bile salts in the ileum and strongly improves hepatic itch. Nevertheless, several observations argue against bile salts as direct pruritogens in cholestasis because no correlation was observed between the intensity of cholestatic pruritus and the levels of bile salts in serum, urine, or skin.[15,16] Women with ICP show only slightly increased total serum bile salt (TBS) levels yet suffer from pruritus. Obstructive cholestasis linked with increased TBS is much less commonly associated with pruritus and the anion exchange resin colesevelam diminished TBS levels by approximately 50% without being superior to placebo in ameliorating pruritus.[17] Thus, bile salts or certain subspecies might instead represent indirect pruritogens in hepatobiliary disorders.

Histamine

Histamine levels have been shown to be elevated in hepatic disorders, in particular in patients suffering from itching and in cholestatic animals. Furthermore, bile salts can trigger histamine release from mast cells. However, also for histamine levels, no correlation with the intensity of pruritus in cholestatic patients could be proven.[13] Typical histamine-specific skin alterations are not observed and treatment with histamine-receptor blockers is typically ineffective.[18]

Serotonin

The neurotransmitter serotonin can cause scratching behavior in mice, as well as itching on intradermal injection in humans. Indeed, hepatic itch was mildly alleviated by selective serotonin reuptake inhibitors (SSRIs), such as sertraline and paroxetine, yet there was no clear evidence for an improvement of pruritus in clinical studies for the 5-hydroxytryptamine type 3 (HT_3)-receptor antagonist ondansetron.[15] Similar to other pruritogens, no correlation between itch intensity and serotonin has been shown.

Endogenous Opioids

Endogenous opioids have been considered potential mediators of pruritus in hepatic disorders for many years. Plasma opioid levels were shown to be increased in cholestatic patients, and the epidural or spinal application of opioids can induce itching in humans.[19] The μ-opioid antagonists naloxone and naltrexone exerted mild antipruritic effects in some cholestatic patients.[20] However, no correlation between itch intensity and endogenous opioids has ever been revealed and, instead, data show an inverse correlation with increased levels of endogenous opioids at later stages of PBC, at which pruritus might ease.[21]

Progesterone Metabolites

The involvement of steroid hormones in cholestatic pruritus[11] was regarded as possible owing to their influence on various ionotropic receptors (eg, transient receptor potential vanilloid 1 [TRPV1]), and the clinical observations that female cholestatic patients experience itch at a higher intensity and frequency than male patients.[22] During pregnancy, steroid hormone levels are exceptionally high and might, therefore, contribute to ICP, of which pruritus is a defining symptom that dissolves within weeks after delivery. Additionally, improvement of pruritus by ursodeoxycholic acid (UDCA) treatment in ICP-patients correlated with reduced levels of urinary disulphated progesterone metabolites, which was not seen for bile salts or other steroid metabolites.[23] Finally, progesterone metabolites were shown to induce scratching behavior in mice on intradermal injection via the bile salt receptor TGR5.[24] Thus, in particular during ICP, progesterone metabolites might represent a major pruritogen.

Lysophosphatidic Acid

LPA has recently been revealed as major neuronal activator in sera of cholestatic pruritic patients.[13] Serum concentrations of the enzyme autotaxin (ATX), which hydrolyzes LPA from its precursor molecule, lysophosphatidylcholine, were elevated in cholestatic pruritic patients compared with those without pruritus[25] and proved as a robust marker to diagnose ICP.[26] As opposed to other suggested pruritogens in cholestasis, ATX activity correlated with itch intensity and response to therapeutic interventions. In mice, intradermal injection of LPA induced dose-dependent scratching behavior.[13,25] Similarly, LPA induced an itch sensation in humans on focal application and is able to activate murine dorsal root ganglion cultures (unpublished data, Robering et al, 2018). Recently, an interesting molecular interaction of ATX and specific natural bile salts was found, possibly linking ATX-LPA signaling to elevated bile salt levels in cholestatic conditions.[27]

Treatment of Cholestatic Pruritus

Therapeutic options of cholestatic itch are based on a few randomized, placebo-controlled trials and cohort studies[28] but also on experimental medical and interventional approaches.[2] General recommendations include the use of emollients and oatmeal extract to ameliorate skin dryness and inflammation, bathing or showering with cold water, the regular application of moisturizing and cooling agents, and the shortening of fingernails to evade skin damage.[1,29] Medical and interventional approaches to alleviate itching might involve the following aspects[1]:

1. Removal of pruritogens from the enterohepatic cycle
   - Anion exchange resins, such as cholestyramine
   - IBAT inhibitors (GSK2330672, maralixibat, A4250)
   - Biliary drainage

2. Altered metabolism and/or secretion of potential pruritogens in the liver or intestine
   • Inducers of hepatic biotransformation enzymes, such as rifampicin
   • Bezafibrate
3. Modulation of itch and pain pathways
   • μ-opioid antagonists, such as naltrexone
   • κ-opioid agonists, such as nalfurafine
   • SSRIs, such as sertraline
4. Removal of potential pruritogens from the body system
   • Anion absorption, plasmapheresis, or extracorporeal albumin dialysis.

All presented drugs, except cholestyramine, are used in an off-label manner. Patients with cholestatic pruritus generally do not respond to antihistaminergic drugs and the commonly observed fatigue in patients with hepatobiliary disorders might be worsened by the central sedative effect, in particular of first-generation antihistamines. Thus, antihistamines should be avoided in hepatic itch.

Ursodeoxycholic Acid

UDCA exerts anticholestatic properties by enhancing hepatobiliary secretory function and reducing bile toxicity. It is, therefore, used to treat patients with hepatobiliary diseases, such as PBC, PSC, or ICP, and cholestatic syndromes in children, to modify the underlying condition. In PBC, it improves overall survival if patients respond to UDCA treatment.[29] In ICP, several trials showed that UDCA at a dosage of 13 to 15 mg/kg/d clearly attenuated itching, improved serum liver test, and had a positive impact on delivery; however, there was no significant improvement of pruritus in chronic hepatic disorders such as PBC or PSC.[30]

Anion Exchange Resins

The anion exchange resin cholestyramine is still the first-line recommendation in current guidelines for hepatic itch.[29] It has been applied in several small, nonplacebo-controlled trials and alleviated pruritus within 14 days. Patients should be advised to take one 4 g sachet of the bile sequestrant 1 hour before and 1 hour after breakfast. The dosage might be increased to 16 g/d. It is important to apply the resin at least 4 hours before any other medication to avoid interference with their intestinal absorption. Aside from its unpalatable taste, patients may experience gastrointestinal adverse effects such as abdominal discomfort, bloating, and malabsorption of fat and fat-soluble vitamins.

Colesevelam, an anion exchange resin with a higher binding affinity for bile salts than cholestyramine, was not superior to placebo in a randomized, placebo-controlled trial.[17] One might speculate that the potential pruritogen is more efficiently bound by cholestyramine, albeit this trial definitely questions bile sequestrants as recommended first-line treatment.

Rifampicin

Rifampicin, a pregnane X receptor (PXR) agonist, can be administered as second-line therapy. In randomized, placebo-controlled trials, rifampicin proved as an effective and safe treatment of hepatic pruritus,[31] which was confirmed in meta-analyses.[30] From a clinical perspective, rifampicin, if well-tolerated, has the strongest antipruritic effect in hepatic itch and can be given for many years. Its method of action in regard to itching has been explained by the induction of various biotransformation enzymes and transporters in liver and intestine, thereby changing the metabolism of potential pruritogens. Rifampicin and phenobarbital induce cytochrome P (CYP)3A4 to a similar extent. Phenobarbital proved to be less effective in alleviation of pruritus in a randomized controlled trial, suggesting that other mechanisms contribute to the antipruritic impact of rifampicin.[32] As antibiotic drug, rifampicin might also alter the intestinal microbiome. Interestingly, rifampicin reduced ATX expression in vitro through a PXR-dependent mechanism.[25] Hepatotoxicity has to be considered as a serious adverse effect, as it was registered in up to 13% of patients, especially in long-term treatment for many months.[31] A close monitoring of laboratory values is, therefore, recommended. Further adverse effects might be nausea and loss of appetite. Finally, patients should be educated about the harmless adverse effect of change in urine or tears to orange-red color.

MODULATORS OF ITCH AND PAIN PATHWAYS
μ-Opioid Antagonists

The μ-opioid antagonist naltrexone can be considered in case treatment with rifampicin was not tolerated or not successful after 2 weeks. Mild antipruritic effects of naltrexone at doses of 25 to 50 mg/d were observed in some small placebo-controlled trials.[2] Naltrexone starting doses should be as low as 12.5 mg/d to avoid opiate withdrawal–like reactions. Another approach can be to start therapy with increasing dosages of intravenous naloxone, then switching to oral naltrexone. To prevent a breakthrough phenomenon (reoccurrence of pruritus during treatment, potentially because of upregulated μ-opioid receptors), naltrexone administration can be interrupted for 2 days per week.[33] In case of continued treatment, opioid antagonists have been reported to increase the risk of a chronic pain syndrome.[34] Furthermore, dizziness, headache, abdominal pain, nausea, and vomiting are commonly reported adverse events, particularly in older patients.

κ-Opioid Agonists

In Japan, the κ-opioid receptor agonist nalfurafine has been licensed for the treatment of hepatic itch. Its mild efficiency and safety was first evaluated in a placebo-controlled study[35] in hemodialysis subjects suffering from uremic pruritus and later in a meta-analysis of 2 placebo-controlled double-blind trials.[36] Recently, a randomized controlled trial indicated a significant but clinically questionable benefit of nalfurafine for chronic hepatic itch at a dosage of (2.5–5 μg/d).[37] Adverse events included pollakiuria (including nycturia), somnolence, insomnia, and constipation. Nalfurafine is currently not available in Europe or the United States. Butorphanol, a κ-opioid receptor agonist and κ-opioid receptor antagonist, with proven antipruritic properties in atopic dermatitis is available in the United States and Europe but has not been investigated in cholestatic pruritus. Further κ-opioid receptor agonists are currently being evaluated in clinical trials for their antipruritic potential in other diseases, such as atopic dermatitis.

Selective Serotonin Reuptake Inhibitors

If naltrexone is ineffective, selective SSRIs such as sertraline or paroxetine may be given as fourth-line therapy. Evidence of a moderate itch-reducing effect is limited to a single placebo-controlled, cross-over trial using sertraline[38] and a few case series.[39]

NEW DRUGS ON THE BLOCK
Bezafibrate

The peroxisome-proliferator activated receptor (PPAR)-agonist bezafibrate has proven anticholestatic effects in many case reports and case series, mainly from Japan. In some of these studies, a significant improvement of itch intensity was also reported in PBC patients. An investigator-initiated, randomized placebo-controlled, 2-year trial (**BEZ**afibrate for the treatment of primary biliary cholangitis in patients with inadequate biochemical response to **URSO**deoxycholic acid therapy [BEZURSO-Trial]) proved strong anticholestatic effects of bezafibrate 400 mg/d in PBC subjects with insufficient response to UDCA.[40] In this trial, subjects on bezafibrate exhibited a 75% reduction in itch intensity.

Currently, the international multicenter the effect of bezaFibrate on cholestatic ITCH (FITCH trial) is investigating the antipruritic effect of bezafibrate in moderate and severe hepatic pruritus.

Ileal Bile Acid Transporter-Inhibitors (Maralixibat, GSK672, A4250)

Interruption of the enterohepatic circulation; for example, by nasobiliary drainage, has proven strong antipruritic effects in PBC and other cholestatic disorders. The IBAT, also known as apical sodium-dependent bile acid transporter (ASBT), represents a highly selective target for interrupting this cycle. Recently, interest in selective IBAT inhibitors has increased. A phase II crossover trial of the IBAT inhibitor GSK2330672 significantly reduced itch intensity within 2 weeks in 21 subjects with PBC suffering from moderate or severe pruritus.[41] The major adverse event was bile salt-induced diarrhea. The currently running GSK2330672 triaL of Ibat inhibition with Multidose Measurement for Evaluation of Response (GLIMMER) phase III trial will provide evidence of the long-term efficacy and safety of this compound. In contrast, maralixibat (elobixibat or LUM001), another IBAT inhibitor, was not superior to placebo in a 3-month phase II trial, albeit there was a comparable reduction in bile salts and ATX levels. A third IBAT inhibitor, A4250, has been investigated in pediatric cholestasis syndromes in a multiple dose, open-label trial. The absolute reduction in visual analog scale scores was comparable to that of the placebo groups of the other 2 trials that are questioning the antipruritic strength of this drug. The different efficacies of these drugs may result from different trial designs, nonstandardized outcome variables for pruritus, and drug potency. These trials clearly indicate the necessity of a placebo control and highlight the need of standardization of clinical trials investigating chronic pruritus.

Patients with chronic hepatic itch should be treated in a stepwise approach (**Table 1**).[29] In case of severe therapy-refractory pruritus, it is advisable to refer patients to a center with experience in experimental approaches. These may include ultraviolet B phototherapy, molecular adsorbent recirculating system (MARS) or Prometheus therapy, plasmapheresis, plasma separation and anion absorption, or nasobiliary drainage. Only if all evidence-based and experimental therapies have failed, liver transplantation may be regarded as the very last therapeutic step; however, this raises issues of organ allocation priority and risks in patients who would otherwise not require transplantation.

Table 1
Therapeutic recommendations for the management of hepatic itch

Approach	Drug[a]	Dosage	Evidence
1st line	Cholestyramine	4–16 g/d (po)	II-2/B1
2nd line	Rifampicin	150–600 mg/d (po)	I/A1
3rd line	Naltrexone	25–50 mg/d (po)	I/B1
4th line	Sertraline	75–100 mg/d (po)	II-2/C2
5th line	Experimental treatments[b]		
Categories of evidence[c]			
I	Randomized controlled trials		
II-1	Controlled trials without randomization		
II-2	Cohort or case-control analytical studies		
II-3	Multiple time series, dramatic uncontrolled experiments		
III	Opinions of respected authorities, descriptive epidemiology		
Evidence grading			
A	High quality: further research is very unlikely to change confidence in the estimate of effect		
B	Moderate quality: further research is likely to have an important impact on confidence in the estimate of effect and may change the estimate		
C	Low quality: further research is very likely to have an important impact on confidence in the estimate of effect and is likely to change the estimate. Any change of estimate is uncertain		
Recommendation			
1	Strong: factors influencing the strength of the recommendation included the quality of the evidence, presumed patient-important outcomes, and cost		
2	Poor: variability in preferences and values, or more uncertainty. Recommendation is made with less certainty, higher cost, or resource consumption		

[a] Except for cholestyramine, all recommended drugs to treat pruritus of cholestasis have an off-label use.
[b] For details see text.
[c] Categories of evidence according to the Grading of Recommendations, Assessment, Development, and Evaluation (GRADE) system.
Adapted from Kremer AE, Beuers U, Oude Elferink RP, et al. Pathogenesis and treatment of pruritus in cholestasis. Drugs 2008;68(15):2172; with permission.

SUMMARY

Chronic pruritus is a bothersome symptom of various hepatobiliary disorders that may strongly reduce the quality of life of affected patients. Although basic pruritus research has increased knowledge on the receptors, cells, and circuits involved in itch signaling, further investigations of the underlying mechanisms of hepatic itch are required to provide causal and more effective treatment strategies in the future. Current recommendations for hepatic itch consist of a stepwise approach, starting with cholestyramine, followed by rifampicin, naltrexone, and sertraline (see **Table 1**). Patients unresponsive to these treatments should be included in currently performed clinical trials or undergo experimental approaches, including bezafibrate or invasive procedures, such as albumin dialysis, plasma separation, or nasobiliary drainage.

REFERENCES

1. Kremer AE, Namer B, Bolier R, et al. Pathogenesis and management of pruritus in PBC and PSC. Dig Dis 2015;33(2):164–75.
2. Kremer AE, Oude Elferink RP, Beuers U. Pathophysiology and current management of pruritus in liver disease. Clin Res Hepatol Gastroenterol 2011; 35(2):89–97.
3. Neuberger J, Jones EA. Liver transplantation for intractable pruritus is contraindicated before an adequate trial of opiate antagonist therapy. Eur J Gastroenterol Hepatol 2001;13(11): 1393–4.

4. Beuers U, Kremer AE, Bolier R, et al. Pruritus in cholestasis: facts and fiction. Hepatology 2014; 60(1):399–407.

5. Bergasa NV, Mehlman JK, Jones EA. Pruritus and fatigue in primary biliary cirrhosis. Baillieres Best Pract Res Clin Gastroenterol 2000;14(4):643–55.

6. Koulentaki M, Ioannidou D, Stefanidou M, et al. Dermatological manifestations in primary biliary cirrhosis patients: a case control study. Am J Gastroenterol 2006;101(3):541–6.

7. Mcphedran NT, Henderson RD. Pruritus and jaundice. Can Med Assoc J 1965;92:1258–60.

8. Chia SC, Bergasa NV, Kleiner DE, et al. Pruritus as a presenting symptom of chronic hepatitis C. Dig Dis Sci 1998;43(10):2177–83.

9. Ghent CN, Bloomer JR. Itch in liver disease: facts and speculations. Yale J Biol Med 1979;52(1):77–82.

10. Bergasa NV. The itch of liver disease. Semin Cutan Med Surg 2011;30(2):93–8.

11. Kremer AE, Beuers U, Oude-Elferink RPJ, et al. Pathogenesis and treatment of pruritus in cholestasis. Drugs 2008;68(15):2163–82.

12. Mells GF, Pells G, Newton JL, et al. Impact of primary biliary cirrhosis on perceived quality of life: the UK-PBC national study. Hepatology 2013;58(1): 273–83.

13. Kremer AE, Martens JJ, Kulik W, et al. Lysophosphatidic acid is a potential mediator of cholestatic pruritus. Gastroenterology 2010;139(3):1008–18.

14. Beuers U, Gerken G, Pusl T. Biliary drainage transiently relieves intractable pruritus in primary biliary cirrhosis. Hepatology 2006;44(1):280–1.

15. Kremer AE, Feramisco J, Reeh PW, et al. Receptors, cells and circuits involved in pruritus of systemic disorders. Biochim Biophys Acta 2014; 1842(7):869–92.

16. Yosipovitch G, Greaves MW, Schmelz M. Itch. Lancet 2003;361(9358):690–4.

17. Kuiper EMM, van Erpecum KJ, Beuers U, et al. The potent bile acid sequestrant colesevelam is not effective in cholestatic pruritus: results of a double-blind, randomized, placebo-controlled trial. Hepatology 2010;52(4):1334–40.

18. Jones EA, Bergasa NV. Evolving concepts of the pathogenesis and treatment of the pruritus of cholestasis. Can J Gastroenterol 2000;14(1):33–40.

19. Ballantyne JC, Loach AB, Carr DB. Itching after epidural and spinal opiates. Pain 1988;33(2): 149–60.

20. Thornton JR, Losowsky MS. Opioid peptides and primary biliary cirrhosis. BMJ 1988;297(6662): 1501–4.

21. Spivey JR, Jorgensen RA, Gores GJ, et al. Methionine-enkephalin concentrations correlate with stage of disease but not pruritus in patients with primary biliary cirrhosis. Am J Gastroenterol 1994;89(11): 2028–32.

22. Lucey MR, Neuberger JM, Williams R. Primary biliary cirrhosis in men. Gut 1986;27(11):1373–6.

23. Glantz A, Reilly S-J, Benthin L, et al. Intrahepatic cholestasis of pregnancy: amelioration of pruritus by UDCA is associated with decreased progesterone disulphates in urine. Hepatology 2008;47(2): 544–51.

24. Abu-Hayyeh S, Ovadia C, Lieu T, et al. Prognostic and mechanistic potential of progesterone sulfates in intrahepatic cholestasis of pregnancy and pruritus gravidarum. Hepatology 2016;63(4): 1287–98.

25. Kremer AE, van Dijk R, Leckie P, et al. Serum autotaxin is increased in pruritus of cholestasis, but not of other origin, and responds to therapeutic interventions. Hepatology 2012;56(4):1391–400.

26. Kremer AE, Bolier R, Dixon PH, et al. Autotaxin activity has a high accuracy to diagnose intrahepatic cholestasis of pregnancy. J Hepatol 2015;62(4): 897–904.

27. Keune W-J, Jens H, Ruth B, et al. Steroid binding to Autotaxin links bile salts and lysophosphatidic acid signalling. Nat Commun 2016;7:11248.

28. European Association for the Study of the Liver. EASL clinical practice guidelines: management of cholestatic liver diseases. J Hepatol 2009;51(2): 237–67.

29. Hirschfield GM, Beuers U, Corpechot C, et al. EASL clinical practice guidelines: the diagnosis and management of patients with primary biliary cholangitis. J Hepatol 2017;67(1):145–72.

30. Tandon P, Rowe BH, Vandermeer B, et al. The efficacy and safety of bile acid binding agents, opioid antagonists, or rifampin in the treatment of cholestasis-associated pruritus. Am J Gastroenterol 2007;102(7):1528–36.

31. Bachs L, Parés A, Elena M, et al. Effects of long-term rifampicin administration in primary biliary cirrhosis. Gastroenterology 1992;102(6):2077–80.

32. Bachs L, Parés A, Elena M, et al. Comparison of rifampicin with phenobarbitone for treatment of pruritus in biliary cirrhosis. Lancet 1989;1(8638): 574–6.

33. Carson KL, Tran TT, Cotton P, et al. Pilot study of the use of naltrexone to treat the severe pruritus of cholestatic liver disease. Am J Gastroenterol 1996; 91(5):1022–3.

34. McRae CA, Prince MI, Hudson M, et al. Pain as a complication of use of opiate antagonists for symptom control in cholestasis. Gastroenterology 2003; 125(2):591–6.

35. Kumagai H, Ebata T, Takamori K, et al. Effect of a novel kappa-receptor agonist, nalfurafine hydrochloride, on severe itch in 337 haemodialysis patients: a Phase III, randomized, double-blind, placebo-controlled study. Nephrol Dial Transplant 2010; 25(4):1251–7.

36. Wikstrom B, Gellert R, Ladefoged SD, et al. Kappa-opioid system in uremic pruritus: multicenter, randomized, double-blind, placebo-controlled clinical studies. J Am Soc Nephrol 2005;16(12):3742–7.

37. Kumada H, Miyakawa H, Muramatsu T, et al. Efficacy of nalfurafine hydrochloride in patients with chronic liver disease with refractory pruritus: a randomized, double-blind trial. Hepatol Res 2017; 47(10):972–82.

38. Mayo MJ, Handem I, Saldana S, et al. Sertraline as a first-line treatment for cholestatic pruritus. Hepatology 2007;45(3):666–74.

39. Browning J, Combes B, Mayo MJ. Long-term efficacy of sertraline as a treatment for cholestatic pruritus in patients with primary biliary cirrhosis. Am J Gastroenterol 2003;98(12):2736–41.

40. Corpechot C, Chazouillères O, Rousseau A, et al. A 2-year multicenter, double-blind, randomized, placebo-controlled study of bezafibrate for the treatment of primary biliary cholangitis in patients with inadequate biochemical response to ursodeoxycholic acid therapy (Bezurso). J Hepatol 2017; 66(1):S89.

41. Hegade VS, Kendrick SFW, Dobbins RL, et al. Effect of ileal bile acid transporter inhibitor GSK2330672 on pruritus in primary biliary cholangitis: a double-blind, randomised, placebo-controlled, crossover, phase 2a study. Lancet 2017;389(10074):1114–23.

Scabies Itch

Arnaud Jannic, MD[a,b,*], Charlotte Bernigaud, MD[a,b], Emilie Brenaut, MD[c,d], Olivier Chosidow, MD, PhD[a,e]

KEYWORDS

- Itch • Pruritus • Scabies • *Sarcoptes scabiei*

KEY POINTS

- Scabies is a parasitic infestation of the skin caused by Sarcoptes scabiei, a mite present worldwide that affects 100 to 130 million people yearly.
- Itch is nearly continuously present during a scabies infestation; it is intense, generalized, and more intense at night time.
- Secondary bacterial infections caused by scratching behavior can have dramatic long-term consequences, especially in tropical areas.
- Psychosocial complications of the itch in scabies are known to have a strong impact on quality of life.
- The latest insights into host-mite interactions open ways to better understand the mechanisms of itch in scabies.
- The itch in scabies is usually controlled after the use of specific treatments but in certain conditions it may persist up to 2-4 weeks.

WHAT IS SCABIES?

Scabies is one of the first human diseases for which the cause was known in the 17th century.[1] It is a contagious parasitic skin infestation caused by a mite, *Sarcoptes scabiei* variety *hominis*. Scabies is present worldwide.[2] According to the Global Burden of Diseases study, 100 to 130 million people are infected yearly,[3] and scabies is responsible for 0.21% of disability-adjusted life-years from all of the 315 conditions studied, a relevant burden (even if scabies-related impetigo was not taken into account).[4,5] Scabies prevalence ranged from 0.2% to 71.4% depending on different populations.[6] Tropical regions with low resources are the most affected regions.[4] In wealthier countries, scabies can occur in both sexes, in all age and in all socioeconomic groups. When it comes to low-resource life conditions, children (mostly under the age of 2) and disadvantaged populations are at greater risk.[6] In both conditions, outbreaks may be frequent, requiring considerable resources to be managed, especially when they occur in collectives or in institutions.[2]

The scabies mite is an obligate human parasite. The female mite burrows into the epidermis

Disclosure Statement: C. Bernigaud reports receiving a research grant from MSD France; a research support from Bioderma Laboratoire Dermatologique and Codexial Dermatologie; and a travel grant from Medicines Development. O. Chosidow reports receiving drugs donated free of charge for research from Codexial Dermatologie and MSD France, lecture fees from Zambon Laboratoire, Codexial Dermatologie, and MSD France. No other potential conflict of interest was reported.

[a] Dermatology Department, AP-HP, Hôpital Henri Mondor, 51 avenue du Maréchal de Lattre de Tassigny, 94010 Créteil, France; [b] Research Group Dynamyc, Ecole nationale vé té rinaire d'Alfort, Maisons-Alfort, Université Paris-Est Créteil, EA7380, Créteil, France; [c] Dermatology Department, University hospital of Brest, 2 avenue Foch, 29200, Brest, France; [d] Laboratory on Interactions Neurons-Keratinocytes (LINK), University of Western Brittany, EA4685, 29238 Brest, France; [e] EpiDermE, Epidé miologie en Dermatologie et Evaluation des Thé rapeutiques, Université Paris-Est Créteil, EA 7379, 9400 Créteil, France

* Corresponding author. Dermatology Department, AP-HP, Hôpital Henri Mondor, 51 avenue du Maréchal de Lattre de Tassigny, 94010 Créteil, France.
E-mail address: arnaud.jannic@aphp.fr

Dermatol Clin 36 (2018) 301–308
https://doi.org/10.1016/j.det.2018.02.009

after mating and lays eggs that hatch into a larvae, followed by a nymph that reaches adulthood in 10 to 14 days.[1] Scabies clinical manifestations are caused by the direct effect of the infestation by the mite, and by the hypersensitivity caused by the mites, their saliva, and other products. Besides an intense itch, classic clinical signs are burrows, vesicles, or papulo-nodular erythematous lesions localized on the finger webs, the wrists, the axillae, the breasts, the buttock, or the genitalia (**Fig. 1**). Atypical forms such as profuse or crusted scabies in immunocompromised patients, or superinfected scabies (impetigo) in children, can be seen among specific populations. Crusted scabies is a rare and severe clinical form, with localized or generalized hyperkeratotic lesions due to a huge mite proliferation.[7] Diagnosis is based on patient history and physical examination. Direct identification of mites, eggs, or feces by microscopy or dermoscopy in characteristic lesions is supportive. The confirmation of the diagnosis can be challenging in classic scabies, as only 5 to 15 adult mites live simultaneously on the host, whereas hundreds, thousands, or even millions live on the host in profuse/crusted scabies. Superinfection of lesions with bacteria may occur as the mite burrow provides an entry point for pathogens into the skin. These bacteria can cause local infections that can become invasive or lead to delayed complications.[8,9] The public health burden caused by scabies, far beyond just a simple itchy rash, was for a long time underappreciated. Recently, a global initiative driven by the International Alliance for the Control of Scabies (IACS, http://www.controlscabies.org), aiming to enhance the agenda for scabies control,[10] fostered the addition of scabies to the World Health Organization list of neglected tropical diseases[11] (http://www.who.int/neglected_diseases/diseases/en/).

SCABIES ITCH: CLINICAL ASPECTS
Characteristics

Itch is the cardinal symptom of scabies and is often used as a major criterion to diagnose scabies.[12] Scabies should be suspected whenever a patient is suffering from itch and should be ruled out by a careful physical examination and parasitology test if needed. Regardless of the clinical type of scabies, having an history of itch within the family members, relatives, or sexual partners is a strong diagnosis criterion. Its absence does not eliminate the diagnosis. Actually, in an article by Boralevi and colleagues,[13] an itch shared within the family was present in only 50% of the cases. The itch is described to be more intense during the night; however, this characteristic seems to not be highly specific, and also described in other dermatoses such as psoriasis or atopic dermatitis.[14–17] There are only a few clinical studies with a limited number of patients included that aimed to characterize the itch in scabies. The primary characteristics are presented in **Table 1**.

Prevalence

In several prospective and retrospective studies, the itch is reported to be affecting more than 90% of classic scabies patients.[18–21] In the pediatric population, Boralevi and colleagues[13] described the clinical characteristics of 323 patients with scabies (divided into 3 age groups: <2 years old, 2 to 15 years old, and >15 years old). Overall, itching was present in 94.5% of the patients, regardless of their age. Looking into subgroups, the itch was less frequent in pediatric cases compared with adults, and increased with age: 90.3% before 2 years old and 95.4% in 2 to 15 years old.[13] In infants, the itch can be expressed by crying, discomfort, irritability or difficulty to eat, making the symptom difficult to assess and define.[2] This may justify the potential underestimation and lower frequency of itch in this population.

In 1976, Mellanby made the observation that "in man it is the active finger nails of the host which keep down the parasite population."[29] This statement may explain the apparition of hyperinfested crusts in anatomic regions that lack cutaneous sensation, and indeed itch sensation (eg, after spinal injury, stroke, leprosy, or syringomyelia) in patients diagnosed with crusted scabies.[26–28] Historically, the itch was

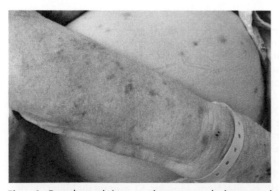

Fig. 1. Papulo-nodular erythematous lesions and scratching lesions observed on the arms and the abdomen of a patient with a confirmed diagnosis of scabies.

Table 1
Primary characteristics of the scabies itch according to the different clinical forms

Clinical Types	Prevalence of the Itch	Characteristics of the Itch	Physical Complications	Psychosocial Complications

Classic scabies	90%–100%[13,18–21]	• Generalized and intense
		• Sparing the head[18]
		• More intense during the night[13,14,18,22,23]
		• Described as stinging, burning or crawling[14,22]
		• Associated with heat sensation, sweating, and pain[22]
		• Increased with heat, sweating, and stress[22]
		• Decreased with cool environment, concentration at work, or having a bath[22]
			• GAS and S aureus superinfections
			  ○ Local (impetigo, excoriations) or invasive infections
			  ○ Acute or delayed poststreptococcal complications
			• Eczematization
				• Disturbed sleep
				• Low work attendance
				• Loss of work productivity, and overall performance
				• Social stigmatization
				• Feeling of shame
				• Sexual life impairment

Scabies affecting infants and children	90.3% in infants <2 y[13] 95.4% in children between 2 and 15 y[13]	• Affects the face and the scalp[13] • In infants, it may be assessed by discomfort or crying • May be more intense during daytime (20% of the cases)[13]		• School absenteeism • Lack of concentration or memory • Fatigue • Loss of performance at school
Crusted scabies	Described as less frequent[24] but present in up to 100% in case series[25,26]	• Hyperkeratosic lesions can be present only in anatomic regions that lack cutaneous sensation[26–28]	• Same complications that in classic scabies • General infectious complications (deeper fissures) and comorbidities • Sepsis • Death	• Severe outbreaks around a case

Abbreviations: GAS, Group A Streptococcus; S aureus, Staphylococcus aureus.

described to be inexistent or less intense in crusted scabies compared with classic scabies, and would decrease with the duration of the infestation. However, in crusted scabies case series, up to 100% of patients suffered from itching.[25,26] It is likely that the itch in crusted scabies may be overlooked. The rationale for the absence of itch in such population could be explained by the incapacity to scratch in patients with neurologic disabilities, or to report the associated feeling (eg, in patients with cognitive disorders).

Complications of Itch in scabies

The main complication of scabies is related to secondary bacterial skin infections. Impetigo is a common complication of itch in scabies, particularly in children, and in patients living in overcrowded conditions in the tropics (eg, Australian Aboriginal communities, the Fijis, and the Solomon islands in the Pacific area where the conditions were well studied).[6,19,30–33] The itch in scabies may cause severe scratching behavior and consequently excoriations of skin lesions that are a port of entry of bacteria penetrating the skin.[19] The most common pathogens known to be involved are group A *Streptococcus* (GAS) and *Staphylococcus aureus*. Scratching lesions seem more frequent in scabies than in any other pruritic skin conditions.[14] Superinfection of the skin can lead to local or general infectious complications (cellulitis, abscesses, lymphadenopathy, bacteremia) or poststreptococcal complications (acute glomerulonephritis, acute rheumatic fever, or rheumatic heart disease).[8,9,34–37] Recent molecular studies have characterized several classes of scabies mite complement inhibitors that counteract the host complement pathways in the mite-infected skin, helping GAS and staphylococcal bacteria to grow mutually.[38–43]

In crusted scabies, infectious complications seem to be more severe. This can be due to patient comorbidities (eg, immunosuppression) and deeper excoriations causing invasive infections leading to severe sepsis.[26,44]

Apart from infectious complications, eczematization of scabies lesions may appear, often misleading the initial diagnosis[25] or delaying treatment efficacy.[45] This misdiagnosis can lead to incorrect prescriptions of topical steroids, initially

Table 2
Hypotheses regarding possible mechanisms involved in scabies itch based on known host-mite interactions

Pathophysiology of Scabies	Possible Involvement in Scabies Itch
Direct scabies mite actions	
TLR pathway activation[56]	Activation of TLR 3, 4, and 7 expressed on primary sensory neurons[57]
Proteases present in mite feces	Activation of protease-activated receptor-2[23]
Direct action on keratinocytes	Release of protease activating protease-activated prurireceptors[52]
Proteins homologous with house dust mite antigens[58]	IgE-mediate allergic response: mast cell activation and histamine release
Immune response against scabies[54]	
Complement system activation	Mast cell activation[59]
Eosinophil dermal infiltrates	Expression of neurotrophins[52]: cutaneous nerve sprouting and myelinization of nerves

Mast cell activation
  Histamine
  TNF-α
  Tryptase
	Activation of histamine H_1 and H_4 prurireceptors[49,50]
	Activation of protease-activated prurireceptor by tryptase[50]

Macrophage implication Prostaglandins and leukotrienes	Itch potentiation[50]

T cell dermal infiltrates
  CD4+ (classic scabies)
  CD8+ (crusted scabies)	

Th1 response (classic scabies)
  CD4+ and CD8+ T cells
  IFN-γ, TNF-α, IL-2
	Activation of cytokine prurireceptors by IFN-γ and IL-2[49]

Th2 response (crusted scabies)
  Nonprotective allergy-like response
  B cell activation
  IL-4, IL-5, IL-13, IL-31
  IgE, IgG
	Increase involvement of eosinophils
	Activation of cytokine prurireceptors by IL-31[23,50]
	Mast cells activation by IgE

Secondary bacterial superinfections
  Staphylococcal superantigens
  TLR activation
	Expression of IL-31 mRNA in the skin[52]
	Activation of TLR 3,4 and 7 expressed on primary sensory neurons[57]

Persistent infestation in absence of treatment	Peripheral sensitization of prurireceptors: decreased threshold for activation, increased responsiveness, and presence of ongoing activity[60]

Abbreviations: Ig, Immunoglobulin; IL, interleukin; TLR, Toll-like receptor.

improving the itch but finally leading to an aggravation of the infestation such as profuse or crusted scabies, or further complications.[25]

In scabies, itch-associated sleep disturbances are common in up to 90% of patients according to several studies,[13,19,46] with a high correlation between the level of itch and disturbed sleep.[32] The absence of sleep results in deleterious effects on health, functionality, and emotional well-being.[23]

Overall, patients with scabies present an altered quality of life assessed by standardized questionnaire (modified Dermatology Quality of Life Index).[18,46,47] Worth and colleagues[46] have demonstrated that the degree of impairment increased in parallel with the itch severity.

The psychosocial and economic burden caused by the scabies itch through the lack of sleep, school absenteeism, or loss of work productivity and performance is considerable and leads to an exacerbation of poverty in affected populations.[48]

PATHOPHYSIOLOGY

There are no specific data available aiming to describe the pathophysiology of itch in scabies, and the molecular pathways linking scabies and itch are still poorly understood. However, considerable progress has been made in understanding mechanisms involving the itch in general.[23,49–53] These mechanisms, including different prurireceptors and itch mediators, are described by Ethan A. Lerner in "Pathophysiology of Chronic Itch," in this issue.

The main immune response steps resulting in scabies mite infestation have been described in recent reviews.[54,55] Briefly, the innate immune system is primarily involved via the complement system, which can be partially inhibited by proteins produced by the mite. Mast cells, activated by the complement system or immunoglobulin E (IgE), and eosinophils are important effectors of the immune response. The T cell-mediated response is different in classic scabies or crusted scabies. In classic scabies, Th1 response is predominant, whereas in crusted scabies it is a nonprotective allergy-like Th2 response. CD8+ T cells are major constituents of T cell dermal infiltrates in crusted scabies and may be responsible for keratinocyte apoptosis, leading to epidermal hyperproliferation. Indeed, several hypotheses have been formulated on how all these mechanisms may lead to the itch sensation in scabies and are presented in **Table 2**.

The establishment of a surrogate experimental porcine model for scabies has facilitated monitoring the itch during the infestation and after treatment.[61] It might be a helpful tool in the future to determine new insights into the pathogenesis and the mechanisms underlying itch in scabies.

TREATMENT
Treatment of Scabies

Scabies itch is generally controlled after specific scabies treatment, but can be persistent in the case of other associated causes. The current available agents for scabies are summarized in

Table 3
Currently available treatments for scabies

Agents	Dose	Notes
Oral treatment		
Ivermectin	200 µg/kg of body weight per os	• Only oral treatment available • Used in mass population treatment[63] • Standard regimen for the CDC and EADV[64]
Topical treatment		
Permethrin	5% cream	• Standard regimen for the CDC and EADV
Benzyl benzoate	10% or 25% lotion	• Standard regimen for the EADV
Malathion	0.5% aqueous lotion	
Ivermectin	1% lotion	
Sulfur	6%–33% cream, ointment or lotion	
Synergized pyrethrins	Foam preparation	• Low level of evidence
Lindane	1% cream or lotion	• Neurotoxicity: no longer distributed in the EU and warning for use by the FDA

Abbreviations: CDC, Centers for Disease Control and Prevention; EADV, European Academy of Dermatology and Venereology; EU, European Union; FDA, US Food and Drug Administration.

Table 4
Main causes of persistent itch after treatment. In case of delusions of parasitosis, experienced dermatologists may also ensure its management

Cause	Management	Prevention
Cutaneous irritation		
Overtreatment	Intensive emollients, with or without mild topical steroids	Limiting quantity prescribed
Severe eczematous scabies		Nonirritant scabicide
Contact dermatitis	Topical steroids	Nonallergic scabicide
Treatment failure		
Low compliance	Further scabicide application	Good instructions and evaluation of comprehension
Resistance	Change scabicide	
Relapse	Further scabicide application (eg, of scalp, new treatment of all contacts at the same time)	Head-to-toe application, treatment of all contacts at the same time
Delusions of parasitosis	Psychiatric referral	
Nonscabietic origin	Treatment of the underlying cause	

From Chosidow O. Scabies and Pediculosis. Lancet 2000;355;9206;822; Reprinted with permission from Elsevier (The Lancet).

Table 3. Both topical treatments and oral ivermectin have to be repeated 7 to 15 days apart. Clothing, bedding, and towels should be decontaminated, and the patient's close contacts should be checked and receive full treatment systematically. In many therapeutic studies, the reduction of the itch has helped assessing treatment efficacy. All recommended scabies treatments have shown equivalent efficiency on the itch even if permethrin has shown a faster efficacy than oral ivermectin.[62]

Other Measures

Nonspecific medications may help reducing the itch in scabies. The use of emollients to restore the skin barrier impaired by the infestation should be widely used, especially in cases with important skin irritation caused by the infestation or the treatment. Antihistamines may help, mainly sedative antihistamines that help patients to sleep, even if histamine is not considered as the main mediator implicated in scabies itch.

Causes of Persistent Itch After Treatment

The itch may persist up to 2 to 4 weeks after an efficient treatment.[2] After this period, different causes should be investigated and are explored in **Table 4**.

Patients suffering from delusional parasitosis are frequently incriminating scabies,[65] but clinical aspects of this condition are distinct from scabies. This condition is described by Jason Reichenberg and Anna Buteaus' article, "Psychogenic Pruritus and Its Management," in this issue.

SUMMARY

Although itch is the cardinal symptom of scabies, causing severe somatic and psychosocial complications, its pathophysiological mechanisms remain underappreciated and poorly understood. Better knowledge on how the infestation with scabies mites leads to the itch feeling may help to manage it better and propose more specific/targeted treatment in the near future.

REFERENCES

1. Arlian LG, Morgan MS. A review of sarcoptes scabiei: past, present and future. Parasit Vectors 2017;10(1):297.
2. Chosidow O. Scabies. N Engl J Med 2006;354(16):1718–27.
3. Hay RJ, Johns NE, Williams HC, et al. The global burden of skin disease in 2010: an analysis of the prevalence and impact of skin conditions. J Invest Dermatol 2014;134(6):1527–34.
4. Karimkhani C, Colombara DV, Drucker AM, et al. The global burden of scabies: a cross-sectional analysis from the Global Burden of Disease Study 2015. Lancet Infect Dis 2017;17(12):1247–54.
5. Chosidow O, Fuller LC. Scratching the itch: is scabies a truly neglected disease? Lancet Infect Dis 2017;17(12):1220–1.

6. Romani L, Steer AC, Whitfeld MJ, et al. Prevalence of scabies and impetigo worldwide: a systematic review. Lancet Infect Dis 2015;15(8):960–7.

7. Mellanby K. The development of symptoms, parasitic infection and immunity in human scabies. Parasitology 1944;35(4):197–206.

8. Streeton CL, Hanna JN, Messer RD, et al. An epidemic of acute post-streptococcal glomerulonephritis among aboriginal children. J Paediatr Child Health 1995;31(3):245–8.

9. Fischer K, Holt D, Currie B, et al. Scabies: important clinical consequences explained by new molecular studies. Adv Parasitol 2012;79:339–73.

10. Engelman D, Kiang K, Chosidow O, et al. Toward the global control of human scabies: introducing the international alliance for the control of scabies. PLoS Negl Trop Dis 2013;7(8):e2167.

11. WHO | Neglected tropical diseases. WHO. Available at: http://www.who.int/neglected_diseases/en/. Accessed September 26, 2017.

12. Hengge UR, Currie BJ, Jäger G, et al. Scabies: a ubiquitous neglected skin disease. Lancet Infect Dis 2006;6(12):769–79.

13. Boralevi F, Diallo A, Miquel J, et al. Clinical phenotype of scabies by age. Pediatrics 2014;133(4): e910–6.

14. Brenaut E, Garlantezec R, Talour K, et al. Itch characteristics in five dermatoses: non-atopic eczema, atopic dermatitis, urticaria, psoriasis and scabies. Acta Derm Venereol 2013;93(5):573–4.

15. Lavery MJ, Stull C, Nattkemper LA, et al. Nocturnal pruritus: prevalence, characteristics, and impact on ItchyQoL in a chronic itch population. Acta Derm Venereol 2017;97(4):513–5.

16. Yosipovitch G, Goon ATJ, Wee J, et al. Itch characteristics in Chinese patients with atopic dermatitis using a new questionnaire for the assessment of pruritus. Int J Dermatol 2002;41(4):212–6.

17. Yosipovitch G, Ansari N, Goon A, et al. Clinical characteristics of pruritus in chronic idiopathic urticaria. Br J Dermatol 2002;147(1):32–6.

18. Nair PA, Vora RV, Jivani NB, et al. A study of clinical profile and quality of life in patients with scabies at a rural tertiary care centre. J Clin Diagn Res 2016; 10(10):WC01–5.

19. Jackson A, Heukelbach J, Filho AF, et al. Clinical features and associated morbidity of scabies in a rural community in Alagoas, Brazil. Trop Med Int Health 2007;12(4):493–502.

20. Hewitt KA, Nalabanda A, Cassell JA. Scabies outbreaks in residential care homes: factors associated with late recognition, burden and impact. A mixed methods study in England. Epidemiol Infect 2015; 143(7):1542–51.

21. Sarwat MA, el Okbi LM, el Sayed MM, et al. Parasitological and clinical studies on human scabies in Cairo. J Egypt Soc Parasitol 1993;23(3):809–19.

22. Shin K, Jin H, You H-S, et al. Clinical characteristics of pruritus in scabies. Indian J Dermatol Venereol Leprol 2017;83(4):492.

23. Lavery MJ, Stull C, Kinney MO, et al. Nocturnal pruritus: the battle for a peaceful night's sleep. Int J Mol Sci 2016;17(3):425.

24. Calnan CD. Crusted scabies. Br J Dermatol Syph 1950;62(2):71–8.

25. Askour M, Bernigaud C, Do-Pham G, et al. [Gales graves hospitalisées en dermatologie et maladies infectieuses en Île-de-France : étude multicentrique rétrospective de 83 patients sur 6 ans]. Ann Dermatol Vénéréologie 2016;143(12, Supplement):S334–5.

26. Roberts LJ, Huffam SE, Walton SF, et al. Crusted scabies: clinical and immunological findings in seventy-eight patients and a review of the literature. J Infect 2005;50(5):375–81.

27. Carslaw RW. Letter: scabies in a spinal injuries ward. Br Med J 1975;2(5971):617.

28. Ram-Wolff C, Mahé E, Saiag P, et al. [Crusted scabies at the spinal injury site of a paraplegic man]. Ann Dermatol Venereol 2008;135(1):68–9 [in French].

29. Mellanby K. Scabies in 1976. R Soc Health J 1977; 97(1):32–6, 40.

30. Romani L, Koroivueta J, Steer AC, et al. Scabies and impetigo prevalence and risk factors in Fiji: a national survey. Plos Negl Trop Dis 2015;9(3): e0003452.

31. Reid HF, Birju B, Holder Y, et al. Epidemic scabies in four Caribbean islands, 1981-1988. Trans R Soc Trop Med Hyg 1990;84(2):298–300.

32. Worth C, Heukelbach J, Fengler G, et al. Acute morbidity associated with scabies and other ectoparasitoses rapidly improves after treatment with ivermectin. Pediatr Dermatol 2012;29(4):430–6.

33. Edison L, Beaudoin A, Goh L, et al. Scabies and bacterial superinfection among american samoan children, 2011–2012. PLoS One 2015;10(10): e0139336.

34. Hay RJ, Steer AC, Engelman D, et al. Scabies in the developing world—its prevalence, complications, and management. Clin Microbiol Infect 2012;18(4): 313–23.

35. Steer AC, Jenney AWJ, Kado J, et al. High burden of impetigo and scabies in a tropical country. Plos Negl Trop Dis 2009;3(6):e467.

36. Mulholland EK, Ogunlesi OO, Adegbola RA, et al. Etiology of serious infections in young Gambian infants. Pediatr Infect Dis J 1999;18(10 Suppl): S35–41.

37. Lawrence G, Leafasia J, Sheridan J, et al. Control of scabies, skin sores and haematuria in children in the Solomon Islands: another role for ivermectin. Bull World Health Organ 2005;83(1):34–42.

38. Swe PM, Fischer K. A scabies mite serpin interferes with complement-mediated neutrophil functions and

promotes staphylococcal growth. Plos Negl Trop Dis 2014;8(6):e2928.

39. Swe PM, Christian LD, Lu HC, et al. Complement inhibition by Sarcoptes scabiei protects Streptococcus pyogenes - An in vitro study to unravel the molecular mechanisms behind the poorly understood predilection of S. pyogenes to infect mite-induced skin lesions. Plos Negl Trop Dis 2017; 11(3):e0005437.

40. Mika A, Reynolds SL, Pickering D, et al. Complement inhibitors from scabies mites promote streptococcal growth–a novel mechanism in infected epidermis? Plos Negl Trop Dis 2012;6(7):e1563.

41. Bergström FC, Reynolds S, Johnstone M, et al. Scabies mite inactivated serine protease paralogs inhibit the human complement system. J Immunol 2009;182(12):7809–17.

42. Mika A, Reynolds SL, Mohlin FC, et al. Novel scabies mite serpins inhibit the three pathways of the human complement system. PLoS One 2012;7(7):e40489.

43. Reynolds SL, Pike RN, Mika A, et al. Scabies mite inactive serine proteases are potent inhibitors of the human complement lectin pathway. Plos Negl Trop Dis 2014;8(5):e2872.

44. Hulbert TV, Larsen RA. Hyperkeratotic (Norwegian) scabies with gram-negative bacteremia as the initial presentation of AIDS. Clin Infect Dis 1992;14(5): 1164–5.

45. Kouotou EA, Nansseu JRN, Sieleunou I, et al. Features of human scabies in resource-limited settings: the Cameroon case. BMC Dermatol 2015;15:12.

46. Worth C, Heukelbach J, Fengler G, et al. Impaired quality of life in adults and children with scabies from an impoverished community in Brazil. Int J Dermatol 2012;51(3):275–82.

47. Jin-gang A, Sheng-xiang X, Sheng-bin X, et al. Quality of life of patients with scabies. J Eur Acad Dermatol Venereol 2010;24(10):1187–91.

48. Feldmeier H, Jackson A, Ariza L, et al. The epidemiology of scabies in an impoverished community in rural Brazil: presence and severity of disease are associated with poor living conditions and illiteracy. J Am Acad Dermatol 2009;60(3):436–43.

49. Misery L. Pruritus: considerable progress in pathophysiology. Med Sci (Paris) 2014;30(12):1123–8 [in French].

50. Azimi E, Xia J, Lerner EA. Peripheral mechanisms of itch. Curr Probl Dermatol 2016;50:18–23.

51. Wong L-S, Wu T, Lee C-H. Inflammatory and noninflammatory itch: implications in pathophysiology-directed treatments. Int J Mol Sci 2017;18(7) [pii: E1485].

52. Raap U, Ständer S, Metz M. Pathophysiology of itch and new treatments. Curr Opin Allergy Clin Immunol 2011;11(5):420–7.

53. LaMotte RH, Dong X, Ringkamp M. Sensory neurons and circuits mediating itch. Nat Rev Neurosci 2014; 15(1):19–31.

54. Bhat SA, Mounsey KE, Liu X, et al. Host immune responses to the itch mite, Sarcoptes scabiei, in humans. Parasit Vectors 2017;10(1):385.

55. Walton SF. The immunology of susceptibility and resistance to scabies. Parasite Immunol 2010; 32(8):532–40.

56. He R, Gu X, Lai W, et al. Transcriptome-microRNA analysis of Sarcoptes scabiei and host immune response. PLoS One 2017;12(5):e0177733.

57. Taves S, Ji R-R. Itch control by Toll-like receptors. Handb Exp Pharmacol 2015;226:135–50.

58. Morgan MS, Rider SD, Arlian LG. Identification of antigenic Sarcoptes scabiei proteins for use in a diagnostic test and of non-antigenic proteins that may be immunomodulatory. Plos Negl Trop Dis 2017;11(6):e0005669.

59. Ricklin D, Hajishengallis G, Yang K, et al. Complement: a key system for immune surveillance and homeostasis. Nat Immunol 2010;11(9):785–97.

60. Potenzieri C, Undem BJ. Basic mechanisms of itch. Clin Exp Allergy 2012;42(1):8–19.

61. Bernigaud C, Fang F, Fischer K, et al. Preclinical study of single-dose moxidectin, a new oral treatment for scabies: efficacy, safety, and pharmacokinetics compared to two-dose ivermectin in a porcine model. Plos Negl Trop Dis 2016;10(10): e0005030.

62. Sharma R, Singal A. Topical permethrin and oral ivermectin in the management of scabies: a prospective, randomized, double blind, controlled study. Indian J Dermatol Venereol Leprol 2011; 77(5):581.

63. Romani L, Whitfeld MJ, Koroivueta J, et al. Mass drug administration for scabies control in a population with endemic disease. N Engl J Med 2015; 373(24):2305–13.

64. Salavastru CM, Chosidow O, Boffa MJ, et al. European guideline for the management of scabies. J Eur Acad Dermatol Venereol JEADV 2017;31(8): 1248–53.

65. Freudenmann RW, Lepping P. Delusional Infestation. Clin Microbiol Rev. 2009;22(4):690–732. https://doi.org/10.1128/CMR.00018-09.

Psychogenic Pruritus and Its Management

Anna Buteau, MD[a], Jason Reichenberg, MD[b],*

KEYWORDS

- Psychogenic itch • Psychiatric itch • Chronic pruritus • Somatic symptom disorder
- Somatoform disorder

KEY POINTS

- Psychogenic pruritus is defined as itch not related to dermatologic or systemic causes.
- Psychogenic pruritus can be categorized as a pruritic disease with psychiatric sequelae, a pruritic disease aggravated by psychosocial factors, or a psychiatric disease–causing pruritus.
- In the work-up of psychogenic pruritus, medical causes must first be ruled out, then medication and behavioral treatment offered.

INTRODUCTION

Chronic itching is a frustrating condition for patients and providers alike, and it can be an even more delicate subject when intertwined with a possible psychiatric source. Psychogenic pruritus is defined as itch not related to dermatologic or systemic causes. Beyond this definition, there is a lack of consensus on how to classify the condition, in part due to the overlap between the fields of dermatology and psychiatry.

The *Diagnostic and Statistical Manual of Mental Disorders* (Fifth Edition) has remained vague on the topic of pruritus. Excoriation falls under the diagnosis of "obsessive-compulsive and related disorders," but psychogenic pruritus could also fall into "somatic symptom disorders," "medically unexplained symptoms," or "impulse control disorders." The *International Classification of Disease, Tenth Revision*, is equally vague: psychogenic pruritus is not defined but could fall into the diagnosis of "other somatoform disorders," a subcategory under the broader diagnosis of "neurotic disorders, stress-linked disorders and other somatoform disorders."

Treating patients with psychogenic pruritus is a challenge for the dermatologist. Although there are tools and criteria to diagnose medical sources of itch, many patients have nonspecific findings. Building a relationship with patients is key, because many patients are not open to hearing that there could be a psychiatric component to their condition. Dermatologists should take a multifaceted approach to working up these patients that includes history and physical examination, laboratory testing for common medical or systemic problems, biopsies as needed, and a thorough psychiatric screen.

SUMMARY/DISCUSSION

Psychogenic pruritus can be divided into 3 broad categories (**Fig. 1**). Some patients present with a primary dermatologic disease with itch (eczema, urticaria, and so forth) and develop psychiatric sequelae as a result. Most commonly, this manifests as depression or unmasks anxiety or obsessive-compulsive disorder (OCD). The second category includes patients who experience an exacerbation of their skin disease (psoriasis or

Disclosure Statement: The authors have nothing to disclose.
a Internal Medicine, Dell Medical School, The University of Texas at Austin, 601 East 15th Street, CEC C2.470, Austin, TX 78701, USA; b Dermatology, Dell Medical School, The University of Texas at Austin, 601 East 15th Street, CEC C2.470, Austin, TX 78701, USA
* Corresponding author.
E-mail address: jreichenberg@ascension.org

Dermatol Clin 36 (2018) 309–314
https://doi.org/10.1016/j.det.2018.02.015

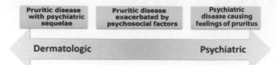

Fig. 1. Spectrum of the source of pruritus.

eczema) in times of stress. Finally, a psychiatric disorder can lead to feelings of pruritus. It can be a challenge to determine whether the skin disease or psychiatric disorder started first. Although the treatment of each of these categories differs, the initial work-up remains the same.

Dermatologists are well versed in how to manage patients who itch due to a known dermatologic problem. In a study of hospitalized psychiatric patients, chronic itch had a prevalence of 32%.[1] In another study, also of hospitalized psychiatric patients, prevalence of itching was 42%, without correlation to a specific psychiatric diagnosis.[2] Patients who are diagnosed as having a psychogenic component to their disorder differ from other patients based on the amount of disability the pruritus causes (**Box 1**). Many skin disorders can negatively affect quality of life, to a degree that may meet or exceed that of patients with diabetes or cystic fibrosis.[3,4] To meet criteria for a psychiatric disorder, however, the disability a patient has must affect social relationships, work, or other daily activities.

Identifying Primary Psychiatric Disease

The management of a dermatology patient with suspected psychiatric disease can be a challenge. The important first step is to assess patients for

---

Box 1
Signs that a patient may have psychogenic itch

History

Disability out of proportion to symptoms

Psychiatric comorbidities

Anxiety, depression correlate with itch intensity

Dysfunctional coping behaviors (helplessness)

High number of doctor visits

Clinical signs

Lack of cutaneous findings

Pruritus of face more likely

Intranasal formication more likely in delusions of parasitosis

Hostility/blame toward provider

Does not follow social cues

---

psychiatric safety. Whether due to the stressors of their skin disease or the prednisone they just received, if patients vocalize concerns about violence (to others) or suicidal thoughts, they require immediate attention. The most helpful questions to ask these patients are the most direct: Do you have thoughts of harming yourself? Of harming others? If patients answer in the affirmative, it is crucial to reach out to local law enforcement or psychiatric services. Asking patients about self-harm does not increase their likelihood of following through on their thoughts.

Screening patients for potential drug and alcohol abuse is also worthwhile because many substances can contribute to the sensation of pruritus. Pruritus is a well-known complication of alcoholic liver disease, particularly in the presence of cholestasis.[5] Cocaine and amphetamine abusers are prone to delusions of parasitosis, sometimes referred to as *meth mites*, often leaving excoriations and prurigo nodules as evidence.[6,7] The use of opioids, either illicit[8] or prescribed,[9] is common in patients with delusions of parasitosis, which may be partially due to histamine release by opioids leading to pruritus.[10] As such, substance abuse can easily confound the work-up of pruritus, and awareness of it early is important. Checking a patient's medication list (current and previous) can be helpful, asking about illicit drug use may yield a benefit, and including a urine drug screen in the work-up of any new patient with pruritus can be enlightening.

Getting patients help from a psychiatrist or psychologist is ideal for these patients. The authors find that it is important to first normalize the idea of psychiatric care, using a statement such as, "I find that many of my patients with severe psoriasis/eczema have a difficult time dealing with their skin disease. Since we know that stress can make the skin disease worse, it is even more important that I don't miss out on any of my patient's symptoms. Have you ever thought you were depressed/anxious?" Many standardized psychiatric screening tools are available for free online and can be completed by patients during check-in. The authors' office uses the Patient Health Questionnaire-15 for patients with depression, because it focuses on physical symptoms of a patient's condition. The Modified Mini screen can look for signs of anxiety, depression, OCD, posttraumatic stress disorder, and psychosis. The advantage of using a standardized tool is that it serves to offer objective evidence of why the provider is concerned, much like a biopsy is sometimes needed to reassure a patient that their physician's clinical diagnosis is correct.

Managing Primary Dermatologic Disease

If it is believed that the skin disease is triggering the psychiatric issue, a dermatologist spends the majority of the time with the patient focusing on the improvement of the skin disease. Intralesional injections can provide significant relief in office, as can wet wraps or other occlusive treatments. Localized treatments for itch, including menthol and cool compresses, can give patients a sense of control over their disorder when prescription medications are unable to help. Dermatologists must remember that the psychiatric consequences of the skin disease may not be proportionate to the extent of disease in these cases. There are reasons to consider systemic medication even for (relatively) minor disease if it is leading to significant disability.

Dermatologists are also well versed in treating the second category of psychogenic pruritus patients—those with known skin diseases, who note their pruritus worsens with psychiatric stress. Stress is well known to cause diseases like psoriasis to flare,[11] so it is not surprising that anxiety, depression, or mania can flare skin disease as well. Those with eczema, chronic urticaria, prurigo nodularis, lichen simplex chronicus, and pruritus of advanced age can be exacerbated with aggravation of latent psychiatric problems.

Patients with known skin diseases who note their pruritus worsens with stress. Dermatologists should work to improve their skin symptoms when possible and help to make patients aware of a potential link between their skin and mental health. Once patients have gained insight into this trigger of their disease, they may be willing to seek treatment. Of all of the patients with psychodermatologic disease, the authors find this group the most rewarding because the improvement of their skin as the mental health improves can be seen. Patients with eczema and pruritus of advancing age often respond to stress reduction treatment, behavioral therapy techniques to limit scratching, or prescription antidepressant treatment.

Managing Primary Psychiatric Disease

The third category of psychogenic pruritus patients, those with a primary psychiatric disorder leading to pruritus, is often the most challenging for a dermatologist to manage. These patients rarely have insight into the psychiatric source of their condition. Patients with depression, anxiety, and psychosis all present differently when dealing with psychogenic pruritus. Often a patient's presenting history aids in differentiating between these causes.

Patients with depression may present with itch much like a patient with fibromyalgia presents with joint pain. These patients may have a more generalized somatic symptom disorder, which involves symptoms that are either very distressing or result in significant disruption of functioning. These patients often complain of fatigue, brain fog, or joint aches in addition to their itching. This condition can be exacerbated by recent trauma and manifest much like posttraumatic stress disorder. The authors have seen several patients present with psychogenic itch after sexual encounters and/or after being a victim of a crime.

Skin picking and trichotillomania are forms of OCD. They are characterized by intrusive thoughts or urges that are experienced as unwanted (obsession), often necessitating repetitive behaviors or rituals to help alleviate the otherwise intolerable anxiety (compulsion).[12] Trichotillomania is characterized by recurrent pulling hair, leading to hair loss in response to tension.[9] Patients experience gratification only after the act is performed.[13] These patients may present with the concern that they "need to get the core out" of an ingrown hair or remove another small skin abnormality.

Patients with bipolar disorder go into manic states which can make them hypervigilant to cutaneous stimuli. They may perceive mild itch as severe and take extraordinary measures to stop the itching. Mania is often accompanied by shopping sprees, increased sexual promiscuity, or prolonged periods of sleeplessness. The authors use 1 patient as an example: a 34-year-old woman presented to the authors' clinic for "itch." She had been preparing for a first date with a man she met online that morning. She spent $500 on cosmetic products at a department store to help her itching and cover up her scratch marks. She was rejected by the man that evening when she made sexual advances. She presented to the office the following day with itching, but by the end of the visit had tried to ask a staff member out as well. On further questioning, she admitted a previous diagnosis of bipolar disorder and having stopped her medications a few months earlier.

Psychoses associated with pruritus include delusions of parasitosis and schizophrenia with tactile hallucinations. Delusions of parasitosis is a monosymptomatic hypochondriacal psychosis characterized by the false belief of being infested with living organisms or innate material.[14] The patients often present with concerns that their infection is causing their itching whereas schizophrenia with tactile hallucinations is polysymptomatic, causing feelings of being touched, burning or tingling, or itch.[15] Patients with delusions rarely present with a chief complaint of itch but instead present with a concern of an infestation. Often they have already made a decision as to the exact organism affecting them. They point out the itch is the "proof": that they are infested and relate changes in itch as various treatments cause the infestation to improve or worsen. Patients with schizophrenia should demonstrate 2 of the following 5 symptoms: (1) *delusions, (2) *hallucinations, (3) *disorganized speech, (4) disorganized or catatonic behavior, and (5) negative symptoms, with 1 of these 5 being 1 of the starred (*) symptoms. Negative symptoms include blunted emotional responses, social withdrawal, or anhedonia. These patients have impaired cognition and a difficult time making logical connections, such as "I used a strong medication to treat the parasite, therefore if the symptoms persist perhaps this is not a parasite." Although patients with delusional disorder can be successfully be treated by a dermatologist,[14] the treatment of schizophrenia should not be attempted in a dermatology office. There is likely a spectrum of presentation for delusions of parasitosis. Although patients with less severe symptoms may be adherent to medication management, those who are in a terminal delusional state are not likely to continue their medications in the long term.

The Workup

For any patient with psychogenic pruritus, it is critical to set expectations at the initial appointment about how the evaluation will proceed and ideally to allocate multiple appointments to the work-up. These patients should receive 1—and only 1—thorough work-up before a provider concludes they have psychogenic pruritus. The work-up of potential psychogenic pruritus is the same as if there were no psychiatric source. It is useful for the first appointment to be used to get to know the patient and review pertinent history. Along with the history, a thorough examination should guide the need for laboratory testing. If time permits and a primary lesion exists, a skin biopsy may be considered, although time often requires this to happen at the second visit. It is advisable to hold off on making a diagnosis unless certain. It may be appropriate to try an empiric treatment (topical or oral) to see how a patient responds. Scheduling a longer follow-up visit within a few weeks of the initial visit allows time for data collection, corroboration from other providers, and time to try any empiric home treatments that may be appropriate.

At a follow-up visit, the physician should review outside records, the laboratory tests, and the results of any review of systems or psychiatric screening test. This may take more than 1 additional visit to complete. The goal is to have a productive conversation about the condition and treatment options. This allows ample time to reassure the patient about the absence of infection or any other skin disease. If appropriate, this is an opportune time to state that the evaluation is complete. At this stage, candor is helpful. If there were no pertinent positives on the work-up, this is the time to discuss the possibility of an idiopathic etiology to the itching. Offering a patient multiple choices on how to proceed can help build rapport and also help assess the patient's level of insight. Some patients choose a hands-off approach once they have been reassured the itch is not caused by cancer or infection. These patients often chose to ignore the itch, live with it, and come back in a period of time to check in. Others continue to seek an "internal" cause for the itch and (unfortunately) seek care elsewhere. The goal is to have patients understand that there is no clear "medical" cause for their pruritus, and they should focus on treating their symptoms. Once dermatologists have built rapport with patients, patients may agree to try trial-and-error treatments, such as oral medications and behavioral treatment, to find a solution.

Treatment Options

Medical and behavioral treatments both play a role in treating psychogenic pruritus. The treatment of localized pruritus or neuropathic pruritus often uses topical therapies, injections, or anticonvulsants.[16,17] For patients with an obsessive-compulsive component to their itch, cognitive behavior therapy (CBT) has been shown most effective.[18] Patients work on techniques to decrease the urge to pick, often by removing triggers and finding alternative coping mechanisms. It is important that providers tell these patients to look specifically for therapists or psychiatrists who perform CBT, because they may differ from other more classically trained therapists.

For any patients with chronic itch, relaxation therapy and CBT can be helpful.[19] It can be even more efficacious to use these treatments in patients with concomitant depression or anxiety.[18] For these patients, it is important that they find a provider they are willing to see and develop a relationship with. For psychosis or significant forms of bipolar disorder, medication management is often needed.

Most dermatologists are already familiar with the first-line medications for patients with psychogenic itch. First-generation antihistamines, such as hydroxyzine and diphenhydramine, are mostly used as sedatives in the evenings. They are generally too sedating for daytime use and their efficacy in treating pruritus specifically is limited. Although second-generation antihistamines are less sedating, unless patients have a histamine-based cause of itch (urticaria,) they are unlikely to respond to this medication. Doxepin is a tricyclic antidepressant (TCA) with strong antihistamine and sedative effects. The benefits of this drug over antihistamines is the longer effect of the drug and its metabolites, so once-daily dosing in the evening may work all day. Doxepin can be started at 10 mg nightly and slowly titrated up to 100 mg.

The medication used to treat psychogenic itch depends on the underlying psychiatric disorder. If the presumed underlying problem is related to depression, anxiety, OCD, or somatoform disorder, selective serotonin reuptake inhibitors (SSRIs) or TCAs are helpful (Table 1). Doxepin certainly can help, as can sertraline and citalopram.[20] Sertraline can be started at 25 mg per day and titrated up to 100 mg slowly to reduce the chance of side effects. Although the mechanisms of gabapentin and pregabalin are not fully understood, case reports have shown it effective in treating prurigo nodularis and other neuropathic itch.[21,22] Gabapentin should be started at 100 mg 3 times per day and can be titrated up to 600 mg 3 times per day. Sedation is usually the limiting factor and can be alleviated by a slowly increased dose. Similarly, pregabalin can be started as low as 75 mg per day, increased by 75 mg per day to 150 mg per day at 1-week intervals to a maximum of 300 mg per day divided in 2 or 3 doses.

If a provider concludes a patient has delusions of parasitosis, antipsychotics are the best choice. It is

important first to develop a rapport of trust with a patient before the idea of starting this medication.[23] It can be helpful to focus on the patient's symptoms of itch and point out that these medications are used for many conditions, including Tourette syndrome (in the case of pimozide) or depression (for aripiprazole). How antipsychotics like olanzapine bind the histamine receptor,[24] which may explain its effectiveness for treating patients with various forms of itch, may be discussed.[25] Aripiprazole has the advantage of approval for both psychosis and depression augmentation and has a lower side-effect profile than the other antipsychotics. For this reason, it is often tried first, even though the literature supporting pimozide is more extensive. The authors have found that adding 5 mg per day of aripiprazole to augment an antidepressant is helpful in patients with somatic symptoms of their delusion. For those patients further along in the "spectrum of delusion," doses between 10 mg per day and 25 mg per day can be helpful.[26] In multiple studies, pimozide has been found to show improvement in symptoms of delusions of parasitosis in 3 weeks to 8 weeks at dosages ranging from 1 mg per day to 6 mg per day.[27]

When to Refer

There are some cases of psychogenic pruritus that dermatologists are simply not equipped to manage. Patients with bipolar disorder or frank

Table 1
Medical treatment options

	Adverse Effects
Antidepressants: depression, anxiety, OCD, somatoform disorder	
TCA: doxepin 6–10 mg po qhs, can increase up to 100 mg qhs	Anticholinergic, antihistiminic, decreased seizure threshold, sexual dysfunction
SSRI: sertraline 25 mg po qd, up to 100 mg qd	Gastrointestinal upset, sexual dysfunction
SSRI: (especially OCD) paroxetine 10 mg po qam, up to 40 mg qam, taper off slowly	Gastrointestinal upset, sexual dysfunction
NaSSA: mirtazapine—7.5 mg po qhs, increase to 15 mg if needed	Dry mouth, sedation, weight gain, avoid in closed-angle glaucoma
Antipsychotics: delusions of parasitosis, psychosis, depression	
Pimozide: 1 mg po qd, increase to 6 mg qd	Extrapyramidal symptoms, QTc prolongation, tardive dyskinesia
Olanzapine: 5 mg po qd, increase to 10 mg qd	Sedation, weight gain
Aripiprazole: 5 mg po qd, increase up to 25 mg qd	Akathisia, restlessness, insomnia
Anticonvulsants: depression, anxiety, OCD, somatoform disorder	
Gabapentin: 100 mg po tid, can increase slowly up to 600 mg po tid, taper off slowly	Sedation
Pregabalin: start 50 mg bid, increase slowly up to 150 bid, taper off slowly	Dizziness, somnolence, ataxia

Abbreviation: NaSSA, noradrenergic and specific serotonergic antidepressant.

schizophrenia need to be referred to a psychiatrist if possible. In other cases, if patients lack insight into their condition and refuse to acknowledge the psychiatric nature of their condition, it may be best for the dermatologist and patient to agree to part ways.

In summary, psychogenic pruritus can be challenging to classify from the outset and may require additional time for proper diagnosis. Once diagnosed, a trusting relationship with the patient along with close follow-up are key to working through possible treatment options. In certain cases, a dermatologist may not be the right person to treat the patient and referral to a psychiatrist is indicated.

REFERENCES

1. Mazeh D, Melamed Y, Cholostoy A, et al. Itching in the psychiatric ward. Acta Derm Venereol 2008;88: 128–31.

2. Kretzmer GE, Gelkopf M, Kretzmer G, et al. Idiopathic pruritus in psychiatric inpatients: an explorative study. Gen Hosp Psychiatry 2008;30(4):344.

3. Hahl J, Hämäläinen H, Sintonen H, et al. Health-related quality of life in type 1 diabetes without or with symptoms of long-term complications. Qual Life Res 2002;11:427–43.

4. Lee Y, Park E, Kwon I, et al. Impact of psoriasis on quality of life: relationship between clinical response to therapy and change in health-related quality of life. Ann Dermatol 2010;22(4):389–96.

5. Liu S, Lien M, Fenske N. The effects of alcohol and drug abuse on the skin. Clin Dermatol 2010;28: 391–9.

6. Brewer J, Meves A, Bostwick M, et al. Cocaine abuse: dermatologic manifestations and therapeutic approaches. J Am Acad Dermatol 2008;59:483–7.

7. Frieden J. Skin Manifestations May Signal Crystal Meth Use: Think 'meth mites' when patients are picking at their skin and think they have insects crawling on them. Family Practice News. 2006. Available at: htttp://www.mdedge.com/sites/default/files/issues/articles/72526_main.pdf. Accessed November 8, 2017.

8. Lepping P, Noorthorn E, Kemperman P, et al. An international study of the prevalence of substance abuse in patients with delusional infestation. J Am Acad Dermatol 2017;77(4):778–9.

9. Zhu T, Nakamura M, Farhnik B, et al. Obsessive compulsive skin disorders: a novel classification based on degree of insight. J Dermatolog Treat 2017;28(4):342–6.

10. Weidman A, Fellner M. Cutaneous manifestations of heroin and other addictive drugs. N Y State J Med 1971;71:2643–6.

11. Seville RH. Stress and psoriasis: the importance of insight and empathy in prognosis. J Am Acad Dermatol 1989;20(1):97–100.

12. American Psychiatric Association. "Obsessive-compulsive and related disorders." Diagnostic and statistical manual of mental disorders: DSM-5. 5th edition. Washington, DC: American Psychiatric Association; 2013.

13. Hautman G, Hercogova J, Lotti T. Trichotillomania. J Am Acad Dermatol 2002;46(6):807–21.

14. Brown G, Sorenson E, Malakouti M, et al. The spectrum of ideation in patients with symptoms of infestation: from overvalued ideas to the terminal delusional state. J Clin Exp Dermatol Res 2014;5:6.

15. Kalamkarian AA, Briun EA, Grebeniuk VN. Skin itching occurring as a type of tactile hallucinosis. Vestn Dermatol Venerol 1978;8:90–2.

16. Oaklander AL. Neuropathic itch. Semin Cutan Med Surg 2011;2:87–92.

17. Elmariah SB, Lerner EA. Topical therapies for pruritus. Semin Cutan Med Surg 2011;30(2): 118–26.

18. Yosipovitch G, Samuel L. Neuropathic and psychogenic itch. Dermatol Ther 2008;21:32–41.

19. Schut C, Mollanazar NK, Kupfer J, et al. Psychologic interventions in the treatment of chronic itch. Acta Derm Venereol 2016;96:157–61.

20. Steinhoff M, Cevikbas F, Ikoma A, et al. Pruritus: management algorithms and experimental therapies. Semin Cutan Med Surg 2011;30(2): 127–37.

21. Dereli T, Karaca N, Inanir I, et al. Gabapentin for the treatment of recalcitrant chronic prurigo nodularis. Eur J Dermatol 2008;18:85–6.

22. Bandelow B, Wedekin D, Leon T. Pregabalin for the treatment of generalized anxiety disorder: a novel pharmacologic intervention. Expert Rev Neurother 2007;7:769–81.

23. Patel V, Koo J. Delusions of parasitosis; suggested dialogue between dermatologist and patient. J Dermatolog Treat 2015;26(5):456–60.

24. Bymaster F, Rasmussen K, Calligaro D, et al. In vitro and in vivo biochemistry of olanzapine: a novel, atypical antipsychotic drug. J Clin Psychiatry 1997; 58(suppl 10):28–36.

25. Hyun J, Gamblicher T, Bader A, et al. Olanzapine therapy for subacute prurigo. Clin Exp Dermatol 2006;31:464–5.

26. Ladizinski B, Busse KL, Bhutani T, et al. Aripiprazole as a viable alternative for treating delusions of parasitosis. J Drugs Dermatol 2010;9:1531–2.

27. Lorenzo CR, Koo J. Pimozide in dermatologic practice: a comprehensive review. Am J Clin Dermatol 2004;5:339–49.

Pruritus Associated with Targeted Anticancer Therapies and Their Management

Check for updates

Jennifer Wu, MD[a,b,c,d], Mario E. Lacouture, MD[e,f],*

KEYWORDS

- Pruritus • Itch • Targeted therapy • Immunotherapy • Cancer • Management

KEY POINTS

- Aberrations in cell signal transduction pathways, including EGFR, MAPK (RAS-RAF-MEK-ERK), and PI3K-Akt-mTOR, play an essential role in tumorigenesis and disease progression. Targeted therapies acting on these signaling pathways cause dermatologic adverse events.
- Immune checkpoints inhibitors targeting CTLA-4, PD-1, or PD-L1 have revolutionized cancer treatments with promising outcomes, yet have collaterally caused immune-related adverse events such as rash and pruritus.
- Pruritus is a common dermatologic adverse event with incidences ranging from 2.2% to 47% across different categories of targeted anticancer therapies, with the highest incidence in patients treated with panitumumab (54.9%) and ipilimumab plus nivolumab combination treatment (33.2%–47%).
- Possible mechanisms of pruritus include alteration of skin barrier function and homeostasis, pruritus preceded by xerosis and skin inflammation, and increasing numbers of dermal mast cells induced by targeted therapies.

INTRODUCTION OF TARGETED ANTICANCER THERAPIES

Aberrations in cell signaling transduction pathways from epidermal growth factor receptor (EGFR) to downstream pathways, including the mitogen-activated protein kinase (MAPK), the phosphatidylinositol-3-OH kinase (PI3K)-Akt (a serine or threonine protein kinase), and the mammalian target of rapamycin (mTOR) pathway, play important roles in tumorigenesis and disease progression.[1] The MAPK pathway has 4 core protein kinases, including rat sarcoma (RAS) virus

---

Disclosure: The authors have nothing to disclose.
[a] Dermatology Service, Department of Medicine, Memorial Sloan Kettering Cancer Center, 16 East 60th Street, Suite 407, Room 4312, New York, NY 10022, USA; [b] Department of Dermatology, Drug Hypersensitivity Clinical and Research Center, Immune-Oncology Center of Excellence, Chang Gung Memorial Hospital, Linkou, No.5, Fuxing Street, Guishan District, Taoyuan City 333, Taiwan; [c] Department of Dermatology, Chang Gung Memorial Hospital, Taipei, No.199, Dunhua North Road, Zhongshan District, Taipei 105, Taiwan; [d] College of Medicine, Chang Gung University, No.159, Wenhua 1st Road, Guishan District, Taoyuan City 333, Taiwan; [e] Oncodermatology Program, Dermatology Service, Department of Medicine, Memorial Sloan Kettering Cancer Center, Outpatient Center, 16 East 60th Street, Suite 407, Room 4312, New York, NY 10022, USA; [f] Department of Medicine, Weill Cornell Medical College, 1320 York Avenue, New York, NY 10021, USA
* Corresponding author. Dermatology Service, Department of Medicine, Memorial Sloan Kettering Cancer Center, 60th Street Outpatient Center, 16 East 60th Street, Suite 407, Room 4312, New York, NY 10022.
E-mail address: lacoutum@mskcc.org

Dermatol Clin 36 (2018) 315–324
https://doi.org/10.1016/j.det.2018.02.010
0733-8635/18/© 2018 Elsevier Inc. All rights reserved.

gene homolog, rapidly accelerated fibrosarcoma (RAF) serine or threonine kinase, mitogen-activated protein kinase (MEK), and extracellular signal-regulated kinase (ERK). In recent years, several anticancer targeted therapies that inhibit the EGFR, RAF, MEK, PI3K-Akt-mTOR, and other pathways have been developed with tumor response.[1–8] Monoclonal antibodies (mAbs; eg, cetuximab, panitumumab) and tyrosine kinase inhibitors (TKIs; eg, erlotinib, gefitinib) targeting EGFR, and multitargeted TKIs (eg, axitinib, pazopanib, sunitinib) targeting vascular endothelial growth factor receptor (VEGFR), platelet-derived growth factor receptor (PDGFR), or Breakpoint cluster region (Bcr)- Abelson tyrosine kinase (Abl) tyrosine kinase are, therefore, indispensable elements of cancer treatment.[3]

Recent developments in cancer immunology have generated a new era of immunotherapy for cancer treatment. The cytotoxic T lymphocyte antigen-4 (CTLA-4) and the programmed death receptor-1 (PD-1)/ programmed death receptor ligand 1 (PD-L1)/ programmed death receptor ligand 2 (PD-L2) signaling pathway are immune checkpoints of tumor-induced immunosuppression. Inhibition of immune checkpoints using anti-CTLA-4, anti-PD-1/PD-L1 agents has revolutionized the treatments of patients for a variety of cancers.[9,10]

DERMATOLOGIC ADVERSE EVENTS TO TARGETED ANTICANCER THERAPIES

Targeted anticancer agents have significantly increased the survival of patients with various malignancies, improved tolerability, prolonged treatment duration, and reduced the risks of systemic toxicities of these agents, such as myelosuppression, infection, nausea, and vomiting, compared with traditional cytotoxic chemotherapy.[2] The increased lifespan and the expanded use of these targeted agents have led to a variety of treatment-related adverse events (AEs). The inhibition of signaling pathways essential for cutaneous homeostasis and functioning leads to specific dermatologic AEs (dAEs).[11] dAEs can involve cosmetically sensitive areas, cause symptoms such as itching and pain, interfere with activities of daily living, and negatively affect quality of life (QoL), all of which may lead to dose reduction and even discontinuation.[3]

PRURITUS IN PATIENTS TREATED WITH TARGETED THERAPIES

Pruritus is a common dAE across different categories of targeted therapies but has received limited attention in the past. A survey conducted by Gandhi and colleagues[12] reported 36% of 379 cancer survivors experienced pruritus during treatments, with 44% having a negative impact on QoL. An analysis reported that rash and pruritus have the greatest negative impact on QoL with dAEs such as alopecia, nail changes, hand-foot syndrome, mucosal changes, and fissures, and that patients may withdraw from anticancer treatment because of intractable pruritus.[7] Clabbers and colleagues[13] examined health-related QoL using questionnaires completed by patients receiving EGFR inhibitors during the first 6 weeks, and reported that xerosis (22.3%) and pruritus (16.9%) were the most impactful AEs. Rash, pruritus, and vitiligo are among the earliest and most common AEs of immune checkpoint inhibitors[9,14–16]

Incidences of Pruritus in Patients Treated with Targeted Anticancer Therapies

A meta-analysis of 17,368 subjects from 141 trials reported the incidence of all-grade pruritus in subjects treated with EGFR, multitargeted tyrosine kinase inhibitor (TKI), B-RAF, mTOR, Bcr-Abl inhibitors, anti-CD 20, and anti-CTLA-4 mAbs ranged between 3.0% to 30.7%, and the overall summary incidence of all-grade pruritus was 17.4%.[7] The overall incidence of high-grade pruritus for all subjects was 1.4%.[7]

The incidences of all-grade and high-grade pruritus associated with targeted anticancer therapies, including novel agents (MEK inhibitors and anti-PD-1 mAbs) are summarized in **Table 1**. The highest incidence of pruritus was 33.2% to 47% in subjects treated with combination therapy consisting of ipilimumab and nivolumab, whereas the lowest incidences were less than 10% in subjects treated with VEGFR inhibitors (axitinib, pazopanib, and vandetanib).[2,7,30]

The incidences of all-grade pruritus in subjects treated with EGFR inhibitors ranged from 18.2 (cetuximab) to 54.9% (panitumumab).[2,7] The incidences of all-grade pruritus in subjects receiving BRAF inhibitors and MEK inhibitors were reported to be 18% and 45%, respectively. And the incidences of pruritus in those treated with immunotherapies including anti-CTLA4 and anti-mAbs ranged from 17% to 47%.[9,10,26,27,30]

The incidence of high-grade pruritus ranged between 0.5% and 2.6%, with the highest incidence in subjects treated with EGFR inhibitors.[2,7] The incidence of high-grade pruritus in subjects receiving immunotherapies ranged from 0.5% to 1.9%.[2,7]

A systemic review and meta-analysis including 24 phase III trials done by Santoni and colleagues[21] found that the relative risk of developing

Table 1
Incidences of all-grade and high-grade pruritus associated with targeted anticancer therapies

Category of Targeted Anticancer Therapy	Drug Names	All-Grade (%)	High-Grade (%)
EGFR inhibitors: mAbs	Cetuximab	18.2	2.1
	Panitumumab	54.9	2.6
EGFR inhibitors: TKIs	Erlotinib	20.8	2.3
	Gefitinib	21.0	1.0
EGFR-HER2 inhibitors	Lapatinib	14.6	1.0
EGFR-VEGFR inhibitors	Vandetanib	9.1	0.5
Multitargeted TKIs (VEGFR, PDGFR, or c-KIT inhibitors)	Axitinib	8.3	3.9
	Pazopanib	2.2	1.1
BRAF plus VEGFR	Sorafenib	18.2	1.0
BRAF inhibitors	Vemurafenib	18.5	1.7
MEK inhibitors	Selumetinib	45	—
mTOR inhibitors	Everolimus	14.3	1.3
	Temsirolimus	37.7	1.0
Bcr-Abl inhibitors	Dasatinib	9.7	0.8
	Imatinib	10.2	0.8
	Nilotinib	17.1	1.0
Anti-CD20 mAbs	Rituximab	10.2	1.2
	Tositumomab	13.7	0.8
Anti-CTLA-4 mAbs	Ipilimumab	24.4–35.4	1.0
	Tremelimumab	30.8	0.9
Anti-PD-1 mAbs	Nivolumab	17–18.8	0.5
	Pembrolizumab	14.1–20.7	1.0
	Ipilimumab plus nivolumab	33.2–47	0–1.9

Abbreviations: HER2, human epidermal growth factor receptor 2; KIT, KIT proto-oncogen receptor kinase.
   Data from Refs.[2,4–7,9,10,13,17–33]

all-grade and high-grade pruritus with targeted therapies compared with that of control groups or placebos were 2.2 and 2.6, respectively.

Possible Pathogenesis of Pruritus Associated with Targeted Anticancer Therapies

The pathogenesis of pruritus remains unclear. Possible pathogenesis of pruritus may involve cutaneous nerve endings, unmyelinated C-fibers ,and neurotransmitters or regulation of various receptors, such as serotonin, neurokinin (NK)-1 receptor, opioid receptors, and gamma-aminobutyric acid (GABA).[2,34–36] Xerosis and skin inflammation (ie, papulopustular eruption resulting from alteration of skin barrier function and increased dermal mast cells) were proposed to be the possible mechanisms of pruritus induced by these targeted therapies.[20] Pruritus was reported to be associated with papulopustular eruption in 62% of cases and xerosis in 50%.[2,7] A study using cell culture and animal models suggested sorafenib induces pruritus via stem cell factor activation of mast cell degranulation and maturation.[20]

Proposed Management Algorithm of Pruritus

Prevention and treatment of papulopustular or maculopapular rash and xerosis induced by targeted therapies have been considered important for pruritus prophylaxis and management.[2,26,27,37–39] The Common Terminology Criteria for Adverse Events grading and proposed management algorithms for pruritus and related skin conditions are summarized in **Table 2**. Prophylactic strategy with gentle skin care, including proper cleaning and moisturizer use, is suggested. Management usually starts from topical antipruritic agents and topical steroids for grades 1 to 2 pruritus. Oral antihistamine can be added for grade 2 pruritus that is not controllable by topical treatments. Systemic treatments, including oral antihistamine, GABA agonist (gabapentin, pregabalin), doxepin, antidepressants, NK-1 receptor antagonist (aprepitant), or corticosteroids are often necessary for grade 3 or intolerable grade 2 pruritus.[2,26,27,37–39]

In patients receiving targeted anticancer therapies, understanding the incidences of pruritus and associated conditions (eg, papulopustular

Table 2
Grading and management algorithms for pruritus and associated skin conditions of targeted therapies

	Common Terminology Criteria for Adverse Events Grading Scale and Management Algorithms for dAEs to Targeted Therapy				
			Grading		
	1	2	3	4	5
AEs	Mild	Moderate	Severe or Medically Significant but not Immediately Life-Threatening	Life-Threatening Consequences	Death
Description	Asymptomatic or mild symptoms; clinical or diagnostic observations only; intervention not indicated	Minimal, local or noninvasive intervention indicated; limiting age-appropriate instrumental ADL[a]	Hospitalization or prolongation of hospitalization indicated; disabling; limiting self-care ADL[b]	Urgent intervention indicated	Death related to AE
General approach	Moisturizer, sunscreen, gentle skin care instructions				
	Continue the drug at current dose and monitor for change in severity	Continue the drug at current dose and monitor for change in severity; continue treatment of skin reaction	Interrupt the drug until severity decreases to grade 1 or 2, modify dose per label, and monitor for change in severity; continue treatment of skin reaction; reassess after 2 wk; if reactions worsen, dose reduction or discontinuation may be necessary	—	
	Reassess after 2 wk (either by health care professional or patient self-report); if reactions worsen or do not improve proceed to next grade therapy				
	Refer to a dermatologist for evaluation and management is considered				

		Mild or localized; topical intervention indicated	Intense or widespread; intermittent; skin changes from scratching (eg, edema, papulation, excoriations, lichenification, oozing or crusts); oral intervention indicated; limiting instrumental ADL[a]	Intense or widespread; constant; limiting self-care ADL[b] or sleep; oral corticosteroid or immunosuppressive therapy indicated	
Pruritus — A disorder characterized by an intense itching sensation	—				—
Management		Topicals: Doxepin 5% cream, menthol 0.5%, topical calcineurin inhibitors (pimecrolimus, tacrolimus), medium to high-potency steroids (triamcinolone acetonide 0.025%, desonide 0.05%, fluticasone propionate 0.05%, alclometasone 0.05%)	Topicals: Medium to high-potency steroids (including clobetasol 0.05%) AND Oral antihistamines	Topicals: Medium to high-potency steroids (including clobetasol 0.05%) AND Oral antihistamines AND Gabapentin, pregabalin, doxepin, aprepitant, or antidepressant AND/OR Prednisone 0.5–1 mg/kg/d for 5 d	—

(continued on next page)

Table 2
(continued)

Common Terminology Criteria for Adverse Events Grading Scale and Management Algorithms for dAEs to Targeted Therapy

AEs	Grading				
	1	2	3	4	5
	Mild	Moderate	Severe or Medically Significant but not Immediately Life-Threatening	Life-Threatening Consequences	Death
Rash acneiform (papulopustular eruption) A disorder characterized by an eruption of papules and pustules, typically appearing in face, scalp, upper chest, and back.	Papules and/or pustules covering <10% BSA, which may or may not be associated with symptoms of pruritus or tenderness	Papules and/or pustules covering 10%–30% BSA, which may or may not be associated with symptoms of pruritus or tenderness; associated with psychosocial impact; limiting instrumental ADL[a]	Papules and/or pustules covering >30% BSA, which may or may not be associated with symptoms of pruritus or tenderness; limiting self-care ADL[b]; associated with local superinfection with oral antibiotics indicated	Papules and/or pustules covering any % BSA, which may or may not be associated with symptoms of pruritus or tenderness and are associated with extensive superinfection with IV antibiotics indicated; life-threatening consequences	Death

Management				
Preemptive treatment of week 1–6	Hydrocortisone 2.5% cream AND Clindamycin 1% gel AND Doxycycline 100 mg bid or minocycline 100 mg bid			—
Reactive treatment	Hydrocortisone 2.5% cream AND Clindamycin 1% gel or dapsone 5% gel	Hydrocortisone 2.5% cream, alclometasone 0.05% cream, or fluocinonide 0.05% cream bid AND Doxycycline 100 mg bid or minocycline 100 mg bid	Hydrocortisone 2.5% cream, alclometasone 0.05% cream, or fluocinonide 0.05% cream bid AND Doxycycline 100 mg bid/minocycline 100 mg qd AND Oral prednisone (0.5 mg/kg/d) for 5 d	—
Rash maculopapular (MPR) A disorder characterized by the presence of macules (flat) and papules (elevated); also known as morbilliform rash, it is among the most common cutaneous AEs, frequently affecting the upper trunk, spreading centripetally and associated with pruritus	Macules or papules covering <10% BSA with or without symptoms (eg, pruritus, burning, tightness)	Macules or papules covering 10%–30% BSA with or without symptoms (eg, pruritus, burning, tightness); limiting instrumental ADL[a]	Macules or papules covering >30% BSA with or without associated symptoms; limiting self-care ADL[b]	—
Management	Hydrocortisone 2.5% cream to face AND Triamcinolone 0.1% cream to body bid	Hydrocortisone 2.5% cream to face AND Fluocinonide 0.1% cream to body bid AND/OR Oral antihistamines	Hydrocortisone 2.5% cream to face AND Fluocinonide 0.1% cream to body AND Oral antihistamines AND Prednisone 0.5–1 mg/kg for 10 d	—
Dry skin A disorder characterized by flaky and dull skin; the pores are generally fine; the texture is a papery thin texture	Covering <10% BSA and no associated erythema or pruritus	Covering 10%–30% BSA and associated with erythema or pruritus; limiting instrumental ADL[a]	Covering >30% BSA and associated with pruritus; limiting self-care ADL[b]	—

(continued on next page)

Table 2
(continued)

Common Terminology Criteria for Adverse Events Grading Scale and Management Algorithms for dAEs to Targeted Therapy

	AEs	Grading				
		1	2	3	4	5
		Mild	Moderate	Severe or Medically Significant but not Immediately Life-Threatening	Life-Threatening Consequences	Death
Management	Preemptive treatment	Bathing techniques; gentle skin care; avoid extreme temperatures and direct sunlight	—	—	—	—
	Reactive treatment	OTC moisturizing cream or ointment to face bid AND Ammonium lactate 12% cream to body	OTC moisturizing cream or ointment to face bid AND Ammonium lactate 12% cream or salicylic acid 6% lactic acid cream 12%, or urea creams 10%–40% to body bid	OTC moisturizing cream or ointment to face bid AND Ammonium lactate 12%, cream or salicylic acid 6%, lactic acid cream 12%, urea creams 10%–40% to body bid AND Mid- to high-potency steroids (triamcinolone acetonide 0.025%, desonide 0.05%, fluticasone propionate 0.05%, alclometasone 0.05%)	—	—

Note: Not all grades are appropriate for all AEs. Therefore, some AEs are listed with fewer than 5 options for grade selection. Grade 5 (death) is not appropriate for some AEs and, therefore, is not an option.

Abbreviations: ADL, activities of daily living; BSA, body surface area; OTC, over-the-counter.

a Instrumental ADL: preparing meals, shopping for groceries or clothes, using the telephone, managing money, and so forth.

b Self-care ADL: bathing, dressing and undressing, feeding self, using the toilet, taking medications, and not bedridden.

Adapted from U.S. Department of Health and Human Services. CTCAE Grading Scale (v4.0: May 28, 2009). Available at: https://evs.nci.nih.gov/ftp1/CTCAE/CTCAE_4.03_2010-06-14_QuickReference_5x7.pdf. Accessed July 27, 2017; with permission; and *Data from* Refs.[1,37,40–50]

eruptions and xerosis), pretreatment patient counseling, proper prophylactic skin care, and management of pruritus are essential to maintain patient QoL.

REFERENCES

1. Lynch TJ Jr, Kim ES, Eaby B, et al. Epidermal growth factor receptor inhibitor-associated cutaneous toxicities: an evolving paradigm in clinical management. Oncologist 2007;12(5):610–21.
2. Fischer A, Rosen AC, Ensslin CJ, et al. Pruritus to anticancer agents targeting the EGFR, BRAF, and CTLA-4. Dermatol Ther 2013;26(2):135–48.
3. Tischer B, Huber R, Kraemer M, et al. Dermatologic events from EGFR inhibitors: the issue of the missing patient voice. Support Care Cancer 2017; 25(2):651–60.
4. Barton-Burke M, Ciccolini K, Mekas M, et al. Dermatologic reactions to targeted therapy: a focus on epidermal growth factor receptor inhibitors and nursing care. Nurs Clin North Am 2017; 52(1):83–113.
5. Macdonald JB, Macdonald B, Golitz LE, et al. Cutaneous adverse effects of targeted therapies: Part II: inhibitors of intracellular molecular signaling pathways. J Am Acad Dermatol 2015;72(2):221–36 [quiz: 237–8].
6. Belum VR, Washington C, Pratilas CA, et al. Dermatologic adverse events in pediatric patients receiving targeted anticancer therapies: a pooled analysis. Pediatr Blood Cancer 2015;62(5):798–806.
7. Ensslin CJ, Rosen AC, Wu S, et al. Pruritus in patients treated with targeted cancer therapies: systematic review and meta-analysis. J Am Acad Dermatol 2013;69(5):708–20.
8. Belum VR, Fontanilla Patel H, Lacouture ME, et al. Skin toxicity of targeted cancer agents: mechanisms and intervention. Future Oncol 2013;9(8):1161–70.
9. Belum VR, Benhuri B, Postow MA, et al. Characterisation and management of dermatologic adverse events to agents targeting the PD-1 receptor. Eur J Cancer 2016;60:12–25.
10. Boutros C, Tarhini A, Routier E, et al. Safety profiles of anti-CTLA-4 and anti-PD-1 antibodies alone and in combination. Nat Rev Clin Oncol 2016;13(8): 473–86.
11. Valentine J, Belum VR, Duran J, et al. Incidence and risk of xerosis with targeted anticancer therapies. J Am Acad Dermatol 2015;72(4):656–67.
12. Gandhi M, Oishi K, Zubal B, et al. Unanticipated toxicities from anticancer therapies: survivors' perspectives. Support Care Cancer 2010;18(11):1461–8.
13. Clabbers JMK, Boers-Doets CB, Gelderblom H, et al. Xerosis and pruritus as major EGFRI-associated adverse events. Support Care Cancer 2016;24(2):513–21.
14. Robert C, Schachter J, Long GV, et al. Pembrolizumab versus ipilimumab in advanced melanoma. N Engl J Med 2015;372(26):2521–32.
15. Wolchok JD, Neyns B, Linette G, et al. Ipilimumab monotherapy in patients with pretreated advanced melanoma: a randomised, double-blind, multicentre, phase 2, dose-ranging study. Lancet Oncol 2010; 11(2):155–64.
16. Larsabal M, Marti A, Jacquemin C, et al. Vitiligo-like lesions occurring in patients receiving anti-programmed cell death-1 therapies are clinically and biologically distinct from vitiligo. J Am Acad Dermatol 2017;76(5):863–70.
17. Choi JN. Dermatologic adverse events to chemotherapeutic agents, Part 2: BRAF inhibitors, MEK inhibitors, and ipilimumab. Semin Cutan Med Surg 2014;33(1):40–8.
18. Balagula Y, Barth Huston K, Busam KJ, et al. Dermatologic side effects associated with the MEK 1/2 inhibitor selumetinib (AZD6244, ARRY-142886). Invest New Drugs 2011;29(5):1114–21.
19. Belum VR, Fischer A, Choi JN, et al. Dermatological adverse events from BRAF inhibitors: a growing problem. Curr Oncol Rep 2013;15(3):249–59.
20. Mizukami Y, Sugawara K, Kira Y, et al. Sorafenib stimulates human skin type mast cell degranulation and maturation. J Dermatol Sci 2017;88(3):308–19.
21. Santoni M, Conti A, Andrikou K, et al. Risk of pruritus in cancer patients treated with biological therapies: a systematic review and meta-analysis of clinical trials. Crit Rev Oncol Hematol 2015;96(2):206–19.
22. Bryce J, Boers-Doets CB. Non-rash dermatologic adverse events related to targeted therapies. Semin Oncol Nurs 2014;30(3):155–68.
23. Rosen AC, Case EC, Dusza SW, et al. Impact of dermatologic adverse events on quality of life in 283 cancer patients: a questionnaire study in a dermatology referral clinic. Am J Clin Dermatol 2013;14(4):327–33.
24. Ebata T. Drug-induced itch management. Curr Probl Dermatol 2016;50:155–63.
25. Reyes-Habito CM, Roh EK. Cutaneous reactions to chemotherapeutic drugs and targeted therapy for cancer: part II. Targeted therapy. J Am Acad Dermatol 2014;71(2):217.e1-11 [quiz: 227–8].
26. de Golian E, Kwong BY, Swetter SM, et al. Cutaneous complications of targeted melanoma therapy. Curr Treat Options Oncol 2016;17(11):57.
27. Collins LK, Chapman MS, Carter JB, et al. Cutaneous adverse effects of the immune checkpoint inhibitors. Curr Probl Cancer 2017;41(2):125–8.
28. Minkis K, Garden BC, Wu S, et al. The risk of rash associated with ipilimumab in patients with cancer: a systematic review of the literature and meta-analysis. J Am Acad Dermatol 2013;69(3):e121–8.
29. Lacouture ME, Wolchok JD, Yosipovitch G, et al. Ipilimumab in patients with cancer and the

management of dermatologic adverse events. J Am Acad Dermatol 2014;71(1):161–9.

30. Sibaud V, Meyer N, Lamant L, et al. Dermatologic complications of anti-PD-1/PD-L1 immune checkpoint antibodies. Curr Opin Oncol 2016;28(4):254–63.

31. Habre M, Habre SB, Kourie HR. Dermatologic adverse events of checkpoint inhibitors: what an oncologist should know. Immunotherapy 2016;8(12):1437–46.

32. Mochel MC, Ming ME, Imadojemu S, et al. Cutaneous autoimmune effects in the setting of therapeutic immune checkpoint inhibition for metastatic melanoma. J Cutan Pathol 2016;43(9):787–91.

33. Ito J, Fujimoto D, Nakamura A, et al. Aprepitant for refractory nivolumab-induced pruritus. Lung Cancer 2017;109:58–61.

34. Pereira MP, Kremer AE, Mettang T, et al. Chronic pruritus in the absence of skin disease: pathophysiology, diagnosis and treatment. Am J Clin Dermatol 2016;17(4):337–48.

35. Wong LS, Wu T, Lee CH. Inflammatory and noninflammatory itch: implications in pathophysiology-directed treatments. Int J Mol Sci 2017;18(7) [pii: E1485].

36. Oetjen LK, Mack MR, Feng J, et al. Sensory neurons co-opt classical immune signaling pathways to mediate chronic itch. Cell 2017;171(1):217–28.e13.

37. Lacouture ME, Anadkat MJ, Bensadoun RJ, et al. Clinical practice guidelines for the prevention and treatment of EGFR inhibitor-associated dermatologic toxicities. Support Care Cancer 2011;19(8):1079–95.

38. Melosky B, Leighl NB, Rothenstein J, et al. Management of egfr tki-induced dermatologic adverse events. Curr Oncol 2015;22(2):123–32.

39. Bergman H, Walton T, Del Bel R, et al. Managing skin toxicities related to panitumumab. J Am Acad Dermatol 2014;71(4):754–9.

40. Common Terminology Criteria for Adverse Events (CTCAE) Version 4.0. Springer (Heidelberg): U.S.Department of Health And Human Services. National Institutes of Health. National Cancer Institute; 2010.

41. Lacouture ME, Maitland ML, Segaert S, et al. A proposed EGFR inhibitor dermatologic adverse event-specific grading scale from the MASCC skin toxicity study group. Support Care Cancer 2010;18(4):509–22.

42. Perez-Soler R, Delord JP, Halpern A, et al. HER1/EGFR inhibitor-associated rash: future directions for management and investigation outcomes from the HER1/EGFR inhibitor rash management forum. Oncologist 2005;10(5):345–56.

43. Eaby B, Culkin A, Lacouture ME. An interdisciplinary consensus on managing skin reactions associated with human epidermal growth factor receptor inhibitors. Clin J Oncol Nurs 2008;12(2):283–90.

44. Melosky B, Burkes R, Rayson D, et al. Management of skin rash during EGFR-targeted monoclonal antibody treatment for gastrointestinal malignancies: Canadian recommendations. Curr Oncol (Toronto, Ont) 2009;16(1):16–26.

45. Jatoi A, Thrower A, Sloan JA, et al. Does sunscreen prevent epidermal growth factor receptor (EGFR) inhibitor-induced rash? Results of a placebo-controlled trial from the North Central Cancer Treatment Group (N05C4). Oncologist 2010;15(9):1016–22.

46. Lacouture ME, Mitchell EP, Piperdi B, et al. Skin toxicity evaluation protocol with panitumumab (STEPP), a phase II, open-label, randomized trial evaluating the impact of a pre-Emptive Skin treatment regimen on skin toxicities and quality of life in patients with metastatic colorectal cancer. J Clin Oncol 2010;28(8):1351–7.

47. Ouwerkerk J, Boers-Doets C. Best practices in the management of toxicities related to anti-EGFR agents for metastatic colorectal cancer. Eur J Oncol Nurs 2010;14(4):337–49.

48. Melosky B, Hirsh V. Management of common toxicities in metastatic NSCLC related to anti-lung cancer therapies with EGFR-TKIs. Front Oncol 2014;4:238.

49. Melosky B, Anderson H, Burkes RL, et al. Pan Canadian rash trial: a randomized phase III trial evaluating the impact of a prophylactic skin treatment regimen on epidermal growth factor receptor-tyrosine kinase inhibitor-induced skin toxicities in patients with metastatic lung cancer. J Clin Oncol 2016;34(8):810–5.

50. Belum VR, Marchetti MA, Dusza SW, et al. A prospective, randomized, double-blinded, split-face/chest study of prophylactic topical dapsone 5% gel versus moisturizer for the prevention of cetuximab-induced acneiform rash. J Am Acad Dermatol 2017;77(3):577–9.

Immunomodulating Agents as Antipruritics

Stephen Erickson, BS[a], Zachary Nahmias, MD[a], Ilana S. Rosman, MD[b,c,d], Brian S. Kim, MD, MTR[a,c,e,f],*

KEYWORDS

- Itch • Pruritus • Immunomodulator • Atopic dermatitis • Urticaria • Prurigo nodularis
- Chronic idiopathic pruritus

KEY POINTS

- Chronic pruritus, or itch lasting longer than 6 weeks, is an increasingly common and debilitating condition.
- Itch involves complex interactions between the skin, immune, and nervous systems.
- Recent studies have implicated type 2–associated cytokines, such as interleukin (IL)-4, IL-13, and IL-31, as critical regulators of itch.
- Blocking the neuroimmune axis has emerged as a novel immunomodulatory approach to treat chronic itch disorders.

INTRODUCTION

Pruritus or itch is defined as any sensation that elicits the desire to scratch. Although scratching may be beneficial by removing pathogens or noxious environmental stimuli from the skin, in its chronic form, itch becomes highly pathologic. Chronic itch, defined as itch lasting greater than 6 weeks, is a symptom that profoundly and negatively affects quality of life.[1–3] Furthermore, chronic itch is common, with an estimated prevalence of 15% and increases with age, affecting 12.3% of those 16 years old to 30 years old and up to 25% of those over 60 years of age.[4–6] Despite its debilitating nature and high prevalence, the biological mechanisms underlying chronic itch remain poorly understood.

It is widely appreciated that skin inflammation leads to itch. Thus, in chronic inflammatory skin disorders, such as atopic dermatitis (AD), chronic itch presents as the central symptom and problem. In both AD and other conditions, such as prurigo nodularis (PN), it has been proposed that inflammation can arise secondary to scratching, which in turn exacerbates the itch-scratch cycle. In the setting of chronic idiopathic pruritus (CIP), it remains even less clear whether immune dysregulation precedes or is secondary to the onset of itch. Regardless of the etiology of inflammatory chronic itch, most therapeutic approaches involve

Disclosure Statement: B.S. Kim has served on advisory boards for Celgene, Regeneron, and Sanofi. He has worked as a consultant for Incyte and has received support for research from Celgene and LEO Pharma. S. Erickson, Z. Nahmias, and I.S. Rosman have nothing to disclose.

[a] Division of Dermatology, Department of Medicine, Washington University School of Medicine, 660 South Euclid Campus Box 8123, St Louis, MO 63110, USA; [b] Division of Dermatology, Department of Medicine, Washington University School of Medicine, St Louis, MO 63110, USA; [c] Department of Pathology and Immunology, Washington University School of Medicine, St Louis, MO, USA; [d] Washington University Dermatopathology Center, Washington University School of Medicine, 660 South Euclid Campus Box 8118, St Louis, MO 63110, USA; [e] Department of Anesthesiology, Washington University School of Medicine, St Louis, MO, USA; [f] Center for the Study of Itch, Washington University School of Medicine, St Louis, MO, USA

* Corresponding author. Division of Dermatology, Department of Medicine, Washington University School of Medicine, 660 South Euclid Campus Box 8123, St Louis, MO 63110.
E-mail address: briankim@wustl.edu

Dermatol Clin 36 (2018) 325–334
https://doi.org/10.1016/j.det.2018.02.014

disrupting the inflammatory process to ultimately limit symptoms of itch. Notwithstanding this, the molecular and cellular mechanisms by which inflammation leads to itch remain to be clearly defined.

Recent seminal discoveries have identified itch-specific receptors, such as the gastrin-releasing peptide receptor and the Mas-related G protein–coupled receptor family, as critical mediators of chronic itch.[7,8] Along these lines, recent studies have also demonstrated that proinflammatory cytokines can function as itch-inducing factors or pruritogens to directly stimulate itch-sensory nerve fibers to evoke symptoms of itch. Collectively, these discoveries have unveiled a new paradigm in which the immune system can directly communicate with the nervous system to mediate itch. Thus, a better understanding of the molecular pathways that regulate the neuroimmunologic interface may offer new therapeutic approaches to treat chronic itch. Herein, by highlighting new studies, this article reviews how proinflammatory responses promote itch and how novel immunomodulatory approaches can be used to treat chronic itch disorders.

THE PATHOGENESIS OF SKIN INFLAMMATION

The immune system is generally divided into 2 broad categories: (1) the innate immune system, which responds directly and rapidly to nonspecific stimuli, such as pathogen-associated molecular patterns, and various inflammatory factors, such as epithelial cell–derived cytokines, and (2) the adaptive immune system, which can form memory and recognize antigens by generating highly specific receptors as on T cells. Innate and adaptive immune cells are present at the skin barrier and can be functionally divided into 3 distinct responses, known as types 1, 2, and 3 immunity (**Fig. 1**). Type 1 immunity involves responses mediated by adaptive cells, such as type 1 helper T (T_H1) cells and cytotoxic T cells, and innate immune cells, such as group 1 innate lymphoid cells (ILC1s) and natural killer (NK) cells. These cells are characterized by the production of interferon (IFN) gamma and tumor necrosis factor (TNF) alpha, which can act on other cells, such as macrophages. Generally, the type 1 immune response is used to protect against intracellular pathogens and tumor cells, but it can also promote chronic inflammatory processes as in autoimmune skin diseases and allergic contact dermatitis (ACD).[9]

Type 2 immunity is mediated by adaptive type 2 helper T (T_H2) cells as well as innate immune cells, including group 2 innate lymphoid cells (ILC2s), basophils, mast cells, and eosinophils. Collectively, these cells produce the effector type 2 cytokines interleukin (IL)-4, IL-5, and IL-13, which promote allergic inflammation and

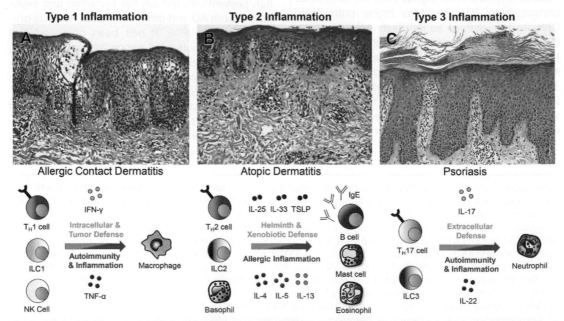

Fig. 1. Distinct immune axes underlie various pruritic inflammatory skin disorders. (*A*) Type 1 inflammation is composed of T_H1, ILC1, and NK cell responses and has been implicated in ACD. (*B*) Type 2 inflammation underlies AD and is composed of pathogenic T_H2 cells, ILC2s, and basophils. (*C*) Type 3 inflammation is associated with T_H17 and ILC3 responses in the setting of psoriasis. Hematoxylin-eosin, ×200 magnification.

immunoglobulin E (IgE) production. Upstream pro-moters of the type 2 inflammatory process include the epithelial cell–derived cytokines IL-25, IL-33, and thymic stromal lymphopoietin (TSLP), which can be directly secreted by keratinocytes. Nor-mally, type 2 immunity functions to bolster barrier immunity and protect against invading helminth parasites and noxious xenobiotics; however, this response can be excessively activated by aller-gens leading to allergic diseases, such as AD (see **Fig. 1**).[9–11]

Type 3 immunity is characterized by the enrich-ment of adaptive type 17 T helper (T_H17) cells and innate immune cells, such as group 3 innate lymphoid cells (ILC3s) and neutrophils, and the production of IL-17 and IL-22. In the steady state, these processes promote epithelial barrier func-tion and help protect against extracellular bacteria and fungi. Similar to type 1 immunity, however, when dysregulated, type 3 immune responses are implicated in the development of autoimmune diseases, such as psoriasis (see **Fig. 1**).[9]

This review highlights new studies that have un-covered previously unrecognized inflammatory factors that specifically drive itch and the potential therapeutic implications. Given the limited litera-ture on type 1 immunomodulating agents in the skin, and the extensive coverage of biologic thera-peutics in psoriasis-associated itch elsewhere, this article focuses on type 2 inflammatory itch.[12]

TYPE 2 INFLAMMATION AND ITCH
Urticaria

Urticaria is characterized by pruritic wheals or hives with individual lesions typically lasting less than 24 hours.[13] Although most cases of acute ur-ticaria are self-resolving, it can become chronic when occurring almost daily for greater than 6 weeks and is often idiopathic. In this setting, it is referred to as chronic idiopathic urticaria or chronic spontaneous urticaria (CSU).[14] The etiol-ogies of urticaria are numerous, including allergic reactions, mechanical stimulation, autoimmunity, and idiopathic.[15] Thus, a deeper understanding of the pathogenesis of urticaria is critical for the development of better therapeutics to address conditions, such as CSU.

The most debilitating aspect of urticaria is its associated itch. It is widely believed that a putative antigen binds IgE on basophils and mast cells, which then results in cross-linking of the high-affinity IgE receptor (FcεRI) and subsequent release of histamine. As a result, histaminergic neural pathways become activated to mediate itch.[16] Although antihistamines can be highly effective in the setting of acute urticaria, they often

fail in the setting of chronic urticaria.[13] Therefore, in severe chronic urticaria, systemic immunomod-ulators are sometimes used to broadly limit inflam-mation in the skin. These clinical observations have provoked the hypothesis that other as-yet unrecognized mediators are likely released from granulocytes, such as basophils and mast cells, to mediate itch. Although the identification of novel granulocyte-derived itch mediators has emerged as an active area of investigation, new therapeutic approaches have already been developed to effectively manage CSU by broadly blocking acti-vation of these cells.

Antihistamines
Antihistamines play a vital role in treating acute ur-ticaria and its associated itch. Of the 4 histamine receptors, H_1R, and more recently H_4R, are known to mediate itch.[17] H_1 antihistamines have long been known to be effective in treating acute urti-carial itch. In CSU, H_1 antihistamines have limited efficacy but remain the first-line therapy.[13] Whether antihistamines work to limit itch predom-inantly through their direct effects on sensory neu-rons or by their effects on other cells remains, however, poorly understood. Beyond H_1R, H_4R represents a new and promising target in itch treatment. Many of the clinically utilized H_1 and H_2 antihistamines have no affinity for H_4R.[18] H_4R is expressed on mast cells and expression on neurons has not been well characterized.[19] A recent clinical trial of an H_4 antihistamine (JNJ 39758979) showed significant reduction in histamine-induced pruritus in patients with no effect on wheal formation.[20] Although H_4 antihista-mines may enter into the clinical realm in the future, H_1R blockade remains a mainstay of ther-apy in acute urticarial itch.

Systemic immunomodulators
Broad immunosuppression, such as the use of systemic corticosteroids, can be effective in the setting of CSU. Short courses of systemic cortico-steroids are widely used and known to be rapidly effective via reduction in the number and function of infiltrating immune cells.[21,22] Cyclosporin A (CsA), a calcineurin inhibitor known to act on T cells to inhibit transcription of inflammatory cyto-kines, also can be effective.[23,24] Additionally, CsA is believed to act on basophils and mast cells to limit the release of histamine and the synthesis of arachidonic acid derivatives.[25] Clinical trials have shown CsA to be an effective add-on therapy to H_1 antihistamines in CSU.[26] Due to multiple adverse effects, however, use of systemic immu-nosuppressants is only recommended in severe, refractory disease for short periods of time.[13]

Omalizumab

Omalizumab has emerged as the first targeted biologic therapy for CSU. It is a recombinant humanized anti-IgE monoclonal antibody (mAb) that blocks IgE binding to FcεRI, thereby preventing the activation of basophils and mast cells.[27] It has been shown to reduce circulating IgE levels and reduce FcεRI expression and function on target cells.[28] In phase 3 clinical trials, omalizumab in patients with moderate to severe CSU, inadequately controlled by H_1 antihistamine therapy, showed significant improvement in itch severity and urticaria. The reductions in itch severity were observed as early as within week 1, and improvements in urticarial lesions were similarly rapid.[29,30] The efficacy of omalizumab, even in patients who fail antihistamine therapy, suggests that IgE blockade likely functions by preventing the release of other unrecognized pruritogens beyond histamine.

Atopic Dermatitis

AD, or atopic eczema, is a chronic, relapsing inflammatory skin disorder characterized by severe pruritus and characteristic skin lesions.[31] Although type 2 immune responses have emerged as central to the pathogenesis of AD, it remains a complex disease composed of both epidermal barrier dysfunction and immune dysregulation (see **Fig. 1**). Additionally, genetic, environmental, and commensal microbial factors are known to contribute to disease pathogenesis.[32–34] Despite recent advances in identifying proinflammatory factors that drive disease, questions remain regarding the precise pathogenic factors that drive pruritus in the setting of AD.

In addition to the proinflammatory cytokines IL-4 and IL-13, the epithelial cell–derived cytokines IL-33 and TSLP have been shown to be critical upstream regulators of the type 2 inflammatory response and AD pathogenesis.[10,35] Beyond proinflammatory functions, other cytokines, such as IL-31, derived from T_H2 cells, have been shown to act as pruritogens by stimulating sensory nerves to promote itch.[36] More recently, IL-33 and TSLP have also been demonstrated to function as pruritogens by directly activating the nervous system.[37,38] Strikingly, the authors demonstrated for the first time that IL-4 directly modulates sensory nerves in both mice and humans and alters responsiveness to a multitude of pruritogens, including histamine, chloroquine, IL-31, and TSLP. The authors found that neuron-restricted deletion of the shared receptor for IL-4 and IL-13 (IL-4Rα) resulted in abatement of itch in vivo in a murine model of AD.[39] Collectively, these studies highlight that targeting pruritogenic cytokines to specifically treat itch apart from inflammation represents a new therapeutic paradigm.

Classically, treatments of AD have centered around targeting skin inflammation. Although emollients help restore the skin barrier and are preventative of flares, they are limited in their efficacy once skin inflammation is triggered. Thus, classic treatments include anti-inflammatories, such as topical corticosteroids (TCSs) and topical calcineurin inhibitors (TCIs), such as tacrolimus and pimecrolimus. In cases of moderate to severe AD, off-label use of systemic immunosuppressants, including systemic corticosteroids, azathioprine, CsA, methotrexate, and mycophenolate mofetil, can also be effective but must be used with caution due to adverse effects. Newer targeted biologic therapeutics have emerged, however, that demonstrate a remarkable combination of safety and efficacy.[31]

Topical immunomodulators

Topical immunomodulators, including TCSs and TCIs have been the mainstay of treatment in AD.[31] Although itch-specific data for TCS treatment are limited, improvement in itch is known to occur concomitantly with improvement of skin inflammation. TCIs have been shown to improve itch symptoms within 48 hours of treatment and have a better side-effect profile than TCSs, with no risk of skin atrophy.[40] Whether the mechanisms of action of TCSs and TCIs are via direct antipruritic effects apart from inflammation remains, however, unclear.

Topical phosphodiesterase 4 (PDE4) inhibitors are a new potential topical therapy for AD. PDE4 is the major enzyme catalyzing cyclic AMP degradation in most immune cells and is also expressed in nonimmune cells, including keratinocytes. PDE4 inhibition affects multiple cytokine pathways and thus likely derives its anti-inflammatory effects by a variety of mechanisms.[41] There is evidence, however, that PDE4 is expressed in sensory neurons, and thus inhibition may have direct antipruritic effects. A topical PDE4 inhibitor rapidly reduced scratching and itch-related cutaneous nerve firing in a mouse model of AD.[42] Phase 3 clinical trials with the topical PDE4 inhibitor crisaborole in patients with mild to moderate AD showed significant improvement in pruritus and skin lesions. Significant itch improvement was seen after 8 days of treatment, the earliest reported time point. On a 4-point itch scale, 63% of patients achieved a score of 0 or 1 and improvement by 1 or more points after 29 days of treatment compared with 53% treated with vehicle alone.[43] It is unclear, however, whether topical crisaborole has unique anti-itch properties compared with other classic topical immunomodulators.

Antihistamines

H$_1$ antihistamines are generally ineffective in treating AD-associated itch.[31] Although histamine seems to promote acute forms of itch, the chronic itch of AD is believed to be driven mainly by nonhistaminergic itch pathways.[16]

Interleukin 4 and interleukin 13 antagonists

Numerous preclinical and translational studies have implicated IL-4 and IL-13 as key cytokines in the pathogenesis of AD.[44] Phase 2 and phase 3 clinical trials using dupilumab, a fully human mAb targeting the IL-4Rα, demonstrated unprecedented efficacy with regard to AD disease severity, quality of life, and itch severity.[45–47] Given that IL-4Rα is present on several immune cells, it is believed that antagonism of this pathway is effective due to its anti-inflammatory effects. Strikingly, the improvement in pruritus was rapid, marked, and significant by 2 weeks into treatment in comparison to the placebo control group.[46] The authors recently found that IL-4Rα is both expressed and functionally active on human sensory neurons from dorsal root ganglia. Using a mouse model of AD, the authors found that deletion of IL-4Rα on only sensory neurons was sufficient to abate AD-associated itch in vivo. In addition, IL-4 promoted neural hypersensitivity to several well-defined pruritogens, including histamine, chloroquine, IL-31, and TSLP, indicating that neuronal IL-4 signaling may be a master regulator of AD-associated itch.[39] Thus, the role of type 2 cytokines in neural hypersensitivity remains an active area of investigation.

Targeting similar pathways to dupilumab, the anti–IL-13 mAbs tralokinumab and lebrikizumab both recently completed phase 2 clinical trials in patients with moderate to severe AD. Tralokinumab showed significant reductions in both itch and skin lesions and is currently undergoing a phase 3 clinical trial (NCT03160885).[48] Lebrikizumab significantly reduced skin lesions.[49,50] Phase 3 clinical trials will likely better characterize the efficacy of IL-13 blockade versus dual IL-4/IL-13 blockade in the setting of dupilumab, particularly with regard to itch symptoms.

Interleukin 31 antagonists

IL-31 has emerged as an important target for itch in the setting of AD.[51] Mainly derived from T$_H$2 cells, IL-31 has been shown to directly stimulate sensory nerves and mediate itch.[36] Its receptor is heterodimeric and composed of the IL-31 receptor alpha (IL-31RA) subunit and oncostatin M receptor.[52] IL-31RA levels are highest in dorsal root ganglia neurons.[53] Transgenic mice overexpressing IL-31 develop an AD-like phenotype characterized by chronic itch, and blockade with anti–IL-31 mAb reduced scratching behavior in a murine model of AD.[52,54] In AD patients, lesional and nonlesional skin shows increased IL-31 expression, and serum levels correlate with disease severity.[53,55] Chronic AD lesions contain increased IL-31–producing T cells, and activated leukocytes from AD patients show increased IL-31 expression.[53,56] Nemolizumab, a humanized anti–IL-31RA mAb, has recently demonstrated unique anti-itch properties. In a phase 2 clinical trial, patients with moderate to severe AD showed significant reduction in pruritus as early as day 2 of treatment. After 12 weeks of treatment, the primary outcome measure of mean percent improvement from baseline score on the pruritus visual analog scale was 63.1% versus 20.9% with placebo.[57] Larger phase 3 clinical trials, however, are required to fully define its widespread efficacy in AD-associated itch.

Epithelial cell–derived cytokine (interleukin 25, interleukin 33, and thymic stromal lymphopoietin) antagonists

Skin barrier dysfunction and its associated immune dysregulation are key features of AD pathogenesis.[58] In the setting of a disrupted skin barrier, the epithelial cell–derived cytokines IL-25, IL-33, and TSLP have been shown to potently promote type 2 immune responses and AD-associated skin inflammation via a variety of cell types, including, but not limited to, T$_H$2 cells, basophils, and ILC2s (see Fig. 1).[10,59–62] All of the epithelial cell–derived cytokines have been implicated in human AD.[63–65] Studies in mice have demonstrated that both IL-33 and TSLP can function as pruritogens by directly stimulating sensory neurons.[37,38] Thus, like IL-31, it seems that these cytokines can act as a direct link between the epithelium and the nerve in mediating itch. Additionally, given that these epithelial cell–derived cytokines act upstream of the effector itch-mediating cytokines, IL-4, IL-13, and IL-31, IL-33, and TSLP may represent unique and potent therapeutic targets in AD-associated itch. A phase 1 clinical trial of an anti–IL-33 mAb was recently completed in healthy adults, and preliminary results from a phase 2 clinical trial showed efficacy in AD.[66] Data are currently limited with regard to the efficacy of these agents in AD-associated itch; however, these biologics remain exciting future therapeutic possibilities.

Janus kinase inhibitors

Janus kinase (JAK) inhibitors are small molecules that selectively target multiple cytokine pathways at once to mediate their anti-inflammatory effects. Cytokine receptors signal via the JAK-STAT pathway and use 1 or more of the 4 JAKs (JAK1, JAK2, JAK3, and TYK2).[67] Oclacitinib most potently targets JAK1, although inhibition of all 4 JAKs has been shown, and inhibits the function of several cytokines, including IL-2, IL-4, IL-13, and IL-31 on leukocytes.[68] Treatment in canines with AD reduced pruritus beginning on day 1 of administration.[69] Similar to oclacitinib, tofacitinib (JAK1/3 selective) reduces signaling across many of the same cytokine pathways.[67] A recent case series showed a good response to oral tofacitinib in 6 patients with AD.[70] A phase 2a clinical trial for topical tofacitinib in patients with mild to moderate AD showed significant reductions in itch starting on day 2 of treatment. At 4 weeks, 68%, compared with 13% of the control subjects, achieved a physician's global assessment (5-point scale) score of clear or almost clear and an improvement of 2 or more points from baseline.[71] A recent phase 2 clinical trial of oral baricitinib (JAK1/2 selective) in patients with moderate to severe AD showed reductions in both itch and skin lesions, and a phase 3 clinical trial is planned.[67,72] In a recent study, the authors identified for the first time that JAK1 is selectively expressed in itch-sensory neurons compared with JAK2 and JAK3. Using neuron-specific genetic deletion of JAK1, the authors found that itch in mice was markedly reduced in the setting of AD-like disease independently of the level of skin inflammation. Furthermore, using the JAK1/2 inhibitor ruxolitinib, the authors found that improvement of itch occurred despite minimal suppression of skin inflammation.[39] In support of this mechanism, a recent phase 2b clinical trial with upadacitinib (ABT-494), an oral JAK1-selective inhibitor, demonstrated improvement of itch as early as 1 week after initiation of therapy.[73] Collectively, these studies suggest that JAK inhibitors may have additional itch-specific effects beyond their anti-inflammatory properties.

Prurigo Nodularis

In patients with chronic itch, a subset develops PN, a condition characterized by multiple intensely pruritic, hyperkeratotic, and lichenified nodules. PN is more common in the elderly but occurs in patients of all ages.[74] The pathogenesis of PN remains largely elusive, and it is unclear whether PN is a unique entity or a common endpoint in chronic itch. Although a history of atopy is present in approximately 50% of patients, PN is a multifactorial disease and a single cause is not usually identified.[75] PN lesions show a nonspecific infiltrate of lymphocytes, eosinophils, neutrophils, and macrophages.[76] Strikingly, IL-31 expression has been shown to be 50-fold and 4.5-fold higher in PN lesions compared with healthy skin and AD lesions, respectively.[53] Additionally, it has been reported that there is an increased density of dermal nerve fibers staining for substance P in PN lesions, indicating that PN may have, in addition to proinflammatory factors, neuropathic processes underlying its pathogenesis.[77]

The treatment of itch in PN is challenging. Initial treatment may include TCSs and TCIs, intralesional corticosteroids, and even systemic immunosuppressants. The immunomodulator thalidomide and its more potent analog lenalidomide have also been used in PN. These drugs have broad immunomodulatory effects; however, mechanistic details with regard to how they work in PN remain unclear.[78–80] Small randomized and retrospective studies have shown thalidomide effective in refractory PN.[79,80] Case studies have shown success with lenalidomide as well.[78]

Targeted immunomodulatory agents are urgently needed for PN. Given the reported high IL-31 expression in PN and strong association with atopy, nemolizumab and other biologics, which have shown promise in AD, may be of use in PN. A phase 2 clinical trial for nemolizumab in patients with PN is planned (NCT03181503).

Chronic Idiopathic Pruritus

CIP, or pruritus of unknown origin, is commonly seen in the elderly. Although many factors are thought to underlie CIP, physiologic changes associated with aging likely contribute, including epidermal barrier dysfunction, sensory neuropathy, and immunosenescence.[81,82] Immunosenescence of aging is characterized by a proinflammatory state with enhanced type 2 immune responses and reduced type 1 immunity.[82] The authors previously showed that elderly patients with CIP display immune dysregulation toward a type 2 immune response in excess of similarly aged peers. Skin biopsies from a subset of CIP patients demonstrated infiltration with eosinophils, suggestive of low-level type 2 skin inflammation.[83] Although primary clinical skin lesions are typically not evident in the setting of CIP, the authors have recently shown that these patients have more severe chronic itch than patients with robustly inflammatory skin lesions in the setting of AD.[39] Based on the identification that JAK1 is expressed in neurons coupled with evidence of type 2 immune responses in CIP, the authors hypothesized that severe, refractory CIP patients would benefit from systemic JAK inhibitors. The authors found that in a small cohort of CIP patients with a baseline numeric rating scale itch score of greater than or equal to 7, all patients improved on oral tofacitinib with a mean overall improvement of approximately 80%.[39] Taken together, it seems that JAK inhibitors may be particularly effective for the treatment of CIP. Larger randomized clinical trials, however, are required in the future to fully determine the efficacy of JAK inhibitors in this context.

SUMMARY

Chronic pruritus, or itch lasting greater than 6 weeks, is a common and debilitating condition. Itch involves complex interactions between the skin, immune, and nervous systems. Exciting advances in understanding of the neuroimmune axis in itch have uncovered several new targets for the treatment of chronic itch. Given the discovery of previously unrecognized cytokines acting directly on cutaneous nerves to promote itch, classic type 2 cytokines, such as IL-4 and IL-13, have emerged as unique factors that can be targeted with the newly arrived biologic agent dupilumab. Additionally, nemolizumab, an IL-31RA antagonist, also demonstrates promise as a therapeutic agent in the setting of AD-associated itch. Finally, JAK inhibitors can also be used to simultaneously target many of these cytokine pathways in AD and other chronic itch disorders. Future clinical trials are required to fully define the efficacy of blocking these pathways in human disease. Collectively, these advances have already revolutionized the treatment of chronic itch disorders, such as AD, and will likely expand into many other pruritic dermatoses including, but not limited to, urticaria, PN, and CIP.

REFERENCES

1. Stander S, Weisshaar E, Mettang T, et al. Clinical classification of itch: a position paper of the international forum for the study of itch. Acta Derm Venereol 2007;87(4):291–4.
2. Kini SP, DeLong LK, Veledar E, et al. The impact of pruritus on quality of life: the skin equivalent of pain. Arch Dermatol 2011,147(10).1153–6.
3. Chrostowska-Plak D, Reich A, Szepietowski JC. Relationship between itch and psychological status of patients with atopic dermatitis. J Eur Acad Dermatol Venereol 2013;27:e239–42.
4. Stander S, Schafer I, Phan NQ, et al. Prevalence of chronic pruritus in Germany: results of a cross-sectional study in a sample working population of 11,730. Dermatology 2010;221(3):229–35.
5. Matterne U, Apfelbacher CJ, Loerbroks A, et al. Prevalence, correlates and characteristics of chronic pruritus: a population-based cross-sectional study. Acta Derm Venereol 2011;91(6):674–9.
6. Valdes-Rodriguez R, Mollanazar NK, González-Muro J, et al. Itch prevalence and characteristics in a Hispanic geriatric population: a comprehensive study using a standardized itch questionnaire. Acta Derm Venereol 2015;95(4):417–21.
7. Sun Y-G, Chen Z-F. A gastrin-releasing peptide receptor mediates the itch sensation in the spinal cord. Nature 2007;448(7154):700–3.
8. Liu Q, Tang Z, Surdenikova L, et al. Sensory neuron-specific GPCR Mrgprs are itch receptors mediating chloroquine-induced pruritus. Cell 2009;139(7):1353–65.
9. Annunziato F, Romagnani C, Romagnani S. The 3 major types of innate and adaptive cell-mediated effector immunity. J Allergy Clin Immunol 2015;135(3):626–35.
10. Gandhi NA, Bennett BL, Graham NMH, et al. Targeting key proximal drivers of type 2 inflammation in disease. Nat Rev Drug Discov 2015;15(1):35–50.
11. Mackay IR, Rosen FS, Kay AB. Allergy and allergic diseases. N Engl J Med 2001;344(1):30–7.
12. Stull C, Grossman S, Yosipovitch G. Current and emerging therapies for itch management in psoriasis. Am J Clin Dermatol 2016;17(6):617–24.
13. Zuberbier T, Aberer W, Asero R, et al. The EAACI/GA2LEN/EDF/WAO guideline for the definition, classification, diagnosis, and management of urticaria: the 2013 revision and update. Allergy 2014;69(7):868–87.
14. Greaves MW. Pathology and classification of urticaria. Immunol Allergy Clin North Am 2014;34(1):1–9.
15. Altman K, Chang C. Pathogenic intracellular and autoimmune mechanisms in urticaria and angioedema. Clin Rev Allergy Immunol 2013;45(1):47–62.
16. Mollanazar NK, Smith PK, Yosipovitch G. Mediators of chronic pruritus in atopic dermatitis: getting the itch out? Clin Rev Allergy Immunol 2016;51(3):263–92.
17. Thurmond RL, Kazerouni K, Chaplan SR, et al. Antihistamines and itch. Handb Exp Pharmacol 2015;226:257–90.
18. Lim HD, van Rijn RM, Ling P, et al. Evaluation of histamine H1-, H2-, and H3-receptor ligands at the human histamine H4 receptor: identification of 4-methylhistamine as the first potent and selective H4 receptor agonist. J Pharmacol Exp Ther 2005;314(3):1310–21.
19. Schneider EH, Seifert R. The histamine H4-receptor and the central and peripheral nervous system: a critical analysis of the literature. Neuropharmacology 2016;106:116–28.

20. Kollmeier A, Francke K, Chen B, et al. The histamine H4 receptor antagonist, JNJ 39758979, is effective in reducing histamine-induced pruritus in a randomized clinical study in healthy subjects. J Pharmacol Exp Ther 2014;350(1):181–7.

21. Asero R, Tedesch A. Usefulness of a short course of oral prednisone in antihistamine-resistant chronic urticaria: a retrospective analysis. J Investig Allergol Clin Immunol 2010;20(5):386–90.

22. Barnes PJ. Molecular mechanisms and cellular effects of glucocorticosteroids. Immunol Allergy Clin North Am 2005;25(3):451–68.

23. Tsuda K, Yamanaka K, Kitagawa H, et al. Calcineurin inhibitors suppress cytokine production from memory T cells and differentiation of naive T cells into cytokine-producing mature T cells. Unutmaz D. PLoS One 2012;7(2):e31465.

24. Kuga K, Nishifuji K, Iwasaki T. Cyclosporine A inhibits transcription of cytokine genes and decreases the frequencies of IL-2 producing cells in feline mononuclear cells. J Vet Med Sci 2008;70(10):1011–6.

25. Harrison CA, Bastan R, Peirce MJ, et al. Role of calcineurin in the regulation of human lung mast cell and basophil function by cyclosporine and FK506. Br J Pharmacol 2007;150(4):509–18.

26. Vena GA, Cassano N, Colombo D, et al. Cyclosporine in chronic idiopathic urticaria: a double-blind, randomized, placebo-controlled trial. J Am Acad Dermatol 2006;55(4):705–9.

27. Chang TW, Wu PC, Hsu CL, et al. Anti-IgE antibodies for the treatment of IgE-mediated allergic diseases. Adv Immunol 2007;93:63–119.

28. Beck LA, Marcotte GV, MacGlashan D, et al. Omalizumab-induced reductions in mast cell FcεRI expression and function. J Allergy Clin Immunol 2004;114(3):527–30.

29. Maurer M, Rosén K, Hsieh H-JJ, et al. Omalizumab for the treatment of chronic idiopathic or spontaneous urticaria. N Engl J Med 2013;368(10):924–35.

30. Saini SS, Bindslev-Jensen C, Maurer M, et al. Efficacy and safety of omalizumab in patients with chronic idiopathic/spontaneous urticaria who remain symptomatic on H1 antihistamines: a randomized, placebo-controlled study. J Invest Dermatol 2015; 135(1):67–75.

31. Wollenberg A, Oranje A, Deleuran M, et al. ETFAD/EADV Eczema task force 2015 position paper on diagnosis and treatment of atopic dermatitis in adult and paediatric patients. J Eur Acad Dermatol Venereol 2016;30(5):729–47.

32. Reynolds LA, Finlay BB. Early life factors that affect allergy development. Nat Rev Immunol 2017;17(8): 518–28.

33. Naik S, Bouladoux N, Linehan JL, et al. Commensal–dendritic-cell interaction specifies a unique protective skin immune signature. Nature 2015; 520(7545):104–8.

34. Kennedy EA, Connolly J, Hourihane JO, et al. Skin microbiome before development of atopic dermatitis: early colonization with commensal staphylococci at 2 months is associated with a lower risk of atopic dermatitis at 1 year. J Allergy Clin Immunol 2017;139(1):166–72.

35. Kim BS. Innate lymphoid cells in the skin. J Invest Dermatol 2015;135(3):673–8.

36. Cevikbas F, Wang X, Akiyama T, et al. A sensory neuron-expressed IL-31 receptor mediates T helper cell-dependent itch: involvement of TRPV1 and TRPA1. J Allergy Clin Immunol 2014;133(2):448–60.

37. Liu B, Tai Y, Achanta S, et al. IL-33/ST2 signaling excites sensory neurons and mediates itch response in a mouse model of poison ivy contact allergy. Proc Natl Acad Sci U S A 2016;113(47):E7572–9.

38. Wilson SR, Thé L, Batia LM, et al. The epithelial cell-derived atopic dermatitis cytokine TSLP activates neurons to induce itch. Cell 2013;155(2):285–95.

39. Oetjen LK, Mack MR, Feng J, et al. Sensory neurons co-opt classical immune signaling pathways to mediate chronic itch. Cell 2017;171(1):217–28.e13.

40. Kaufmann R, Bieber T, Helgesen AL, et al. Onset of pruritus relief with pimecrolimus cream 1% in adult patients with atopic dermatitis: a randomized trial. Allergy 2006;61(3):375–81.

41. Bäumer W, Hoppmann J, Rundfeldt C, et al. Highly selective phosphodiesterase 4 inhibitors for the treatment of allergic skin diseases and psoriasis. Inflamm Allergy Drug Targets 2007;6(1):17–26.

42. Andoh T, Yoshida T, Kuraishi Y. Topical E6005, a novel phosphodiesterase 4 inhibitor, attenuates spontaneous itch-related responses in mice with chronic atopy-like dermatitis. Exp Dermatol 2014; 23(5):359–61.

43. Paller AS, Tom WL, Lebwohl MG, et al. Efficacy and safety of crisaborole ointment, a novel, nonsteroidal phosphodiesterase 4 (PDE4) inhibitor for the topical treatment of atopic dermatitis (AD) in children and adults. J Am Acad Dermatol 2016;75(3):494–503.

44. Brandt EB, Sivaprasad U. Th2 cytokines and atopic dermatitis. J Clin Cell Immunol 2011;2(3):110.

45. Beck LA, Thaçi D, Hamilton JD, et al. Dupilumab treatment in adults with moderate-to-severe atopic dermatitis. N Engl J Med 2014;371(2):130–9.

46. Simpson EL, Bieber T, Guttman-Yassky E, et al. Two phase 3 trials of dupilumab versus placebo in atopic dermatitis. N Engl J Med 2016;375(24):2335–48.

47. Thaçi D, Simpson EL, Beck LA, et al. Efficacy and safety of dupilumab in adults with moderate-to-severe atopic dermatitis inadequately controlled by topical treatments: a randomised, placebo-controlled, dose-ranging phase 2b trial. Lancet 2016;387(10013):40–52.

48. Wollenberg A, Birrell C, Dawson MA, et al. A phase 2b dose-ranging efficacy and safety study of tralokinumab in adult patients with moderate to severe

atopic dermatitis. Presented at: 75th Annual AAD Meeting. Orlando (FL), March 3–7, 2017. [abstract: 4496].

49. Gandhi NA, Pirozzi G, Graham NMH. Commonality of the IL-4/IL-13 pathway in atopic diseases. Expert Rev Clin Immunol 2017;13(5):425–37.

50. Simpson E, Flohr C, Eichenfield L, et al. Efficacy and safety of lebrikizumab in patients with atopic dermatitis: a phase II randomized, controlled trial (TREBLE). Presented at: 25th EADV Congress. Vienna (Austria), September 28–October 2, 2016.

51. Han L, Dong X. Itch mechanisms and circuits. Annu Rev Biophys 2014;43(1):331–55.

52. Dillon SR, Sprecher C, Hammond A, et al. Interleukin 31, a cytokine produced by activated T cells, induces dermatitis in mice. Nat Immunol 2004;5(7): 752–60.

53. Sonkoly E, Muller A, Lauerma AI, et al. IL-31: a new link between T cells and pruritus in atopic skin inflammation. J Allergy Clin Immunol 2006;117(2): 411–7.

54. Grimstad O, Sawanobori Y, Vestergaard C, et al. Anti-interleukin-31-antibodies ameliorate scratching behaviour in NC/Nga mice: a model of atopic dermatitis. Exp Dermatol 2009;18(1):35–43.

55. Raap U, Wichmann K, Bruder M, et al. Correlation of IL-31 serum levels with severity of atopic dermatitis. J Allergy Clin Immunol 2017;122(2):421–3.

56. Szegedi K, Kremer AE, Kezic S, et al. Increased frequencies of IL-31-producing T cells are found in chronic atopic dermatitis skin. Exp Dermatol 2012; 21(6):431–6.

57. Ruzicka T, Hanifin JM, Furue M, et al. Anti–interleukin-31 receptor A antibody for atopic dermatitis. N Engl J Med 2017;376(9):826–35.

58. Boguniewicz M, Leung DY. Atopic dermatitis: a disease of altered skin barrier and immune dysregulation. Immunol Rev 2011;242:233–46.

59. Kim BS, Siracusa MC, Saenz SA, et al. TSLP elicits IL-33-independent innate lymphoid cell responses to promote skin inflammation. Sci Transl Med 2013; 5(170):170ra16.

60. Kim BS, Wang K, Siracusa MC, et al. Basophils promote innate lymphoid cell responses in inflamed skin. J Immunol 2014;193(7):3717–25.

61. Mashiko S, Mehta H, Bissonnette R, et al. Increased frequencies of basophils, type 2 innate lymphoid cells and Th2 cells in skin of patients with atopic dermatitis but not psoriasis. J Dermatol Sci 2017; 88(2):167–74.

62. Kim BS, Artis D. Group 2 innate lymphoid cells in health and disease. Cold Spring Harb Perspect Biol 2015;7(5):a016337.

63. Soumelis V, Reche PA, Kanzler H, et al. Human epithelial cells trigger dendritic cell mediated allergic inflammation by producing TSLP. Nat Immunol 2002;3(7):673–80.

64. Savinko T, Matikainen S, Saarialho-Kere U, et al. IL-33 and ST2 in atopic dermatitis: expression profiles and modulation by triggering factors. J Invest Dermatol 2012;132(5):1392–400.

65. Wang Y-H, Angkasekwinai P, Lu N, et al. IL-25 augments type 2 immune responses by enhancing the expansion and functions of TSLP-DC–activated Th2 memory cells. J Exp Med 2007;204(8):1837–47.

66. Londei M, Kenney B, Los G, et al. A phase 1 study of ANB020, an anti-IL-33 monoclonal antibody, in healthy volunteers. J Am Acad Dermatol 2017; 76(6, Supplement 1):AB20.

67. Winthrop K. The emerging safety profile of JAK inhibitors in rheumatic disease. Nat Rev Rheumatol 2017;13:234–43.

68. Gonzales AJ, Bowman JW, Fici GJ, et al. Oclacitinib (APOQUEL) is a novel Janus kinase inhibitor with activity against cytokines involved in allergy. J Vet Pharmacol Ther 2014;37(4):317–24.

69. Little PR, King VL, Davis KR, et al. A blinded, randomized clinical trial comparing the efficacy and safety of oclacitinib and ciclosporin for the control of atopic dermatitis in client-owned dogs. Vet Dermatol 2015;26(1):23–30. e7-8.

70. Levy LL, Urban J, King BA. Treatment of recalcitrant atopic dermatitis with the oral Janus kinase inhibitor tofacitinib citrate. J Am Acad Dermatol 2017;73(3): 395–9.

71. Bissonnette R, Papp KA, Poulin Y, et al. Topical tofacitinib for atopic dermatitis: a phase IIa randomized trial. Br J Dermatol 2016;175(5):902–11.

72. Eli Lilly and Company Inc. Baricitinib meets primary endpoint in phase 2 study of patients with moderate-to-severe atopic dermatitis. 2017. Available at: http://www.prnewswire.com/news-releases/baricitinib-meets-primary-endpoint-in-phase-2-study-of-patients-with-moderate-to-severe-atopic-dermatitis-300518896.html. Accessed September 15, 2017.

73. AbbVie Inc. AbbVie's Upadacitinib (ABT-494) meets primary endpoint in phase 2b study in atopic dermatitis. 2017. Available at: https://news.abbvie.com/news/abbvies-upadacitinib-abt-494-meets-primary-endpoint-in-phase-2b-study-in-atopic-dermatitis.htm. Accessed September 11, 2017.

74. Zeidler C, Stander S. The pathogenesis of prurigo nodularis - "super-itch" in exploration. Eur J Pain 2016;20(1):37–40.

75. Iking A, Grundmann S, Chatzigeorgakidis E, et al. Prurigo as a symptom of atopic and non-atopic diseases: aetiological survey in a consecutive cohort of 108 patients. J Eur Acad Dermatol Venereol 2013; 27(5):550–7.

76. Weigelt N, Metze D, Stander S. Prurigo nodularis: systematic analysis of 58 histological criteria in 136 patients. J Cutan Pathol 2010;37(5):578–86.

77. Haas S, Capellino S, Phan NQ, et al. Low density of sympathetic nerve fibers relative to substance

P-positive nerve fibers in lesional skin of chronic pruritus and prurigo nodularis. J Dermatol Sci 2010; 58(3):193–7.

78. Kanavy H, Bahner J, Korman NJ. Treatment of refractory prurigo nodularis with lenalidomide. Arch Dermatol 2012;148(7):794–6.

79. Andersen TP, Fogh K. Thalidomide in 42 patients with prurigo nodularis hyde. Dermatology 2011; 223(2):107–12.

80. Maurer T, Poncelet A, Berger T. Thalidomide treatment for prurigo nodularis in human immunodeficiency virus-infected subjects: efficacy and risk of neuropathy. Arch Dermatol 2004;140(7): 845–9.

81. Valdes-Rodriguez R, Stull C, Yosipovitch G. Chronic pruritus in the elderly: pathophysiology, diagnosis and management. Drugs Aging 2015;32:201–15.

82. Berger TG, Steinhoff M. Pruritus in elderly patients – eruptions of senescence. Semin Cutan Med Surg 2011;30:113–7.

83. Xu AZ, Tripathi SV, Kau AL, et al. Immune dysregulation underlies a subset of patients with chronic idiopathic pruritus. J Am Acad Dermatol 2017;74(5): 1017–20.

Drugs on the Horizon for Chronic Pruritus

Matthew W. McEwen, BS[a], Elizabeth M. Fite, MD[b], Gil Yosipovitch, MD[c],
Tejesh Patel, MD[d],*

KEYWORDS

- Chronic pruritus • Chronic itch • Atopic dermatitis • Psoriasis • Uremic pruritus
- Cholestatic pruritus • Novel therapies

KEY POINTS

- The elucidation of itch signaling pathways has led to the development of novel therapeutic agents.
- Emerging systemic therapies include neurokinin 1 antagonists, drugs acting on the k- and μ-opioid receptors, interleukin antagonists, janus kinase inhibitors, histamine antagonists, leukotriene receptor antagonists, and bile acid transporter inhibitors.
- Emerging topical and local therapies include drugs acting on transient receptor potential vanilloid 1, tropomyosin-receptor-kinase A inhibitors, phosphodiesterase-4 inhibitors, analgesics, cannabinoids, and botulinum toxin type A.

INTRODUCTION

Chronic pruritus, which is defined as a greater than 6-month duration of sensations that lead to the desire to scratch,[1,2] is a common condition with an estimated point prevalence of 8.4% to 13.5%.[3,4] Diseases associated with chronic pruritus can be divided into 4 broad categories: dermatologic (eg, atopic dermatitis [AD], psoriasis, chronic urticaria, lichen planus, scabies), systemic (eg, chronic renal disease, cholestatic disease, hyperthyroidism, myeloproliferative disorders), neuropathic (eg, notalgia paresthetica, brachoradial pruritus, post-herpetic neuralgia), and psychogenic (eg, depression, obsessive-compulsive disorder).[5] Chronic pruritus is known to have a detrimental impact on quality of life and is associated with depressive symptoms, sleep impairment, agitation, impaired concentration, and sexual dysfunction.[6–8]

Itch is primarily mediated by unmyelinated, slow-conducting C-fibers, which are found at the dermal–epidermal junction with free nerve endings extending into the epidermis.[9] When a pruritogen is encountered, G-protein coupled receptors or ion channels initiate itch signaling. G-protein coupled receptor signaling may be induced by proteases such as tryptase, cathepsin S, and kallikreins, neuropeptides such as substance P, prostaglandins, and histamines.[9,10] Ion channels in the transient receptor potential (TRP) family play a role in itch signaling and include TRP vanilloid 1 (TRPV1), which is a receptor for capsaicin, and TRPA1.[9,11] Several

---

Disclosure Statement: G. Yosipovitch is a member of the scientific advisory board and consultant for Opko, TREVI, Menlo, Eli Lilly, Sanofi Regeneron, Galderma, Novartis, Sienna, Pfizer; and a PI for GSK, LEO, Pfizer, Vanda, Menlo, Kiniksa, and Allergen. M.W. McEwen, E.M. Fite, and T. Patel have nothing to disclose.
[a] Kaplan-Amonette Department of Dermatology, College of Medicine, University of Tennessee Health Science Center, 930 Madison Avenue, Suite 840, Memphis, TN 38163, USA; [b] Department of Dermatology, University of Tennessee Health Science Center, 930 Madison Avenue, Suite 840, Memphis, TN 38163, USA; [c] Department of Dermatology, Miami Itch Center, University of Miami, Miller School of Medicine, 1600 Northwest 10th Avenue, Rosenstiel Medical Science Building – Room 2023, Miami, FL 33136, USA; [d] Kaplan-Amonette Department of Dermatology, University of Tennessee Health Science Center, 930 Madison Avenue, Suite 840, Memphis, TN 38163, USA
* Corresponding author.
E-mail address: tpatel3@uthsc.edu

Dermatol Clin 36 (2018) 335–344
https://doi.org/10.1016/j.det.2018.02.016

cytokines can induce itch including interleukin (IL)-31, which is highly associated with pruritus in AD, prurigo nodularis, lichen amyloidosis, and cutaneous T-cell lymphoma.[12–15] Tropomyosin receptor kinase A, which responds to nerve growth factor by stimulating the growth of small diameter nerves expressing tropomyosin receptor kinase A and TRPV1, is also implicated in itch signaling.[16] Finally, opioid receptors are thought to play a role in itch pathogenesis, with μ-opioid receptors having an excitatory effect on itch signaling and κ-opioid receptors having an inhibitory effect.[10,17] Decreased numbers of κ-opioid receptors are observed in patients with AD[18] and psoriasis patients suffering from pruritus,[19] suggesting a role for κ-opioid receptors in the normal suppression of pruritus.

Current therapies for chronic pruritus include topical glucocorticoids, topical calcineurin inhibitors, topical capsaicin, antidepressants, antihistamines, gabapentin, cyclosporine, methotrexate, naloxone, naltrexone, and phototherapy.[20] As the molecular pathogenesis of itch continues to be elucidated, novel therapies are being developed to disrupt itch pathways. Herein, we review the drugs that have been recently approved or are under investigation for the treatment of chronic pruritus (**Table 1**).

SYSTEMIC THERAPIES
Drugs Targeting the Neural System

Neurokinin antagonists
Neurokinin 1, which is the receptor for substance P, plays a significant role in chronic itch.[21] Aprepitant is an oral neurokinin-1 receptor antagonist that is reported to be effective in reducing pruritus of various etiologies including cutaneous T-cell lymphoma,[22] biological therapies for solid tumor

Table 1
Emerging therapies for chronic pruritus listed by class

Drug Class	Drug Name	Route
Neurokinin antagonists	Aprepitant	Oral
	Serlopitant	Oral
	Tradipitant	Oral
κ-Opioid receptor agonists	Nalfurafine hydrochloride	Oral
	Difelikefalin (CR845)	Intravenous
	Asimadoline	Oral
Mixed κ-opioid receptor agonist/μ-opioid receptor antagonists	Nalbuphine hydrochloride	Oral
Interleukin antagonists	Nemolizumab	Subcutaneous
	Dupilumab	Subcutaneous
	Secukinumab	Subcutaneous
	Ixekizumab	Subcutaneous
Janus kinase inhibitors	Tofacitinib	Oral
	Upadacitinib	Oral
Histamine antagonists	Bilastine	Oral
	JNJ-39758979	Oral
	ZPL-389	Oral
Leukotriene receptor antagonists	Montelukast	Oral
Bile acid transporter inhibitors	GSK2330672	Oral
	A4250	Oral
Drugs acting on TRPV1	PAC-14028	Topical
	Capsaicin	Topical
TrkA inhibitors	Pegcantratinib (CT327)	Topical
PDE-4 inhibitors	Crisaborole	Topical
	OPA-15406/MM36	Topical
Analgesics	Ketamine-amitriptyline-lidocaine	Topical
Cannabinoids	PEA	Topical
	AEA	Topical
Botulinum toxin	Botulinum toxin type A	Intradermal

Abbreviations: AEA, N-acetylethanolamine; PDE-4, phosphodiesterase-4; PEA, N-palmitoylethanolamine; TrkA, tropomyosin-receptor-kinase A; TRPV1, transient receptor potential vanilloid 1.

malignancies,[23] renal, multifactorial,[24] and idiopathic pruritus.[24,25] However, aprepitant's usefulness in chronic itch is limited owing to its many drug–drug interactions and high price.[26]

Serlopitant is another oral neurokinin-1 receptor antagonist that, in a randomized, double-blinded, placebo-controlled phase II clinical trial of 127 patients with prurigo nodularis, reduced average pruritus visual analog scale (VAS) scores by 48% in an 8-week period at a dose of 5 mg daily, compared with a 26% decrease with placebo.[27,28] In another randomized, double-blinded, placebo-controlled phase II study of 257 patients with chronic pruritus of various etiologies, serlopitant was given at doses of 0.25, 1.00, and 5.00 mg once daily for 6 weeks. Significant decreases in VAS pruritus scores of 41.4% and 42.5% were seen in the 1- and 5-mg treatment groups, respectively, compared with a 28.3% decrease with placebo.[29] Treatment-emergent adverse effects seen in these trials were mild to moderate and included somnolence, diarrhea, fatigue, and nasopharyngitis.[28,29]

Tradipitant is another neurokinin-1 receptor antagonist. In a randomized, placebo-controlled study of 69 patients with AD, it was shown to be ineffective compared with placebo in reducing pruritus when taken by mouth at night. However, in a post hoc analysis, it was found that patients surveyed in the morning had a significant reduction in pruritus compared with placebo, which was not observed in patients surveyed in the afternoon. The authors suggest that this correlated with increased serum drug concentration and may provide evidence for tradipitant's efficacy.[30] In another randomized, placebo-controlled phase II study, 168 patients with moderate AD and chronic pruritus received 85 mg tradipitant or placebo twice daily for 8 weeks. Treatment was associated with a 44.2-point decrease in worst itch VAS, which was statistically significant compared with a 30.6-point decrease with placebo.[31]

Drugs targeting opioid receptors

In chronic uremic pruritus, an imbalance was found between μ-opioid receptor overexpression and κ-opioid receptor downregulation. This finding led to the development of nalfurafine hydrochloride, an oral κ-opioid receptor agonist that is approved in Japan for uremic pruritus.[32] In a randomized, double-blinded, placebo-controlled trial of 337 patients on hemodialysis with refractory pruritus, 2.5 or 5.0 μg daily of oral nalfurafine hydrochloride was shown to cause a significant decrease in pruritus of 23 or 22 points, respectively, compared with a 13-point decrease in placebo as measured using a VAS, which ranges from 0 to 100.[33] More recently, 2.5 μg daily of

oral nalfurafine hydrochloride improved pruritus associated with chronic liver disease as assessed by patient surveys and VAS scores.[34] In a randomized, double-blinded, placebo-controlled trial of 318 patients with cholestatic pruritus, oral nalfurafine hydrochloride given at 2.5 or 5.0 μg daily was associated with a 28.56- or 27.46-mm decrease in VAS itch scores, respectively, compared with a 19.25-mm decrease with placebo.[35] Reported adverse drug reactions in these studies included insomnia, somnolence, constipation, and pollakiuria.[33,35]

Difelikefalin (CR845) is a κ-opioid receptor agonist[36] that was studied in a randomized, double-blinded, placebo-controlled phase II/III clinical trial of 174 patients on hemodialysis for chronic kidney disease with moderate to severe uremic pruritus. Patients given IV difelikefalin at doses of 0.5, 1.0, or 1.5 μg/kg 3 times weekly had a 68% decrease in mean worst itch compared with placebo. Additionally, improvement in quality of life was observed in the treatment arm. Adverse effects included transient paresthesias and dizziness.[37]

Asimadoline is an oral κ-opioid receptor agonist that is used in the treatment of irritable bowel syndrome.[38] It is currently being evaluated at a dose of 2.5 mg twice daily for efficacy in pruritus associated with AD in phase II clinical trials.[39]

Nalbuphine hydrochloride is a mixed κ-opioid receptor agonist and μ-opioid receptor antagonist that is currently marketed for the treatment of chronic pain. In an open-label study of 15 hemodialysis patients with pruritus, an oral, extended release formulation of nalbuphine hydrochloride in doses escalating from 30 mg daily to 240 twice daily over 15 days was shown to reduce VAS pruritus scores in a dose-dependent fashion from a mean of 4.0 to 1.2 or 0.4 with 180 mg or 240 mg twice daily, respectively, on a scale from 0 to 10.[40] Currently, phase II/III clinical trials of nalbuphine hydrochloride extended release in doses from 90 to 180 mg twice daily are underway to examine its efficacy in prurigo nodularis[41,42] and in doses from 60 to 120 mg twice daily for uremic pruritus.[43,44]

Drugs Targeting the Immune System

Interleukin antagonists

IL-31 has been coined an itchy cytokine owing to its role in pruritus associated with AD, prurigo nodularis, cutaneous T-cell lymphoma, lichen amyloidosis, and uremic pruritus.[12–15] Nemolizumab is an IL-31 receptor A antagonist that was recently studied in a randomized, double-blinded, placebo-controlled phase II trial of

264 adults with moderate to severe AD. Nemolizumab in doses of 0.1, 0.5, or 2.0 mg/kg administered subcutaneously every 4 weeks was shown to decrease pruritus by 43.7% to 63.1% in a dose-dependent fashion over a 12-week period as measured using a VAS, compared with a 20.9% decrease with placebo. Treatment was also associated with a dose-dependent decrease in sleep disturbance. Adverse effects more commonly observed with treatment than with placebo included AD exacerbation and peripheral edema.[45]

Dupilumab is an IL-4 receptor A antagonist that blocks IL-4 and IL-13 signaling that was recently approved for use in adults with AD.[46] In 2 identical, randomized, double-blinded, placebo-controlled studies of 1379 adults with moderate to severe AD, doses of 300 mg administered subcutaneously either weekly or every other week were associated with a 44.3% to 51.0% decrease in pruritus as measured by a numerical rating scale (NRS) after 16 weeks, compared with a 15.4% to 26.1% decrease with placebo. The major adverse effects included conjunctivitis and injection site reactions.[47]

In patients with psoriasis, several of the novel biologic therapies decrease pruritic symptoms. Secukinumab is an IL-17a antagonist that was examined in 2 randomized, double-blinded, placebo-controlled studies that included a total of 2044 adults with psoriasis. Patients were randomized to receive subcutaneous injections of 150 mg secukinumab, 300 mg secukinumab, biologic active control, or placebo in a 1:1:1:1 ratio at weeks 0, 1, 2, 3, and 4 followed by once every 4 weeks, and a symptom diary was used to rate daily symptoms on a scale of 0 to 10. Patients on secukinumab had a 4.90- to 5.14-point decrease in itching compared with a 0.4-point decrease with placebo, and 78.2% to 83.0% of patients reported at least a 2.2-point reduction in itching, compared with 16.9% of those receiving placebo.[48] Ixekizumab is another IL-17a antagonist that has been studied in adults with chronic plaque psoriasis. In 3 parallel phase III randomized, double-blinded, placebo-controlled trials, a total of 3866 patients with psoriasis were randomized in a 2:2:2:1 ratio to receive either 80 mg of ixekizumab every 2 weeks after a 160-mg starting dose, 80 mg of ixekizumab every 4 weeks after a 160-mg starting dose, 50 mg of etanercept twice weekly (in 2 of the 3 parallel trials), or placebo subcutaneously. Ixekizumab was found to significantly decrease pruritus by 4.9 to 5.4 points from baseline as measured by the Itch NRS, which is a scale from 0 to 10, compared with etanercept and placebo, which were associated with decreases of 3.5 to 3.9 points and 0.2 to 0.6 points, respectively.[49] More patients on ixekizumab were found to have a 4-point or greater decrease in pruritus than etanercept (hazard ratio, 2.1–2.2) or placebo (hazard ratio, 5.4–5.7), and this decrease was achieved more rapidly (2.1 weeks) than with etanercept (8.1 weeks) or placebo (>12 weeks).[50] Other emerging antipsoriatic biologic agents such as guselkumab, an IL-23 antagonist, and brodalumab, an IL-17 receptor-a antagonist, reduce psoriatic symptoms as measured by indices that include itch as a component,[51–54] but further examination of the data is needed to determine the specific effect on pruritus.

Janus kinase inhibitors

Tofacitinib is an oral janus kinase inhibitor that is used for the treatment of rheumatoid arthritis[55] and shows promise in the treatment of ulcerative colitis,[56] psoriasis,[57,58] and alopecia areata.[59] In 2 identical, randomized, double-blinded, placebo-controlled phase III studies of tofacitinib with a total of 1861 patients with moderate to severe psoriasis,[57] pruritus was measured using the Itch Severity Item, which ranges from 0 signifying no itch to 10 signifying worst itch.[60] Analyzing data from the same studies, Feldman and colleagues[61] found that at 16 weeks decreases in Itch Severity Item scores in the treatment groups of 2.9 to 3.2 points with 5 mg twice daily and 3.8 to 4.0 points with 10 mg twice daily were observed, compared with a 0.2- to 0.3-point decrease in the placebo group. This decrease in pruritus was maintained for the entire 52-week duration of treatment. Adverse effects seen in the same studies and in a long-term, open-label extension of these studies included serious infections, herpes zoster, nonmelanoma skin cancer, nasopharyngitis, upper respiratory tract infection, increased blood creatine phosphokinase, headache, and hypercholesterolemia.[62]

Upadacitinib is an oral, selective JAK1 inhibitor. In a randomized, double-blinded, placebo-controlled phase IIb study, adults with moderate to severe AD refractory to topical therapy were given 7.5, 15, or 30 mg of upadacitinib daily or placebo in a 1:1:1:1 ratio for 16 weeks. Significant reductions in pruritus were seen within 1 week of treatment, and pruritus NRS scores were reduced by 40% to 69% in the treatment group in a dose-dependent fashion, compared with a 10% reduction with placebo. Adverse effects included upper respiratory tract infections, AD, and acne.[63]

Other Systemic Drugs

Histamine antagonists

Although most H1 antihistamines have shown limited efficacy in most types of chronic itch,[64] bilastine is a nonsedating, second-generation H1 antihistamine that was studied in a phase III, open-label, single-arm study of 198 patients with chronic spontaneous urticaria or dermatologic disease-associated pruritus. Patients received 20 mg of bilastine once daily, and significant decreases in total symptom score and itch score were seen, along with a significant improvement in quality of life. Bilastine-related adverse effects included somnolence and nocturia, observed in 2 and 1 patients, respectively.[65]

JNJ-39758979 is an H4 histamine receptor antagonist. In a randomized, double-blinded, placebo-controlled study of 88 patients with moderate AD, patients in the treatment arms were given 100 or 300 mg of JNJ-39758979 daily by mouth. A significant decrease in pruritus severity and duration was seen with 300 mg JNJ-39758979 compared with placebo. There was also a trend toward significance in improved sleep and decreased impact of pruritus on daily living in the 300-mg group. However, the study was terminated early owing to the development of severe agranulocytosis by 2 study participants, which was thought to be due to an idiosyncratic drug reaction.[66]

ZPL-389 is an oral selective H4 histamine receptor antagonist that is being studied as a potential treatment for AD. In a phase IIa randomized, double-blinded, placebo-controlled study, 98 adults with moderate to severe AD were given 30 mg ZPL-389 or placebo daily for 8 weeks. Treatment with ZPL-389 was associated with significantly decreased Eczema Area and Severity Index scores, which include excoriations as a component. Although treatment was associated with a 42% decrease in NRS pruritus scores, this was not significant compared with the 37% reduction seen with placebo. ZPL-389 was well-tolerated, with similar rates of adverse effects between placebo and treatment groups.[67,68]

Leukotriene receptor antagonists

Montelukast is an oral leukotriene receptor antagonist. Previously, it was shown to be ineffective in reducing pruritus in patients with AD at a dose of 10 mg daily.[69] More recently, its effect on uremic pruritus was studied in a randomized, double-blinded, placebo-controlled trial of 80 patients on hemodialysis with refractory pruritus lasting longer than 3 months. In the treatment arm, patients received 10 mg of montelukast daily. VAS pruritus scores decreased significantly by 3.70 points compared with 0.53 points with placebo, and on a detailed pruritus scale, a significant 5.65-point decrease was seen in the treatment group, compared with a 0.73-point decrease with placebo.[70]

Bile acid transporter inhibitors

GSK2330672 is an oral ileal bile acid transport inhibitor that underwent a phase IIa randomized, double-blinded, placebo-controlled crossover study of 22 adult patients with primary biliary cirrhosis and pruritus. During treatment periods, patients received 45 mg twice daily on days 1 to 3 and 90 mg twice daily on days 4 to 14. Three scales were used to measure pruritus outcomes, including an NRS ranging from 0 to 10, the primary biliary cholangitis-40 itch domain, and the 5-D itch scale. Treatment was associated with a decrease in pruritus by 57% as measured by NRS scores, 31% as measured by the primary biliary cholangitis-40 domain, and 35% as measured by the 5-D itch scale, which were significant compared with reductions of 23%, 14%, and 20% with placebo, respectively. Reported adverse effects included diarrhea, abdominal distention, abdominal pain, nausea, and vomiting.[71]

A4250 is another ileal bile acid transport inhibitor. A phase IIa clinical study of 1.5 to 3.0 mg of oral A4250 daily in adult patients with primary biliary cirrhosis and pruritus was terminated owing to side effects. Study results are not yet reported.[72] In an open-label study of pediatric patients with cholestatic liver disease, doses of A4250 ranging from 0.01 to 0.20 mg/kg were found to decrease VAS scores in 14 of 19 patients by a mean of 2.86 points, on a scale from 0 to 10, which correlated with an overall decrease in serum bile acid concentration. Minor adverse effects such as increased transaminases were observed, but they were deemed to be unrelated to A4250 treatment.[73]

TOPICAL AND LOCAL THERAPIES
Drugs Acting on TRPV1

PAC-14028 is a TRPV1 antagonist that was found to attenuate pruritus, decrease serum immunoglobulin E, and decrease mast cell degranulation in mice with AD in a topical formulation.[74] A phase II study of PAC-14028 cream in strengths of 0.1%, 0.3%, and 1.0% in adult patients with mild to moderate AD was completed, but study results are not yet reported.[75]

Capsaicin, which is derived from plants of the genus *Capsicum*, acts in itch by depolarizing TRPV1-positive pruritus and nociceptive C-fibers leading to desensitization.[76,77] It is also thought to eradicate abnormal epidermal nerve fibers and promote the regrowth of normal nerves.[78] In a case series of 7 patients with brachoradial pruritus, notalgia paresthetica, or small fiber neuropathy, treatment with 8% capsaicin patches led to full remission of itch within 1 week with no relapses reported at 6 or 12 months of follow-up. In this study, prilocaine-lidocaine cream was successfully used before treatment to avoid pain or discomfort with patch administration.[79] The efficacy of topical 8% capsaicin patches was also examined in 44 patients with notalgia paresthetica and brachoradial pruritus. Patches were applied to cover the entire pruritic area at study initiation, and at 3 and 6 months, additional patch treatment was given if needed. At 6 months after initial patch application, significant decrease in itch VAS and NRS scores were seen.[78] Adverse effects of 8% capsaicin reported in a separate study of patients with postherpetic neuralgia included erythema and pain at the patch application site.[80]

Tropomyosin Receptor Kinase A inhibitors

Pegcantratinib (CT327) is a tropomyosin receptor kinase A inhibitor. A topical formulation at concentrations of 0.05%, 0.10%, and 0.50% used twice daily was evaluated in a phase II, randomized, double-blinded, vehicle-controlled study of 160 patients with mild to moderate psoriasis. Of 108 patients with baseline pruritus, a statistically significant decrease of 31.5 to 37.1 mm on the pruritus VAS, a scale from 0 to 100 mm, was seen in the treatment group, compared with a 16.1-mm decrease with vehicle alone. No significant improvement in psoriasis severity was observed. Treatment was well-tolerated, with similar rates of minor adverse events seen in treatment and vehicle groups.[16]

Phosphodiesterase Inhibitors

Crisaborole is a boron-based, topical phosphodiesterase-4 inhibitor that has been approved for the treatment of mild to moderate AD.[81] In 2 identical, randomized, double-blinded, vehicle-controlled phase III studies, a total of 1522 patients aged 2 years and older with mild to moderate AD were randomized 2:1 to receive 2% crisaborole ointment or vehicle twice daily for 28 days. Pruritus was assessed using a scale from 0 to 3 with 0 signifying no pruritus and 3 signifying severe pruritus. In the treatment group, significant improvement in pruritus, as defined as a pruritus score of 0 or 1 with a 1-grade or greater decrease from baseline, was seen in 58% of patients by day 8% and 63% by day 29, compared with 42% and 53% with vehicle, respectively. Improvement in pruritus was achieved in 1.37 days with treatment, compared with 1.7 days with placebo. Treatment-related adverse effects were minimal and included application site pain that usually resolved within 1 day and had a decreased incidence with extended use.[82,83]

OPA-15406/MM36 is a topical phosphodiesterase-4 inhibitor that is selective for phosphodiesterase-4 subtype B. In a phase II randomized, double-blinded, vehicle-controlled study, 121 patients ranging in age from 10 to 70 years with mild to moderate AD were treated with 0.3% or 1.0% ointment twice daily for 8 weeks. In the 1.0% OPA-15406 group, a significant 36.4% decrease in mean VAS pruritus scores was seen within the first week, which resulted in improved quality of life as measured by the Dermatology Life Quality Index and Children's Dermatology Life Quality Index. Treatment was well-tolerated, with minimal treatment-related adverse effects.[84] In a separate phase II study of 32 patients with moderate to severe AD, twice daily application of MM36 was shown to cause a sustained reduction in pruritus by a median of 60% as assessed by VAS. This improvement was rapidly achieved, with a median of 5.76 hours from drug application to itch improvement.[85]

ANALGESICS

Topical analgesics such as ketamine, amitriptyline, and lidocaine act by blocking N-methyl-D-aspartate receptors and sodium channels[86,87] and are thought to decrease peripheral nerve hypersensitivity.[88] A combination of 10% ketamine, 5% amitriptyline, and 5% lidocaine in a lipoderm cream was used in 96 patients with chronic pruritus of various etiologies including neuropathic and prurigo nodularis. Sixteen of these patients received a formulation with 5% ketamine replacing 10% ketamine. After application to areas of severe pruritus up to 3 times daily, patients had a mean reduction in pruritus severity of 4.61 on an NRS, a scale from 0 to 10. Relief of pruritus was achieved by an average of 4.18 minutes after topical administration. Adverse effects included mild burning and erythema at the site of application.[88]

CANNABINOIDS

Endocannabinoids, which are naturally found in the central and peripheral nervous systems of humans, have been suggested as a potential treatment for chronic pruritus.[89,90] N-Acetylethanolamines, are thought to mediate downregulation of inflammatory responses through cannabinoid receptors.[91] N-Palmitoylethanolamine (PEA) is in this family, and it is thought to act by stimulating endocannabinoid activation of cannabinoid 1 receptors.[90] In 21 patients on hemodialysis with uremic pruritus, a cream containing PEA and N-acetylethanolamine was applied twice daily for

3 weeks. Treatment was associated with a significant decrease in VAS pruritus scores from an average of 6.24 at baseline to 1.29 after 21 days, and in 8 patients, treatment led to complete resolution of pruritus.[92] In another study of 22 patients with pruritus of various etiologies, treatment with PEA cream had a therapeutic effect in 14 patients with an 86.4% average decrease in itch.[93] In a study of 2456 patients from 2 to 70 years old with mild to moderate AD, PEA cream was applied at least twice daily for 4 to 6 weeks. On an itch scale of 0 to 3, with 0 signifying absence of itch and 3 signifying severe itch, average scores were significantly decreased from 1.98 to 0.84 with treatment. Pruritus VAS scores also decreased significantly from 4.89 to 1.97, on a scale from 0 to 10. Adverse effects found to be causally related to treatment included pruritus, burning, and erythema.[91]

BOTULINUM TOXIN

Botulinum toxin type A is thought to act on itch through the inhibition of pruritic factors such as acetylcholine, substance P, and glutamate. In a randomized, single-blinded, placebo-controlled study of 35 healthy subjects, 10 units of botulinum toxin type A were injected intradermally into a 4 × 4-cm area on the volar arm, and 10 units of saline were injected contralaterally as a control. Cowhage, which induces itch via the nonhistaminergic pathway, was applied, and itch intensity was examined at 1 week, 1 month, and 3 months. Significant decreases in itch intensity, including peak itch intensity, were seen at all time points.[94]

SUMMARY

Chronic pruritus is a common condition that adversely affects quality of life of those patients affected. As the pathophysiology of itch is elucidated, novel treatments that target itch pathways in different disease states are being evaluated. These drugs, in particular the neurokinin 1 antagonists, κ-opioid agonists, IL antagonists, and janus kinase inhibitors, show promising results in treating pruritus of various etiologies. Further studies comparing these agents, particularly within classes that act through similar mechanisms, are needed to determine optimal therapy for patients suffering from chronic pruritus.

REFERENCES

1. Stander S, Weisshaar E, Mettang T, et al. Clinical classification of itch: a position paper of the International Forum for the Study of Itch. Acta Derm Venereol 2007;87(4):291–4.

2. Savin JA. How should we define itching? J Am Acad Dermatol 1998;39(2 Pt 1):268–9.

3. Dalgard F, Svensson A, Holm JO, et al. Self-reported skin morbidity in Oslo. Associations with sociodemographic factors among adults in a cross-sectional study. Br J Dermatol 2004;151(2):452–7.

4. Matterne U, Apfelbacher CJ, Loerbroks A, et al. Prevalence, correlates and characteristics of chronic pruritus: a population-based cross-sectional study. Acta Derm Venereol 2011;91(6):674–9.

5. Yosipovitch G, Bernhard JD. Clinical practice. Chronic pruritus. N Engl J Med 2013;368(17):1625–34.

6. Zachariae R, Zachariae CO, Lei U, et al. Affective and sensory dimensions of pruritus severity: associations with psychological symptoms and quality of life in psoriasis patients. Acta Derm Venereol 2008; 88(2):121–7.

7. Yosipovitch G, Goon A, Wee J, et al. The prevalence and clinical characteristics of pruritus among patients with extensive psoriasis. Br J Dermatol 2000; 143(5):969–73.

8. Sheehan-Dare RA, Henderson MJ, Cotterill JA. Anxiety and depression in patients with chronic urticaria and generalized pruritus. Br J Dermatol 1990; 123(6):769–74.

9. Garibyan L, Rheingold CG, Lerner EA. Understanding the pathophysiology of itch. Dermatol Ther 2013; 26(2):84–91.

10. Stander S, Raap U, Weisshaar E, et al. Pathogenesis of pruritus. J Dtsch Dermatol Ges 2011;9(6):456–63.

11. Mollanazar NK, Smith PK, Yosipovitch G. Mediators of chronic pruritus in atopic dermatitis: getting the itch out? Clin Rev Allergy Immunol 2016;51(3):263–92.

12. Sonkoly E, Muller A, Lauerma AI, et al. IL-31: a new link between T cells and pruritus in atopic skin inflammation. J Allergy Clin Immunol 2006;117(2):411–7.

13. Dousset L, Seneschal J, Boniface K, et al. A Th2 cytokine interleukin-31 signature in a case of sporadic lichen amyloidosis. Acta Derm Venereol 2015;95(2):223–4.

14. Singer EM, Shin DB, Nattkemper LA, et al. IL-31 is produced by the malignant T-cell population in cutaneous T-cell lymphoma and correlates with CTCL pruritus. J Invest Dermatol 2013;133(12):2783–5.

15. Nattkemper LA, Martinez-Escala ME, Gelman AB, et al. Cutaneous T-cell lymphoma and pruritus: the expression of IL-31 and its receptors in the skin. Acta Derm Venereol 2016;96(7):894–8.

16. Roblin D, Yosipovitch G, Boyce B, et al. Topical TrkA kinase inhibitor CT327 is an effective, novel therapy for the treatment of pruritus due to psoriasis: results from experimental studies, and efficacy and safety of CT327 in a phase 2b clinical trial in patients with psoriasis. Acta Derm Venereol 2015;95(5):542–8.

17. Phan NQ, Bernhard JD, Luger TA, et al. Antipruritic treatment with systemic mu-opioid receptor antagonists: a review. J Am Acad Dermatol 2010;63(4):680–8.

18. Tominaga M, Ogawa H, Takamori K. Possible roles of epidermal opioid systems in pruritus of atopic dermatitis. J Invest Dermatol 2007;127(9):2228–35.

19. Taneda K, Tominaga M, Negi O, et al. Evaluation of epidermal nerve density and opioid receptor levels in psoriatic itch. Br J Dermatol 2011;165(2):277–84.

20. Pereira MP, Stander S. Chronic pruritus: current and emerging treatment options. Drugs 2017;77(9): 999–1007.

21. Stander S, Luger TA. NK-1 antagonists and itch. Handb Exp Pharmacol 2015;226:237–55.

22. Song JS, Tawa M, Chau NG, et al. Aprepitant for refractory cutaneous T-cell lymphoma-associated pruritus: 4 cases and a review of the literature. BMC Cancer 2017;17(1):200.

23. Santini D, Vincenzi B, Guida FM, et al. Aprepitant for management of severe pruritus related to biological cancer treatments: a pilot study. Lancet Oncol 2012; 13(10):1020–4.

24. Stander S, Siepmann D, Herrgott I, et al. Targeting the neurokinin receptor 1 with aprepitant: a novel antipruritic strategy. PLoS One 2010;5(6):e10968.

25. Huh JW, Jeong YI, Choi KH, et al. Treatment for refractory pruritus using oral aprepitant. Ann Dermatol 2016;28(1):124–5.

26. Stull C, Lavery MJ, Yosipovitch G. Advances in therapeutic strategies for the treatment of pruritus. Expert Opin Pharmacother 2016;17(5):671–87.

27. Menlo therapeutics announces successful pruritus reduction results from phase 2 serlopitant trial (TCP-102) in 127 subjects with prurigo nodularis [press release]. 2017. Results presented at the 2017 American Academy of Dermatology (AAD) meeting. Orlando, March 3-7, 2017.

28. Stander S, Kwon P, Luger T. Randomized, double-blind, placebo-controlled phase 2 clinical trial of serlopitant effects on multiple measures of pruritus in patients with prurigo nodularis. Acta Derm Venereol 2017;97(8):1014.

29. Yosipovitch G, Stander S, Kerby M, et al. Serlopitant for treatment of chronic pruritus: results of a randomized, multicenter, double-blind, placebo-controlled phase 2 clinical trial. Acta Derm Venereol 2017;97(8):1015.

30. Stander S, Perry CA, Heitman A, et al. An investigational study of tradipitant for the treatment of chronic pruritus in patients with atopic dermatitis. Acta Derm Venereol 2015;95(7):875–912.

31. Vanda's tradipitant improves itch and disease severity in patients with atopic dermatitis [press release]. 2017. Available at: http://phx.corporate-ir.net/phoenix.zhtml?c=196233&p=irol-newsArticle&ID=2300433. Accessed September 21, 2017.

32. Cowan A, Kehner GB, Inan S. Targeting itch with ligands selective for kappa opioid receptors. Handb Exp Pharmacol 2015;226:291–314.

33. Kumagai H, Ebata T, Takamori K, et al. Effect of a novel kappa-receptor agonist, nalfurafine hydrochloride, on severe itch in 337 haemodialysis patients: a phase III, randomized, double-blind, placebo-controlled study. Nephrol Dial Transplant 2010;25(4):1251–7.

34. Kamimura K, Yokoo T, Kamimura H, et al. Long-term efficacy and safety of nalfurafine hydrochloride on pruritus in chronic liver disease patients: patient-reported outcome based analyses. PLoS One 2017;12(6):e0178991.

35. Kumada H, Miyakawa H, Muramatsu T, et al. Efficacy of nalfurafine hydrochloride in patients with chronic liver disease with refractory pruritus: a randomized, double-blind trial. Hepatol Res 2017; 47(10):972–82.

36. Keppel Hesselink JM. CR845 (Difelikefalin), a kappa receptors agonist in phase III by CARA therapeutics: a case of 'spin' in scientific writing? Journal of Pharmacology & Clinical Research 2017;2(3):1–10.

37. Cara therapeutics announces positive top-line data from part A of a phase 2/3 trial of I.V. CR845 in chronic kidney disease-associated pruritus [press release]. 2017.

38. Foxx-Orenstein AE. New and emerging therapies for the treatment of irritable bowel syndrome: an update for gastroenterologists. Therap Adv Gastroenterol 2016;9(3):354–75. Available at: http://ir.caratherapeutics.com/news-releases/news-release-details/cara-therapeutics-announces-positive-top-line-data-part-phase-23. Accessed August 6, 2017.

39. McGuire D. Safety, pharmacokinetics and preliminary efficacy of asimadoline in pruritus associated with atopic dermatitis. Available at: https://clinicaltrials.gov/show/NCT02475447.

40. Hawi A, Alcorn H Jr, Berg J, et al. Pharmacokinetics of nalbuphine hydrochloride extended release tablets in hemodialysis patients with exploratory effect on pruritus. BMC Nephrol 2015;16:47.

41. Sciascia T. Study of nalbuphine HCl ER tablets in patients with prurigo nodularis. Available at: https://clinicaltrials.gov/show/NCT02174419.

42. Sciascia T. Open label extension study of nalbuphine HCl ER in patients with prurigo nodularis. Available at: https://clinicaltrials.gov/show/NCT02174432.

43. Sciascia T. Study of nalbuphine HCl ER tablets in hemodialysis patients with uremic pruritus. Available at: https://clinicaltrials.gov/show/NCT02143648.

44. Sciascia T. Open label extension study of nalbuphine HCl ER in hemodialysis patients with uremic pruritus. Available at: https://clinicaltrials.gov/show/NCT02143973.

45. Ruzicka T, Hanifin JM, Furue M, et al. Anti-interleukin-31 receptor a antibody for atopic dermatitis. N Engl J Med 2017;376(9):826–35.

46. Shirley M. Dupilumab: first global approval. Drugs 2017;77(10):1115–21.

47. Simpson EL, Bieber T, Guttman-Yassky E, et al. Two phase 3 trials of dupilumab versus placebo in atopic dermatitis. N Engl J Med 2016;375(24):2335–48.

48. Strober B, Sigurgeirsson B, Popp G, et al. Secukinumab improves patient-reported psoriasis symptoms of itching, pain, and scaling: results of two phase 3, randomized, placebo-controlled clinical trials. Int J Dermatol 2016;55(4):401–7.

49. Kimball AB, Luger T, Gottlieb A, et al. Impact of ixekizumab on psoriasis itch severity and other psoriasis symptoms: results from 3 phase III psoriasis clinical trials. J Am Acad Dermatol 2016;75(6): 1156–61.

50. Leonardi CL, Blauvelt A, Sofen HL, et al. Rapid improvements in health-related quality of life and itch with ixekizumab treatment in randomized phase 3 trials: results from UNCOVER-2 and UNCOVER-3. J Eur Acad Dermatol Venereol 2017;31(9):1483–90.

51. Papp KA, Reich K, Paul C, et al. A prospective phase III, randomized, double-blind, placebo-controlled study of brodalumab in patients with moderate-to-severe plaque psoriasis. Br J Dermatol 2016;175(2):273–86.

52. Langley RG, Tsai TF, Flavin S, et al. Efficacy and safety of guselkumab in patients with psoriasis who have an inadequate response to ustekinumab: results of the randomized, double-blind, Phase 3 NAVIGATE trial. Br J Dermatol 2018;178(1):114–23.

53. Reich K, Armstrong AW, Foley P, et al. Efficacy and safety of guselkumab, an anti-interleukin-23 monoclonal antibody, compared with adalimumab for the treatment of patients with moderate to severe psoriasis with randomized withdrawal and retreatment: results from the phase III, double-blind, placebo- and active comparator-controlled VOYAGE 2 trial. J Am Acad Dermatol 2017;76(3):418–31.

54. Blauvelt A, Papp KA, Griffiths CE, et al. Efficacy and safety of guselkumab, an anti-interleukin-23 monoclonal antibody, compared with adalimumab for the continuous treatment of patients with moderate to severe psoriasis: results from the phase III, double-blinded, placebo- and active comparator-controlled VOYAGE 1 trial. J Am Acad Dermatol 2017;76(3):405–17.

55. Fleischmann R, Mysler E, Hall S, et al. Efficacy and safety of tofacitinib monotherapy, tofacitinib with methotrexate, and adalimumab with methotrexate in patients with rheumatoid arthritis (ORAL Strategy): a phase 3b/4, double-blind, head-to-head, randomised controlled trial. Lancet 2017;390(10093):457–68.

56. Sandborn WJ, Su C, Sands BE, et al. Tofacitinib as induction and maintenance therapy for ulcerative colitis. N Engl J Med 2017;376(18):1723–36.

57. Papp KA, Menter MA, Abe M, et al. Tofacitinib, an oral Janus kinase inhibitor, for the treatment of chronic plaque psoriasis: results from two randomized, placebo-controlled, phase III trials. Br J Dermatol 2015;173(4):949–61.

58. Abe M, Nishigori C, Torii H, et al. Tofacitinib for the treatment of moderate to severe chronic plaque psoriasis in Japanese patients: subgroup analyses from a randomized, placebo-controlled phase 3 trial. J Dermatol 2017;44(11):1228–37.

59. Ibrahim O, Bayart CB, Hogan S, et al. Treatment of alopecia areata with tofacitinib. JAMA Dermatol 2017;153(6):600–2.

60. Mamolo CM, Bushmakin AG, Cappelleri JC. Application of the itch severity score in patients with moderate-to-severe plaque psoriasis: clinically important difference and responder analyses. J Dermatolog Treat 2015;26(2):121–3.

61. Feldman SR, Thaci D, Gooderham M, et al. Tofacitinib improves pruritus and health-related quality of life up to 52 weeks: results from 2 randomized phase III trials in patients with moderate to severe plaque psoriasis. J Am Acad Dermatol 2016;75(6): 1162–70.e3.

62. Papp KA, Krueger JG, Feldman SR, et al. Tofacitinib, an oral Janus kinase inhibitor, for the treatment of chronic plaque psoriasis: long-term efficacy and safety results from 2 randomized phase-III studies and 1 open-label long-term extension study. J Am Acad Dermatol 2016;74(5):841–50.

63. AbbVie's upadacitinib (ABT-494) meets primary endpoint in phase 2b study in atopic dermatitis [press release]. 2017. Available at: https://news.abbvie.com/news/abbvies-upadacitinib-abt-494-meets-primary-endpoint-in-phase-2b-study-in-atopic-dermatitis.htm. Accessed September 23, 2017.

64. Tey HL, Yosipovitch G. Targeted treatment of pruritus: a look into the future. Br J Dermatol 2011; 165(1):5–17.

65. Yagami A, Furue M, Togawa M, et al. One-year safety and efficacy study of bilastine treatment in Japanese patients with chronic spontaneous urticaria or pruritus associated with skin diseases. J Dermatol 2017;44(4):375–85.

66. Murata Y, Song M, Kikuchi H, et al. Phase 2a, randomized, double-blind, placebo-controlled, multicenter, parallel-group study of a H4 R-antagonist (JNJ-39758979) in Japanese adults with moderate atopic dermatitis. J Dermatol 2015;42(2):129–39.

67. Werfel T, Lynch V, Asher A, et al. A phase 2a proof of concept clinical trial to evaluate ZPL-3893787 (ZPL-389), a potent, oral histamine H4 receptor antagonist for the treatment of moderate to severe atopic dermatitis (AD) in adults. Allergy 2016;71(S102):95.

68. Ziarco reports positive phase 2a study results with ZPL-389 in moderate to severe atopic dermatitis patients [press release]. 2016. Available at: https://globenewswire.com/news-release/2016/06/13/847881/10163430/en/Ziarco-Pharma-Ltd-Ziarco-reports-positive-Phase-2a-study-results-with-ZPL-389-in-moderate-to-severe-atopic-dermatitis-patients.html. Accessed October 1, 2017.

69. Friedmann PS, Palmer R, Tan E, et al. A double-blind, placebo-controlled trial of montelukast in adult

atopic eczema. Clin Exp Allergy 2007;37(10): 1536–40.

70. Mahmudpour M, Roozbeh J, Raiss Jalali GA, et al. Therapeutic effect of montelukast for treatment of uremic pruritus in hemodialysis patients. Iran J Kidney Dis 2017;11(1):50–5.

71. Hegade VS, Kendrick SF, Dobbins RL, et al. Effect of ileal bile acid transporter inhibitor GSK2330672 on pruritus in primary biliary cholangitis: a double-blind, randomised, placebo-controlled, crossover, phase 2a study. Lancet 2017;389(10074):1114–23.

72. Marschall HU. IBAT inhibitor A4250 for cholestatic pruritus. Available at: https://clinicaltrials.gov/show/NCT02360852.

73. Baumann U, Lacaille F, Sturm E, et al. The Ileal Bile Acid Transport inhibitor A4250 decreases pruritus and serum bile acids in cholestatic liver diseases - an ongoing multiple dose, open-label, multicentre study. J Hepatol 2017;66(1):S91.

74. Yun JW, Seo JA, Jeong YS, et al. TRPV1 antagonist can suppress the atopic dermatitis-like symptoms by accelerating skin barrier recovery. J Dermatol Sci 2011;62(1):8–15.

75. Kim B. A study to evaluate the safety and efficacy of PAC-14028 cream in adults with atopic dermatitis. Available at: https://clinicaltrials.gov/show/NCT02757729.

76. O'Neill J, Brock C, Olesen AE, et al. Unravelling the mystery of capsaicin: a tool to understand and treat pain. Pharmacol Rev 2012;64(4):939–71.

77. Andersen HH, Sand C, Elberling J. Considerable variability in the efficacy of 8% capsaicin topical patches in the treatment of chronic pruritus in 3 patients with notalgia paresthetica. Ann Dermatol 2016;28(1):86–9.

78. Steinke S, Gutknecht M, Zeidler C, et al. Cost-effectiveness of an 8% capsaicin patch in the treatment of brachioradial pruritus and notalgia paraesthetica, two forms of neuropathic pruritus. Acta Derm Venereol 2017;97(1):71–6.

79. Misery L, Erfan N, Castela E, et al. Successful treatment of refractory neuropathic pruritus with capsaicin 8% patch: a bicentric retrospective study with long-term follow-up. Acta Derm Venereol 2015; 95(7):864–5.

80. Backonja M, Wallace MS, Blonsky ER, et al. NGX-4010, a high-concentration capsaicin patch, for the treatment of postherpetic neuralgia: a randomised, double-blind study. Lancet Neurol 2008;7(12): 1106–12.

81. FDA approves eucrisa for eczema [press release]. 2016. Available at: https://www.fda.gov/newsevents/newsroom/pressannouncements/ucm533371.htm. Accessed September 11, 2017.

82. Paller AS, Tom WL, Lebwohl MG, et al. Efficacy and safety of crisaborole ointment, a novel, nonsteroidal phosphodiesterase 4 (PDE4) inhibitor for the topical treatment of atopic dermatitis (AD) in children and adults. J Am Acad Dermatol 2016;75(3):494–503.e6.

83. Eichenfield LF, Call RS, Forsha DW, et al. Long-term safety of crisaborole ointment 2% in children and adults with mild to moderate atopic dermatitis. J Am Acad Dermatol 2017;77(4):641–9.e5.

84. Hanifin JM, Ellis CN, Frieden IJ, et al. OPA-15406, a novel, topical, nonsteroidal, selective phosphodiesterase-4 (PDE4) inhibitor, in the treatment of adult and adolescent patients with mild to moderate atopic dermatitis (AD): a phase-II randomized, double-blind, placebo-controlled study. J Am Acad Dermatol 2016;75(2):297–305.

85. AD breakthrough? Medimetriks' MM36 achieves rapid itch relief, safety in phase 2 study [press release]. 2017. Available at: http://practicaldermatology.com/dermwire/2017/09/06/ad-breakthrough-medimetriks-mm36-achieves-rapid-itch-relief-safety-in-phase-2-study. Accessed September 11, 2017.

86. Pancrazio JJ, Kamatchi GL, Roscoe AK, et al. Inhibition of neuronal Na+ channels by antidepressant drugs. J Pharmacol Exp Ther 1998;284(1): 208–14.

87. Sawynok J. Topical and peripherally acting analgesics. Pharmacol Rev 2003;55(1):1–20.

88. Lee HG, Grossman SK, Valdes-Rodriguez R, et al. Topical ketamine-amitriptyline-lidocaine for chronic pruritus: a retrospective study assessing efficacy and tolerability. J Am Acad Dermatol 2017;76(4): 760–1.

89. Mounessa JS, Siegel JA, Dunnick CA, et al. The role of cannabinoids in dermatology. J Am Acad Dermatol 2017;77(1):188–90.

90. Liszewski W, Farah RS. Response to: "the role of cannabinoids in dermatology". J Am Acad Dermatol 2017;77(3):e87–8.

91. Eberlein B, Eicke C, Reinhardt HW, et al. Adjuvant treatment of atopic eczema: assessment of an emollient containing N-palmitoylethanolamine (ATOPA study). J Eur Acad Dermatol Venereol 2008;22(1): 73–82.

92. Szepietowski JC, Szepietowski T, Reich A. Efficacy and tolerance of the cream containing structured physiological lipids with endocannabinoids in the treatment of uremic pruritus: a preliminary study. Acta Dermatovenerol Croat 2005;13(2):97–103.

93. Stander S, Reinhardt HW, Luger TA. Topical cannabinoid agonists. An effective new possibility for treating chronic pruritus. Hautarzt 2006;57(9):801–7 [in German].

94. Nattkemper L, Stull C, Lavery M, et al. Prolonged antipruritic effect of botulinum toxin type A on cowhage-induced itch. Acta Derm Venereol 2017; 97(8):1021.

Moving?

Make sure your subscription moves with you!

To notify us of your new address, find your **Clinics Account Number** (located on your mailing label above your name), and contact customer service at:

Email: journalscustomerservice-usa@elsevier.com

800-654-2452 (subscribers in the U.S. & Canada)
314-447-8871 (subscribers outside of the U.S. & Canada)

Fax number: 314-447-8029

Elsevier Health Sciences Division
Subscription Customer Service
3251 Riverport Lane
Maryland Heights, MO 63043

ELSEVIER

Moving?

Make sure your subscription moves with you!

To notify us of your new address, find your Clinics Account Number (located on your mailing label above your name), and contact customer service at:

Email: journalscustomerservice-usa@elsevier.com

800-654-2452 (subscribers in the U.S. & Canada)
314-447-8871 (subscribers outside of the U.S. & Canada)

Fax number: 314-447-8029

Elsevier Health Sciences Division
Subscription Customer Service
3251 Riverport Lane
Maryland Heights, MO 63043

To ensure uninterrupted delivery of your subscription, please notify us at least 4 weeks in advance of move.

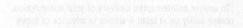